The Year in Endocrinology
1977

The Year in Endocrinology

Editor-in-Chief: SIDNEY H. INGBAR • Boston, Massachusetts

The Year in Endocrinology

1977

Edited by

Sidney H. Ingbar, M. D.

Professor of Medicine, Harvard Medical School
Director, Thorndike Laboratory
of Harvard Medical School
at the
Beth Israel Hospital
Boston, Massachusetts

SPRINGER SCIENCE+BUSINESS MEDIA, LLC

The Library of Congress cataloged the first volume of this work as follows:

Main entry under title:

The Year in endocrinology, 1975-1976.

 Includes bibliographical references and index.
 1. Endocrinology. I. Ingbar, Sidney H. [DNLM: 1. Endocrinology—Yearbooks.
W1 YE39]

QP187.Y44	612'.4	76-46325

Library of Congress Catalog Card Number 76-46325

ISBN 978-1-4684-2504-8 ISBN 978-1-4684-2502-4 (eBook)
DOI 10.1007/978-1-4684-2502-4

© 1978 Springer Science+Business Media New York
Originally published by Plenum Publishing Corporation in 1978
Softcover reprint of the hardcover 1st edition 1978

227 West 17th Street, New York, N. Y. 10011

Plenum Medical Book Company is an imprint of Plenum Publishing Corporation

Contributors

Edward G. Biglieri, M.D. • Chief of Endocrinology Division of the Medical Service and Director of the Clinical Study Center, San Francisco General Hospital; and Professor of Medicine, University of California, San Francisco, California

Lewis E. Braverman, M.D. • Professor of Medicine; Director of Endocrinology and Metabolism, University of Massachusetts Medical School, Worcester, Massachusetts

William H. Daughaday, M.D. • Professor of Medicine; Director, Metabolism Division, Department of Medicine, Washington University School of Medicine, St. Louis, Missouri

Daniel D. Federman, M.D. • Professor of Medicine, Harvard Medical School, Boston, Massachusetts

John Gwynne, M.D. • Assistant Professor of Medicine, University of North Carolina School of Medicine, Chapel Hill, North Carolina

Charles R. Kleeman, M.D. • Professor of Medicine; Chief, Division of Nephrology, UCLA School of Medicine and Center for the Health Sciences, Los Angeles, California

Karen Kleeman, M.D. • Department of Medicine, Beth Israel Hospital, Boston, Massachusetts

Dorothy T. Krieger, M.D. • Professor of Medicine; Director, Division of Endocrinology and Metabolism, The Mount Sinai School of Medicine of the City University of New York, New York, New York

Lewis Landsberg, M.D. • Associate Professor of Medicine at Beth Israel Hospital, Harvard Medical School; Associate Chief, Department of Medicine, Beth Israel Hospital, Boston, Massachusetts

Mortimer B. Lipsett, M.D. • Director, Clinical Center, National Institutes of Health, Bethesda, Maryland

Robert L. Ney, M.D. • Professor of Medicine and Physiology; Chairman, Department of Medicine, University of North Carolina School of Medicine, Chapel Hill, North Carolina

Gary L. Robertson, M.D. • Professor of Medicine, Indiana University School of Medicine, and Chief, Endocrinology and Metabolism Section, Medical Service, Veterans Administration Hospital, Indianapolis, Indiana

Griff T. Ross, M.D. • Deputy Director, Clinical Center, National Institutes of Health, Bethesda, Maryland

Jay Silverberg, M.D. • Endocrinology Research Laboratory, The Wellesley Hospital, and Department of Medicine, University of Toronto, Toronto, Ontario, Canada

Robert Volpé, M.D. • Physician-in-Chief, Endocrinology Research Laboratory, The Wellesley Hospital; Professor of Medicine, University of Toronto, Toronto, Ontario, Canada

Kenneth A. Woeber, M.D. • Professor of Medicine, University of California; Chief of Medicine, Mount Zion Hospital and Medical Center, San Francisco, California

Preface

This has been a year of substantial change for *The Year in Endocrinology*. The first change, though perhaps only a semantic one, nevertheless represents a landmark. Although last year's volume was designated as the first of an annual series, that seemed to me at the time merely a hope—a realistic hope, perhaps, but a hope, nevertheless. With the publication of this year's volume, however, this can accurately be said to be an annual series, one that we trust will fulfill a need and will therefore continue for years to come.

Among other changes from last year's volume are some that were originally intended and others that were unintended. In the former category is the substitution of a chapter on water metabolism and vasopressin, excellently prepared by Dr. Gary L. Robertson, for the chapter on paraendocrine syndromes that appeared last year. Chapters on these two topics will continue to appear on alternate years. Obviously, the nonrecurring chapter on a topic of special interest has also changed, and this year's comprises a comprehensive review of autoimmune endocrine disease by Drs. Jay Silverberg and Robert Volpé. The unexpected change results from the inability of Dr. Louis Avioli to continue as a member of the Editorial Board. Most fortunately, however, we have persuaded Dr. Charles R. Kleeman to join the Board and to be responsible for the chapter on the parathyroid gland and mineral metabolism. Dr. Kleeman has been assisted on the preparation of this chapter by his daughter, Dr. Karen Kleeman, a highly talented young physician. Readers of this year's volume will agree, I am sure, that a little nepotism can sometimes, as in this instance, be a very fine thing.

With all this, the greatest and most important change that has occurred during the past year is the continuing, incredibly rapid, growth of knowledge in all aspects of endocrinology; this is both exemplified and specified in each of the chapters in this year's volume. As indicated in the Preface to last year's volume, it was our desire to assist interested members of the biomedical community in coping with this change that originally motivated this annual series, and it is this desire that continues to do so.

Sidney H. Ingbar, M.D.

Contents

Chapter 1
Hypothalamus
Dorothy T. Krieger

Chapter 2
Anterior Pituitary
William H. Daughaday

Chapter 5
The Adrenal Cortex
John T. Gwynne and Robert L. Ney

Chapter 6
Aldosterone and the Renin–Angiotensin System
Edward G. Biglieri

Chapter 7
Vasopressin and Water Metabolism
Gary L. Robertson

Chapter 8
The Ovary
Mortimer B. Lipsett and Griff T. Ross

Chapter 9
The Testis
Daniel D. Federman

Chapter 10
The Sympathoadrenal System
Lewis Landsberg

Chapter 11

Autoimmunity in Endocrine Disease

Jay Silverberg and Robert Volpé

Hypothalamus

Dorothy T. Krieger

1.1. Hormones in Brain

Reports of the presence and presumed synthesis in brain of peptides first demonstrated in the GI tract (gastrin, vasoactive intestinal polypeptide, Substance P),* kidney (renin), and pituitary (ACTH, α-MSH, growth hormone, endorphin), the isolation of previously uncharacterized peptides from brain for which metabolic functions have now been described (i.e., neurotensin), and the demonstration of nonendocrine effects of the "hypothalamic" releasing and inhibiting hormones have opened new vistas and raised new question with regard to the role of such peptides in CNS function.

1.1.1. 'Gastrointestinal Peptides'

1.1.1.1. Gastrin

Immunoreactive gastrin has been isolated from human, canine, avian, piscine, and amphibian brain.[1] The highest concentration was found in cortex, in contrast to the low levels of releasing factors in this

---

*There is a recent report[99] of cortical localization of a peptide resembling the COOH-terminal octapeptide of cholecystokinin.

DOROTHY T. KRIEGER • Division of Endocrinology and Metabolism, Department of Medicine, Mount Sinai School of Medicine, New York, New York 10029.

area. Dose–response curves obtained with dilutions of brain extract were not identical to those obtained with unlabeled gastrin 2–17. The molecular weight of the brain peptide appears to be less than that of gastrin 2–17. To date, no studies have been performed with regard to its physiological significance and regulatory mechanisms.

1.1.1.2. Vasoactive Intestinal Polypeptide

Vasoactive intestinal polypeptide (VIP) is structurally related to secretin and glucagon, and is found throughout the GI tract of mammals and birds. Both immunoassayable and bioassayable VIP are present in dog neural tissue,[2] with the highest concentration also seen in cortex. Such concentrations were higher per gram of wet weight than concentrations in the GI tract.

1.1.1.3. Substance P

Substance P was originally isolated from both brain and intestine, and was characterized by its hypotensive effects and contractile activity in intestine. Its structure was determined only recently, allowing for detection by both immunohistochemistry[3] and immunoassay.[4] Cell bodies containing Substance P have been demonstrated by immunohistochemistry in only one area in the rat CNS—the medial habenula—whereas fiber systems were present in the periaqueductal central gray, substantia nigra, medial amygdaloid nucleus, medial preoptic area, and substantia gelatinosa trigemini. High concentrations were also seen in spinal cord, spinal ganglia, and peripheral nerve, similar to reported somatostatin distribution, but dissimilar to reported gastrin and VIP distribution. Quantitation by immunoassay revealed the highest concentrations in hypothalamus, preoptic area, mesencephalon, and brainstem. When individual nuclei in these regions were examined, all had higher concentrations than the average for whole brain, those in the reticular part of the substantia nigra and the interpeduncular nucleus being the highest. The medial forebrain bundle appears to be progressively depleted of Substance P as it moves caudally from the preoptic area into the mesencephalon. The specificity of the antibodies developed in both these studies remains to be determined, as does the role of substance P in the CNS.

1.1.2. Neurotensin

During the course of purification of Substance P from bovine hypothalamic extracts, a new peptide was detected, sequenced, and synthesized. This has been termed *neurotensin*. Its sequence is: Glu-Leu-Tyr-Glu-Asn-Lys-Pro-Arg-Arg-Pro-Tyr-Ile-Leu-OH; that of Substance P is: H-Arg-Pro-Lys-Pro-Gln-Gln-Phe-Phe-Gly-Leu-Met-NH_2. Neurotensin has been found to cause hypotension, increased vascular permeability, cyanosis, increased secretion of ACTH, LH, and FSH, and marked hyperglycemia on intravenous injection into anesthetized rats.[5] Its hyperglycemic effect is not seen *in vitro*. The hyperglycemic response is not blocked by α- or β-blocking agents or morphine sulfate, is presumably not secondary to an increase in plasma glucagon concentration, and does not require the presence of the pituitary, adrenal, or vasopressin. The highest concentrations are in gray matter and in synaptosomal fractions. Immunoassay reveals the highest concentrations in hypothalamus, caudate nucleus, and globus pallidus, whereas receptor binding studies show some disparity, with the highest concentrations in thalamus, hypothalamus, and cerebral cortex.[6] Its mechanism of action and physiological significance remain to be elucidated.

1.1.3. Renin

The presence of an angiotensin-forming enzyme of nonrenal origin, characterized as "reninlike," in extracts of various CNS areas and pituitary of several species, including the human, was first described in 1971.[7] Cathespin D, a pepsinlike acid protease found in brain, can also form angiotensin from renin substrate under appropriate conditions. A recent study[8] demonstrated parallel distribution of renin and cathepsin D activity in different brain regions, as well as similar molecular weight estimates, isoelectric focusing patterns, and subcellular localization—with different pH optima, however, such pH optima also differing from that described for renal renin. Angiotensinogen,[9] but not renin,[6] has been detected in CSF, and angiotensin receptors have been described in choroid plexus and various brain regions.[8] It would therefore appear that there is a separate renin–angiotensin system within the CNS with effects on blood pressure, drinking behavior, and vasopressin secretion, but its physiological significance requires further characterization.

1.1.4. Pituitarylike Peptides

1.1.4.1. ACTH, MSH, Growth Hormone, and Endorphin in Hypophysectomized Animals

Immunoreactive and bioreactive ACTH-like activity has been demonstrated in extracts of median eminence and medial basal hypothala-

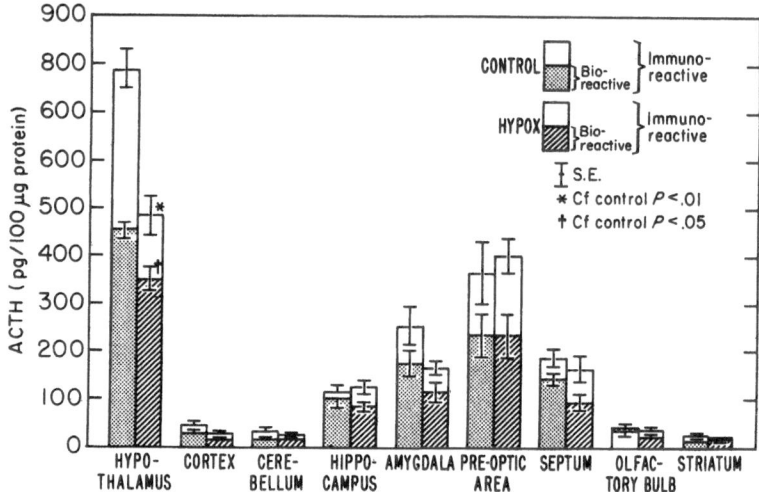

Fig. 1. Distribution of immunoreactive and bioreactive ACTH-like activity in selected areas of rat brain. In addition to the areas depicted, analysis of midbrain, medulla, caudate nucleus, and globus pallidus revealed no detectable ACTH-like activity, while that of pons was approximately equivalent to that of cerebellum. (Reproduced from Krieger *et al.*[11])

mus,[10] (Fig. 1), as well as in portions of the limbic system[11] of intact and hypophysectomized animals. Hypophysectomy does not produce any significant alteration in such concentrations, save in hypothalamus. Concentrations in the median eminence and medial basal hypothalamus are approximately $\frac{1}{25}$ and $\frac{1}{30}$, respectively, of those reported for whole pituitary. Since plasma ACTH is undetectable and adrenal weight and adrenal function are not maintained in hypophysectomized animals, it may well be that such ACTH present in brain has extrapituitary actions (see *The Year in Endocrinology 1975–1976,* Chapter 1).

Immunoreactive[12] and bioreactive[13] α-MSH has also been reported to be present in rat brain after hypophysectomy. These reports do not state whether the concentrations were similar to those found in intact animals. Growth hormone,[14] bioassayable melanotropic and lipolytic activity,[15] endorphinlike activity,[16] and immunocytochemically identified α- and β-endorphin[16] have also been demonstrated in brain tissue from hypophysectomized animals. These findings suggest that nonpituitary cells can either synthesize these hormones or cleave their precursor molecules. To quote Guillemin[17]: "The recent hypotheses about the ontogenic commonality between all the pituitary elements and the central nervous system[18] make such a statement somewhat less of a challenge than it would have been a couple of years ago."

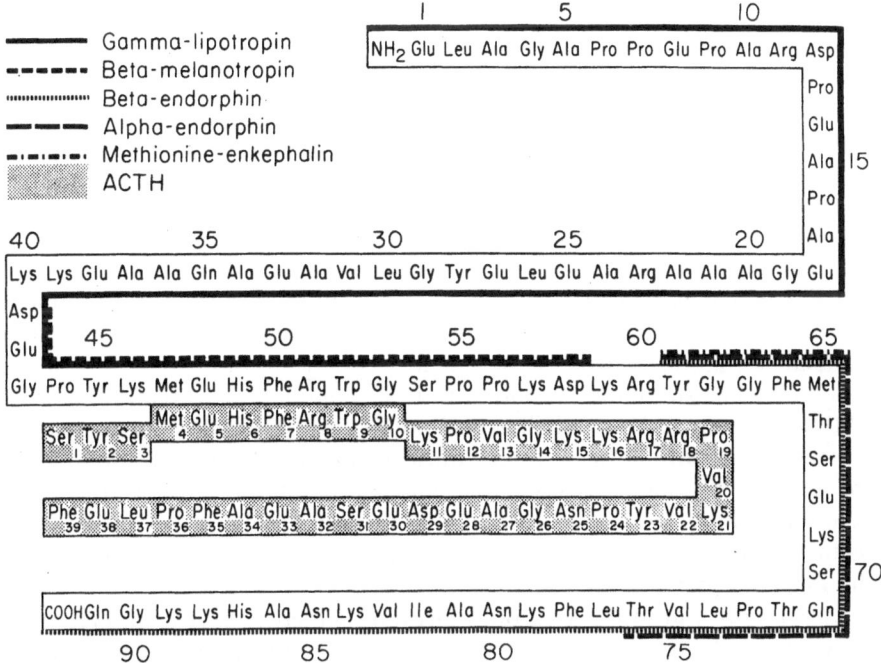

Fig. 2. β-Lipotropin, a pituitary peptide hormone 91 amino acids long, has amino acid sequences with several distinct physiological functions. The peptide chain as a whole induces the metabolism of fat, as does the segment termed γ-lipotropin (amino acid units 1–58). The sequence 41–58 is that of the hormone β-melanotropin, which plays a role in skin pigmentation. The sequence 61–91 is that of β-endorphin, a pituitary peptide that has analgesic effects when it is injected intravenously or is injected directly into the brain. A second pituitary peptide, designated α-endorphin (61–76), has similar but less potent effects. The β-lipotropin sequence 61–65 is identical with that of methionine-enkephalin, a morphinelike peptide found in the brain, the spinal cord, and the intestines. The relationship between the opiatelike peptides and β-lipotropin is not known. The homologous sequence with ACTH$_{4-10}$ is also indicated. (Reproduced from Snyder[19] with modifications.)

1.1.4.2. β-Lipotropin, Endorphin, and Enkephalin

The demonstration that β-lipotropin (β-LPH) contains within it the sequences of β-MSH, methionine-enkephalin, and endorphin has led to many studies seeking to characterize the distribution of these diverse peptides, the precursor role of β-LPH in the formation of these other fragments (see Fig. 2), and the physiological role of these fragments. To date, β-LPH has been demonstrated only in pituitary,* while α- and β-

*There is a recent report[100] demonstrating the presence of β-LPH in bovine brain and spinal cord.

endorphin have been demonstrated in both pituitary and brain; in the latter, as noted above, it has also been found in hypophysectomized animals. Opiate receptors have been demonstrated in brain (substantia gelatinosa of the spinal trigeminal nucleus, periaqueductal gray, locus caeruleus, striatal area, basolateral nucleus of amygdala, and portions of the habenula).[20] The greatest abundance of such receptors occurs in the amygdala and in the pituitary. In the pituitary, opiate receptor binding is localized predominantly in the posterior pituitary, most likely in the pars intermedia in those species in which this anatomical division occurs. Enkephalins have been isolated from brain, but not from pituitary. Immunohistochemical mapping reveals a distribution of enkephalin nerve terminals similar to that described for the opiate receptor. Still to be characterized are opiatelike substances reported in brain, pituitary, and blood that are different from the enkephalins and endorphins thus far characterized. Interpretation of all these studies must be tempered with considerations of whether the methods used for tissue preparation or extraction may allow for either local enzymatic action or chemical alteration so that the compounds that are found do not correspond to their natural occurrence in a given region.

β-Lipotropin itself has no morphinomimetic activity in bioassay (myenteric plexus–longitudinal muscle of guinea pig ileum) or in opiate-binding assays (rat brain synaptosome preparations).[21] There is one study reporting that intraventricular administration[22] is associated with moderate analgesic activity, in contrast to other studies in which β-LPH administration produced no behavioral effects. However, intracerebrospinal fluid administration[23] or microinjection into the periaqueductal gray[24] of β-endorphin, α-endorphin, methionine-enkephalin, and leucine-enkephalin is associated with marked behavioral effects, β-endorphin leading to profound sedation and catalepsy (Fig. 3). Administration of the other peptides produces lesser and diverse effects on this and other measures of CNS activity.

Initial studies indicate that incubation of β-LPH with homogenates of porcine pituitary glands results in specific cleavage between residues 77 and 78,[25] as well as between 60 and 61. The enzymes responsible for this presumably do not occur in brain. Incubation of β-LPH at neutral pH with supernatant aqueous extracts of rat brain[21] generates opioid activity, which disappears after 2 hr; the primary structure of the fragments produced has thus far not been characterized. When methionine- and leucine-enkephalins were incubated with brain homogenates, both peptides were found to undergo breakdown within 1–5 min, whereas the C-fragment (61–91) was found to be more stable.[24] It would therefore appear that the more prolonged effect of endorphin as compared with that of enkephalin is accounted for by its greater stability, and that the inactivity of β-LPH may be explained by postulating that it serves as a

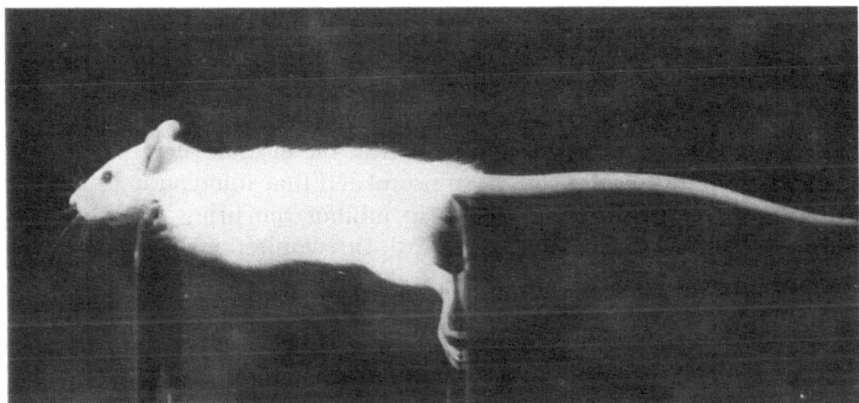

Fig. 3. Rat 30 min after intracisternal injection of β-endorphin. The rat exhibited sufficient rigid immobility to remain totally self-supporting when placed across metal bookends that were in contact only at the upper neck and base of the tail. Such postures were maintained for prolonged periods. (Reproduced from Bloom et al.[23])

"prohormone" for opiatelike peptides, which are derived from it by the action of specific proteases present in brain or pituitary, or both. The relationship between the brain and pituitary system is unclear at present.

The physiological role of the LPH–endorphin–enkephalin system remains to be characterized. It may well be that the endorphins and enkephalins function as neurotransmitters or modulators of the function of other neurotransmitters. Enkephalins have been shown to have depressant effects on the firing of brainstem neurons of rats[26] and cats[27] similar to that produced by morphine; only in the former species, however, is the effect reversed by naloxone, a specific opiate antagonist. The extra-CNS distribution of enkephalin appears to be confined chiefly to the GI tract, similar to that noted above for gastrin, VIP, and Substance P, as well as that of somatostatin. In addition to the endocrine effects reported for these foregoing peptides, it was recently shown that somatostatin acutely inhibits the release of acetylcholine by the myenteric plexus of the guinea pig ileum.[28]

A behavioral role for the endorphins and the enkephalins has been suggested. To date, there is no consensus on the effect of opiate antagonists in schizophrenia. Last year's review cited the effect of $ACTH_{4-10}$ and $ACTH_{4-7}$ to increase the rate of acquisition of avoidance behavior (memory retention) and to delay the extinction of such avoidance behavior (persistence of a learned response). β-LPH_{61-69}, β-LPH_{51-76}, and β-LPH_{61-91} have been demonstrated to be, on a weight basis, 10 times as active as $ACTH_{4-10}$ in this regard.[29] Desglycinamide$_9$-lysine$_8$-vasopressin (DG-LVP), which was reported to have a longer-term effect on such responses than $ACTH_{4-10}$, is now also reported to facilitate physical dependence on the analgesic action of morphine, without itself binding to opiate receptors. Oxytocin is even more effective than DG-LVP in this regard.

It has also been suggested that endogenous opiates function in response to painful stimuli and may play a role in some of the symptoms of narcotic withdrawal. It has been postulated that stimulation of centers in the central gray area of the brain inhibits the firing of the nerves carrying pain signals into the spinal cord. Direct injections of morphine or endorphin into these central areas produce similar effects. The analgesia produced by electrical stimulation of these areas can be partially blocked by naloxone. It remains to be shown, however, that electrical stimulation results in endorphin release. There is a recent report[30] that acupuncture analgesia is abolished by naloxone, and that hypophysectomy abolishes acupuncture analgesia in mice. The role of endogenous opiates in addiction to, or withdrawal from, opiates is unclear. Acute exposure of neuroblastoma–glioma clones to opiates results in inhibition of basal levels of adenylate cyclase. Chronic exposure of these clones[31] to either morphine or enkephalin increases basal levels of adenylate cyclase, so that concentrations of opiates that would decrease levels of cAMP in untreated cells no longer do so in these opiate-treated cells. Decreases in cAMP in the treated cells are effected only by increased concentrations of opiates. When opiates are removed from these treated cells, concentrations of cAMP rise markedly. It has been suggested that these phenomena represent "tolerance" and "withdrawal," respectively. There is one report[32] of development of "tolerance" in *in vivo* studies in rats, in which repeated injections of human β-endorphin induced tolerance to analgesic response, catatonia, and hypothermia; cross-tolerance to morphine was also observed. Whether suppression of endogenous opiate release by administration of exogenous opiates is the basis for the syndrome that occurs when such exogenous opiates are withdrawn is speculative at present.

It has long been known that morphine has stimulatory effects on ACTH, growth hormone, and prolactin release. Intravenous or intracisternal administration of β-endorphin stimulates both growth hormone and prolactin release *in vivo*,[33] endorphin being 20 times more potent on a molar basis than morphine. The effects of β-endorphin are reversible by naloxone. In the doses employed *in vivo*, met-enkephalin was not effective, although in another study,[34] stimulatory effects of enkephalin on prolactin secretion were seen both *in vitro* and *in vivo*. No stimulatory effects were seen when endorphin was incubated with short-term-cultured dispersed pituitary cells,[33] suggesting a CNS site of action of endorphin, despite the known presence of pituitary opiate receptors. These studies further point out the complexity of the pituitary–brain interrelationships with regard to endorphins.

1.2. Hormones in Pituitary Blood

1.2.1. Demonstration of Releasing Factors and Pituitary Hormones in Portal Blood: Newer Studies on the Pituitary Portal System

The actual demonstration of releasing factors, i.e., TRH[35] and GnRH,[36] in pituitary portal blood is not surprising. Even the vasopressin in portal blood[37] can be accounted for as emanating from projections of the supraoptic and paraventricular nuclei to the external layer of the median eminence with consequent access to the pituitary portal circulation. The very recent finding[38] of marked elevations in the concentration of immunoreactive LH, TSH, prolactin, ACTH, α-MSH, and vasopressin in pituitary portal plasma of anesthetized male rats, and the differential effects of anterior and posterior pituitary lobectomy on the portal blood concentrations of these hormones (see Fig. 4) suggest that pituitary hormones are transported retrograde in certain vascular channels of the pituitary stalk, perhaps other than the long portal veins, toward the hypothalamus. It is postulated that, additionally, connections exist allowing hormones in these retrograde channels to enter into the long portal vessels going to the anterior pituitary (see Fig. 5). If such findings are confirmed, and shown not to be artifacts of the method used for portal vein cannulation, and if subsequent blood–brain transport can be demonstrated, they may explain in part the reported presence (see Section 1.1.3) of pituitary hormones and pituitary hormone fragments in the brains of intact animals. The findings may also shed light on the mechanism of postulated pituitary hormone "short-loop" feedback in brain. These findings would not explain, however, the presence of such hormones and hormone fragments in brains of hypophysectomized animals.

An anatomical basis for such retrograde flow was presented by Page et al.[39] These authors demonstrated, in the dorsum of the rabbit pituitary stalk: (1) the presence of vessels that connected the posterior pituitary gland to the hypothalamus (Fig. 6); (2) the presence of connections between these vessels and the long portal vessels; (3) a common capillary bed between the posterior and anterior pituitary; and (4) routes for the delivery of blood from the posterior pituitary to the ventricular surface of the median eminence.

1.3. Factors Involved in Brain Androgenization

1.3.1. Sexual Dimorphism of Brain

Sexual dimorphism has been demonstrated neuroanatomically, neurophysiologically, behaviorally (sexual and nonsexual), and hormonally

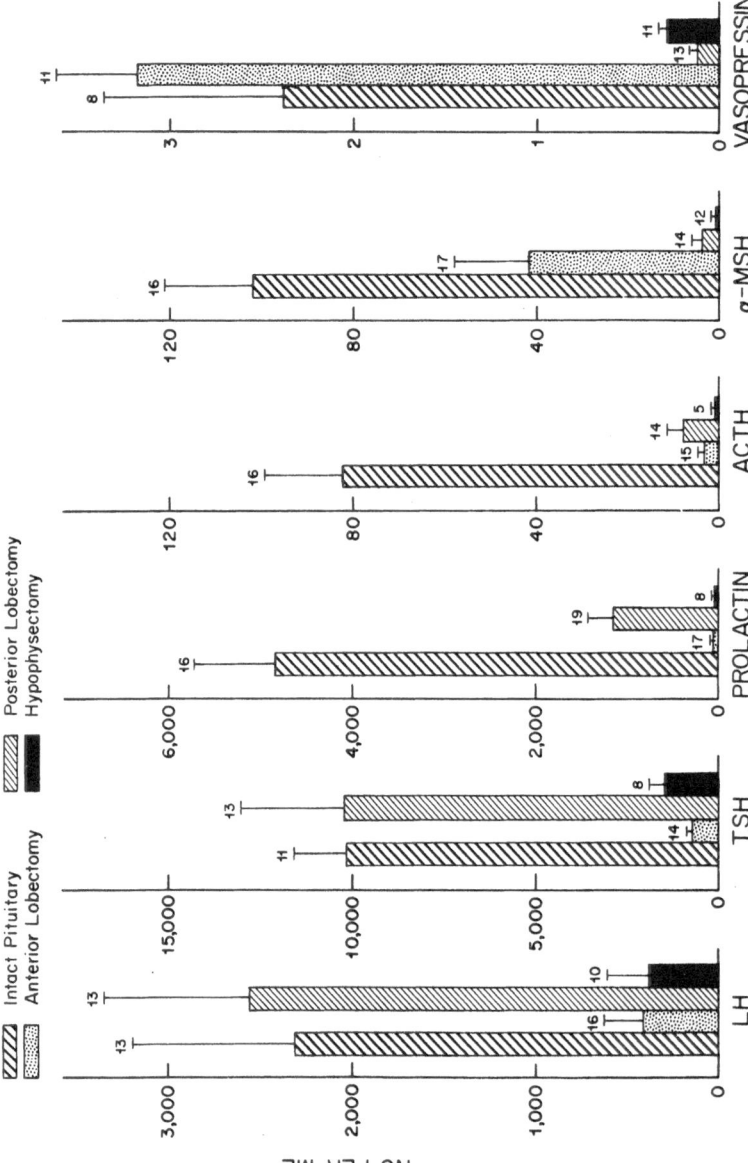

Fig. 4. Concentrations of LH, TSH, prolactin, ACTH, α-MSH, and vasopressin in plasma from hypophyseal portal vessel blood from anesthetized male rats with intact pituitaries and from anterior lobectomized, posterior lobectomized, and hypophysectomized animals. The heights of the bars denote means; the vertical lines represent the magnitude of the standard error. The number of animals is given above each bar. (Reproduced from Oliver et al.[38])

(with regard to both hormone level and pattern). Male rats have fewer nonamygdaloid synapses on dendritic spines in the preoptic area than do female animals. Castration of male animals within 12 hr of birth is associated with an increase to the female number of spine synapses, while testosterone treatment of female animals on the fourth day of life decreases the number of such synapses to the male range.[40] Electrophysiological studies show that more of the cells projecting to the medial basal hypothalamus receive synaptic connections from the amygdala in males than in normal female animals or neonatally castrated males, while female animals treated with testosterone have an intermediate number. Additionally, other neurons, not influenced by medial basal hypothalamic stimulation, fire twice as fast in normal female and neonatally castrate males as do these same cell types in normal males and females neonatally treated with testosterone.[41] Neonatal female rats have much higher titers of plasma LH and FSH than do males of equivalent age[42] and show increased staining of LHRH fibers in arcuate–median eminence and prechiasmatic region than do male animals, as well as increased brain immunoreactive LHRH content.[43] (It is problematical whether this increase is related to the later onset of steroidogenesis in the rat ovary than in the testes.)[44]

It has long been known that in the rodent, exposure to neonatal androgen (endogenous in the male, exogenous in the female) is associated with male type of pituitary gonadotropin release and male type of behavior, whereas the absence of such androgen or exposure of neonatal males (especially castrates) to estrogen results in female patterns of hormone release and behavior. "Androgen-insensitive" rats, while refractory to adult administration of testosterone with regard to mating performance, can, in the untreated condition, manifest some evidence of masculine sexual behavior, but are no more sensitive to estrogen with regard to facilitation of lordosis response than are normal males.[45] This may be, however, an expression of the reported partial androgen insensitivity in Tfm/Y mutants, compatible with some residual androgen binding present in these animals. Human patients with the androgen insensitivity syndrome appear to have a normal female gender identity.[46]

As can be seen, most of the studies cited above were done on rodents, and it is not clear that similar considerations apply to primate and human models. Female primates exposed to perinatal androgen[47] or human female patients with congenital adrenal hyperplasia (who have been exposed to high androgen concentrations *in utero*) can display (subsequent to treatment in the latter group) cyclic gonadotropin release and female sexual behavior. In the human, however, a sexual dimorphism in neural organization underlying cognition has been demonstrated in tests of spatial processing; boys perform in a manner consistent with right hemi-

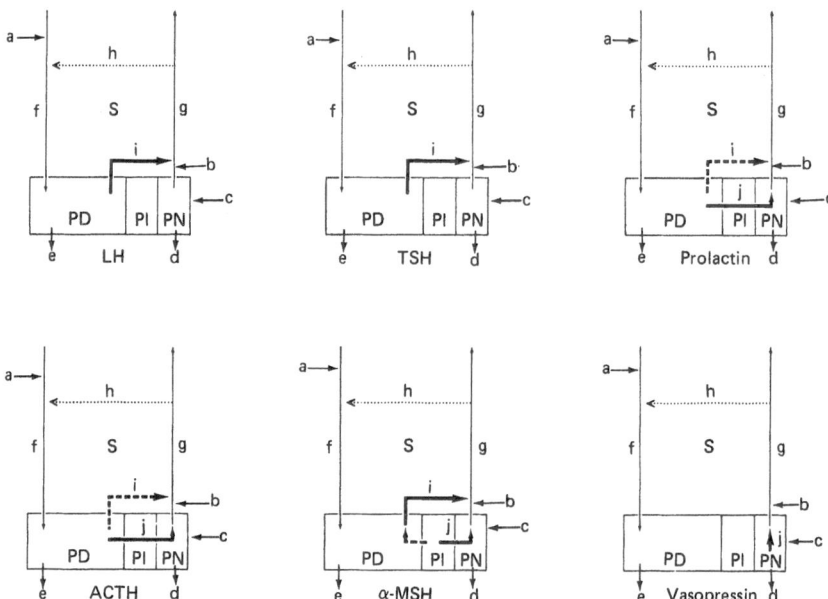

Fig. 5. Diagrammatic representations of the directions of blood flow and transport of pituitary hormones in the hypothalmic–hypophyseal vasculature. The model proposed for a given hormone is indicated below each scheme. Arrows denote the direction of blood flow. (PD), Pars distalis; (PI), pars intermedia; (PN), pars nervosa; (S), pituitary stalk; (a) superior hypophyseal arteries; (b), peduncular artery(ies); (c), inferior hypophyseal arteries; (d), venous outflow of the pars nervosa; (e), venous outflow of the pars distalis; (f), long portal vessels; (g), retrograde vascular channels; (h), diffusional or vascular connections, or both, between the retrograde vascular channels and the long portal vessels; (i), venous flow from the pars distalis not involving the pars nervosa; (j), diffusional or vascular connections, or both, between the pars distalis, pars intermedia, pars nervosa, and the retrograde vascular channels. (Reproduced from Oliver et al.[38])

⎯⎯⎯⎯⎯⎯⎯⎯⎯⎯⎯⎯⎯⎯⎯⎯⎯⎯⎯⎯⎯⎯⎯⎯⎯⎯⎯⎯⎯⎯⎯⎯⟶

Fig. 6. (35) Sagittal view of pituitary-median eminence complex. Vessels of the infundibular process (IP) overlie those of pars distalis (PD). These vascular beds are joined by short portal vessels (x). White vertical arrowhead designates anterior hypophyseal artery. Hollow white horizontal arrowhead designates venous drainage. ×20. (36) Sagittal view of infundibular process (IP) and pars distalis (PD). Short portal vessels (white arrow) cross between neural and glandular pituitary. ×32. (37) Sagittal view of infundibular process. Higher magnification of area designated by arrow in (36). Short portal vessel (white arrowhead) courses between infundibular process on left and pars distalis on right. ×75. (38) Dorsal view of pars distalis. In this specimen there was no filling of vessels in the infundibular process. Capillaries of the pars distalis unite to form venous trunks on the surface of glandular pituitary. The posterior aspect of the cast is at the bottom. (39) Sagittal view of infundibular process (IP) and pars distalis (PD). The arterial supply is seen superiorly (black arrow), coursing to the infundibular process. Venous trunks (white arrow) drain infundibular process as well as pars distalis. ×30.

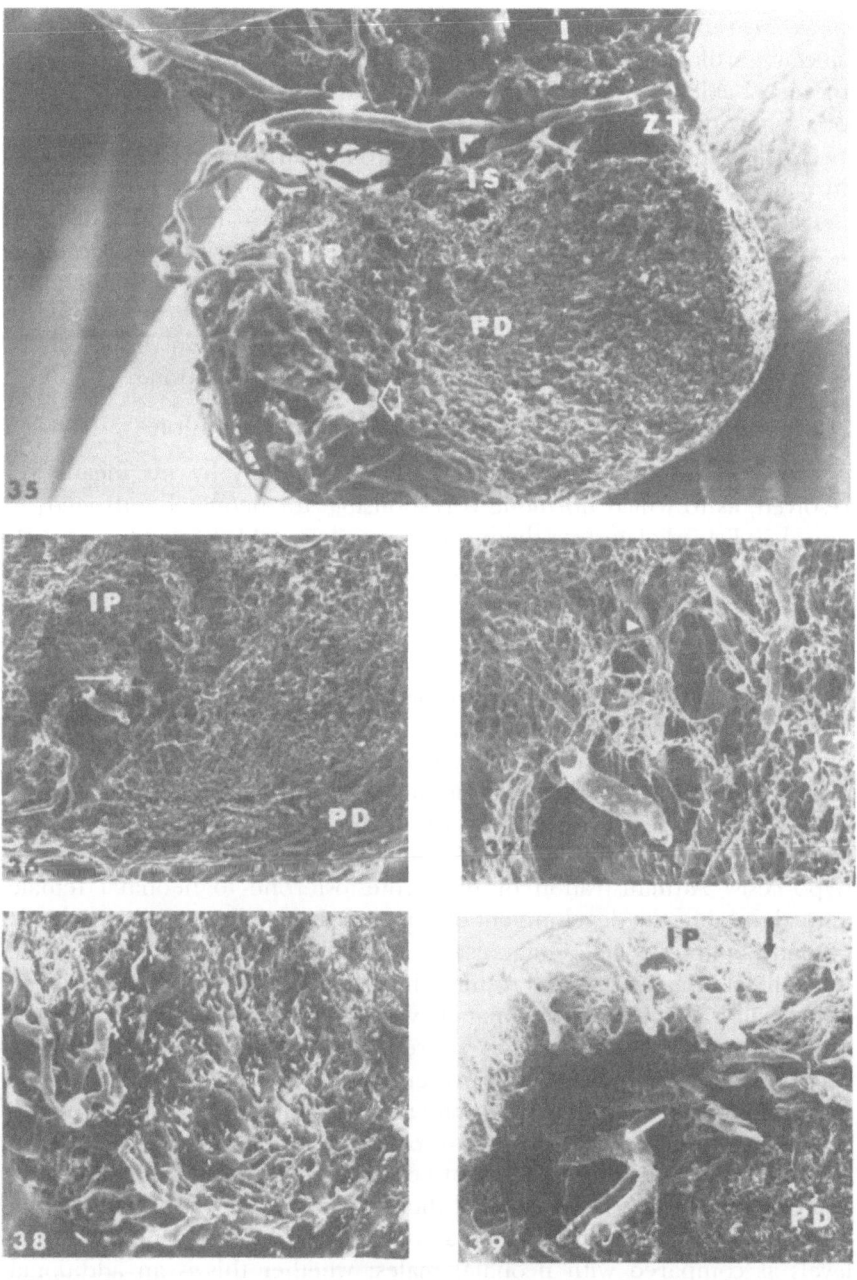

sphere specialization as early as 6 years of age, whereas girls show evidence of bilateral representation until age 13.[48] Such differences may, however, reflect differences in the rate of attainment of sexual maturity, since regardless of sex, early-maturing adolescents perform better in tests of verbal abilities than in tests of spatial abilities, whereas late-maturing ones show the opposite pattern.[49] In monkeys, orbital prefrontal lesions performed in infancy were associated with impairment in behavioral tests in male animals at $2\frac{1}{2}$ months of age, whereas similar defects were not detected in females with comparable lesions until 15–18 months of age.[50] Lesions made in juvenile animals were not associated with sex differences on subsequent testing of such animals. These studies therefore suggest that even in the primate species, a sex-dependent difference in brain organization is present, although obviously no studies on the effects of neonatal castration or hormone replacement have been done.

1.3.2. Hormones Involved in Neonatal Androgenization

In the rat, there is considerable controversy, by no means yet resolved, as to which hormone is responsible for neonatal androgenization. 17β-Estradiol and synthetic estrogens are capable of producing such androgenization; only aromatizable androgens (i.e., not 5α-dihydrotestosterone) are also effective, Since rat brain tissue can aromatize androgens,[51] this has led to the suggestion that aromatization of androgens may be a prerequisite for their action in masculine sex differentiation. Androgen can also block estradiol binding to the estrogen receptor.[52] Additionally, the high circulating levels of α-fetoprotein present in the neonate serve to bind maternal and fetal estrogen, making it unavailable for interaction with brain receptors. These considerations all emphasize the primary role of androgen in sexual differentiation of the brain.

There are several observations seemingly at variance with this hypothesis. Administration of dihydrotestosterone to neonatal female animals inhibits the development of female behavior.[53] Intrahypothalamic implants of an estrogen antagonist do not block the effects of testosterone in neonatal female rats[54] and result in high levels of female sex behavior in adult male rats implanted neonatally with cyproterone.[55] (These findings can be construed, however, as representing other than antiandrogen actions of cyproterone; i.e., cyproterone is a weak antagonist of the aromatizing enzyme system in human placental microsomes[56] and can also reduce hypothalamic uptake of testosterone.[57]) Neonatal progesterone treatment antagonizes the effects of both neonatal testosterone and estrogen treatment on androgenization; there is a recent report[58] that neonatal female animals have greatly increased serum and adrenal progesterone levels as compared with neonatal males; whether this is an additional mechanism to protect the developing female brain from endogenous estrogen and androgen, or whether progesterone has a direct effect on female differentiation, remains to be seen. Last, phenoxybenzamine, but not propanolol, can prevent the masculinizing action of testosterone.[59] The possible interrelationship of monoamines and receptor concentrations or affinity remains to be explored.

It is apparent that interpretation of whether the hormonal effects associated with brain sexual differentiation are secondary to androgen or estrogen hinges on the demonstration and the nature of hormone-binding proteins (receptors?) present in neonatal brain. Nuclear localization would be more significant than cytosol retention in this regard.

Cytosol estrogen "receptors"[60] and aromatizing enzymes[51] have been demonstrated in neonatal brain, the former throughout the forebrain, the latter localized in hypothalamus and limbic system, with higher activity in male tissues. Estrogen receptors are not detectable in adult rat cortex, but available evidence[61] reveals that the cellular binding mechanisms in neonatal and adult brain (whatever their location) have similar properties. Cytosol androgen-binding macromolecules with high affinity for dihydrotestosterone and testosterone have also been demonstrated in male and female neonatal brain, these macromolecules having different specificities and developmental patterns than those of estrogen receptors.[62] It should be recognized that there are considerable technical difficulties in demonstrating and characterizing androgen "receptors" in brain because of their low concentration, in contrast to those found in other androgen-responsive tissues. In neonatal brain, estradiol, but not diethylstilbestrol, competes effectively with androgens for receptor binding. Nuclear translocation of the estrogen receptor was present in hypothalami of 4-day-old males and in female animals treated with testosterone, but was absent in female and castrate male animals.[63] Since nuclear translocation was not evident in cortical tissue from such animals under these conditions, but could be demonstrated in both cortical and hypothalamic tissue from male or female animals treated with diethylstilbestrol, this would suggest different functions for these two types of receptors. That in the hypothalamus would be responsive to aromatized androgens, whereas that in cortex would represent a more diffuse system, perhaps of importance at a time of high estrogen levels (i.e., prenatally or after the tenth day of life in the female).

These data indicate that there are several components that affect sexual differentiation of the brain: estradiol receptors (cytoplasmic and nuclear), an estradiol neonatal binding protein, aromatizing enzymes for converting androgens to estrogens, a cytosol androgen-binding macromolecule, levels of circulating progesterone, and possible neurotransmitter modulation. The interrelationships of these factors remains to be explored.

1.4. Melatonin

There has been further confirmation of a circadian rhythm of serum melatonin concentrations in the rat,[64] sheep,[65] human,[66] and calf,[67] with the highest concentrations in all species (nocturnal or diurnal) occurring during darkness. A similar circadian cycle is present in calf CSF.[67] In ewes, the plasma rhythm is abolished in constant light (all levels being equal to the trough levels seen with light–dark alternation),[65] but persists in constant dark. Human subjects, however, maintain a normal circadian pattern of serum melatonin levels in constant light.[66] The serum rhythm disappears following pinealectomy in rats,[68] although in such animals, blood and urine levels of melatonin are detectable, being approximately 20% of those seen in intact animals.

A possible variation in serum melatonin concentrations related to the menstrual cycle may also exist, with the highest concentrations at the time of menses and the lowest at the time of the LH peak.[69] This would be in agreement with the report that melatonin can significantly reduce the stimulatory effect of LRF on LH secretion from neonatal rat anterior pituitary glands in organ culture.[70] A similar inhibitory effect of melatonin was not seen in *in vivo* human studies; whether this was a function of the dose administered remains to be determined.[71]

1.5. Clinical Neuroendocrinology

1.5.1. Endocrine Effects of Pituitary–Hypothalamic Irradiation for Nonpituitary or Hypothalamic Tumors

Radiotherapy has frequently been employed in the treatment of chromophobe pituitary tumors, alone or in association with surgery. There is a general consensus that such treatment (doses up to 4500 r) is not associated with any endocrine deficit in those patients with normal indices prior to treatment, or with worsening of any deficits already present; indeed, there are reports of normal pregnancies following such treatment in patients with evidence of prior hypogonadism.[72] There have been occasional reports[73] of the development of postradiation sarcoma following such pituitary irradiation for either chromophobe or eosinophilic adenomata. In 10 cases in which the irradiation dosage was known, this exceeded 4500 r in 7; in 2 of the 3 cases receiving a lesser total amount, the dose was administered over two different time periods.

The hypothalamus is considered to be more radiosensitive than the pituitary.[74,75] Several recent reports of "hypothalamic–hypopituitarism" following irradiation of nonpituitary, noncranial tumors are therefore of interest.

Of 15 adult patients who received radiotherapy for nasopharyngeal tumors, 14 had evidence of some endocrine abnormality 5–20 years subsequently.[76] The estimated dose to the hypothalamic–pituitary area ranged from 5040 to 8305 r. Basal prolactin concentrations were elevated in all but 1 patient, and virtually all patients showed a rise in such levels following TRF, with only 4 manifesting significant rises following chlorpromazine administration. Five patients had low TSH levels and failed to respond to TRF (3 of these had prolactin responsiveness to TRF). All but 2 of these 5 patients responded to LRF, while only 2 responded with an increase in growth hormone levels following insulin-induced hypoglycemia. On the basis of current knowledge regarding responses to releasing factors, it is difficult to interpret the localizing value of a positive response to LRF compared with a negative response to TRF in a given patient. Such a pattern of results might be more compatible with hypothalamic rather than pituitary dysfunction ("priming" by additional TRF perhaps being necessary for a positive response). In only 1 patient could tests be interpreted as being associated with a primary pituitary defect. These findings are in agreement with another study of 7 patients (including 3 children) who received irradiation (the hypothalamic–pituitary area being in the radiotherapy field) for nasal or nasopharyngeal tumors or brain tumors distant from the hypothalamus.[77] (One case in this report of a sarcoma of the left optic nerve sheath is excluded because its anatomical location alone might be associated with some evidence of endocrine abnormality.) The dose to the hypothalamic–pituitary area was less than 4500 r in only 2 patients (ages 1 and 8 years). In 3 patients whose plasma cortisol responses to both vasopressin and insulin-induced hypoglycemia were determined, normal responses were present in the former and absent in the latter test; none showed a growth hormone response to the latter stimulus. (In the 4 patients who had been irradiated in childhood, growth failure was noted.) Evidence of responsiveness to TRH was present in all patients, and prolactin levels were elevated in only 2 of 5 patients tested.

The findings cited above suggest that irradiation of tumors of the head in children can be associated with growth failure. This is confirmed by two other studies,[78,79] again suggestive of a hypothalamic effect of irradiation in this regard. These reports emphasize the necessity of shielding the hypothalamic–pituitary area in patients receiving such irradiation, and the need for frequent growth measurements to anticipate the possibility of growth hormone deficiency, so as to be able to institute appropriate replacement therapy should the primary tumor be controlled. There are not sufficient data to suggest that children are more susceptible to the effects of such irradiation with regard to growth hormone suppression: it may be that the clinical manifestations of such deficiency are more apparent in children.

1.5.2. Selective Removal of Hypersecreting Pituitary Microadenomas

1.5.2.1. Theoretical and Pathological Considerations

Although there have been isolated reports of pituitary tumors associated with hypersecretion of the glycoprotein hormones FSH[80] and TSH,[81] the three main endocrine conditions associated with such hypersecretion are the galactorrhea–amenorrhea syndrome, acromegaly, and Cushing's disease. These three clinical states may be associated with roentgen findings of a normal or enlarged sella turcica, or with pituitary microadenomata—some of the latter visible with the technique of pituitary polytomography, others evident only on surgical exploration.

The incidence of microadenomata in these disease categories is difficult to estimate. As judged from conventional radiographic techniques, there is no evidence of sellar enlargement in 25–30% of patients with acromegaly. Of 29 untreated patients with hyperprolactinemic amenorrhea, 12 were found to have pituitary tumors on radiological examination; whether the tumors were gross or microscopic was not stated,[82] although correlation between tumor size and serum prolactin levels was noted. Approximately 10% of patients presenting with Cushing's disease (bilateral adrenocortical hyperplasia) manifest gross sellar enlargement at the time of diagnosis. A 65% incidence of pituitary adenomata was reported in autopsied cases of Cushing's disease (tumor size was not stated nor correlated with X-ray evidence of sellar enlargement).[83] These findings are challenged by a recent report[84] of pathological findings in 15 cases of Cushing's disease explored by transphenoidal hypophysectomy. In only 2 cases were discrete adenomas alone found. In 9 additional cases in which adenomata were found, these were associated with evidence of diffuse ACTH cell hyperplasia in 2, and with evidence of nodular ACTH cell hyperplasia in 7; in 2 instances each, either diffuse ACTH cell hyperplasia or nodular ACTH cell hyperplasia alone was found. In this last report, the apparent incidence of eosinophilic cell hyperplasia in acromegaly, in contrast to that of adenoma alone, was much lower than in the cases of Cushing's disease, although precise data were not presented. It should also be noted that pathological examination of pituitaries containing microadenomata has revealed absence of a capsule around such adenomas in all instances, these adenomas being imbedded in normal pituitary tissue and surrounded by normal pituitary cells.[85] Last, a recent case report[86] of precocious puberty in association with a hypothalamic hamartoma, in which the pituitary was normal on roentgen examination (no pathological studies were done), is of extreme interest. This 19-month-old child had adult levels of FSH, LH, and testosterone. The excised tissue from the hamartona contained neurons with neurosecretory granules, similar to those described in hypothalamus and median eminence. Immunofluorescence studies using specific antibody to LHRH demonstrated staining throughout the tumor tissue. These findings would suggest that functional or neoplastic overactivity of cells that produce releasing hormone could result in evidence of pituitary hypersecretion. It will be of interest to ascertain whether such changes are seen in the case of tumors associated with hypersecretion of other pituitary hormones. To date, there has been no detailed pathological study of the hypothalamus–median eminence area in such cases.

The reports cited above are pertinent to a consideration of the etiology of hypersecreting pituitary tumors and the type of treatment to be employed. There is controversy as to whether acromegaly[87] and Cushing's disease[88] represent primary pituitary disease or are secondary to hyperstimulation by CNS releasing hormones. If the former theory is correct, permanent cure should result following *selective* removal of the pituitary tumor. (Cases in which total hypophysectomy has been performed cannot be considered in this regard.) If the second theory is correct, remission might or might not occur, in this latter instance representing residual adenomatous or hyperplastic tissue. Even should remission occur, prolonged follow-up would be necessary to determine its permanence. It should be recognized that in a given instance, one or the other etiology might be present.

1.5.2.2. Results of Treatment

1.5.2.2.a. Acromegaly and Galactorrhea. Hardy *et al.*[89] reported cure (growth hormone levels <5 ng/ml, or slightly elevated above this and falling to this level following glucose administration) in 46 of 57 previously untreated cases of acromegaly, utilizing selective transphenoidal hypophysectomy. The exact duration of follow-up was not stated. These results can be further subdivided as representing cure in 12 of 13 cases with microadenomata, 15 of 18 cases in which the sella was enlarged but the sellar floor was intact, 10 of 11 cases in which sellar enlargement was accompanied by evidence of local erosion of the sellar floor, and 9 of 13 cases with suprasellar extension. An additional 8 cases in the entire group were described as improved (significant reduction in basal growth hormone, but no suppression of growth hormone release by hyperglycemia). There were no postoperative changes in other pituitary hormone functions. In another series,[84] cure was also reported in 70 of 80 patients in whom transphenoidal hypophysectomy was performed; selective adenomectomy could be performed in only 53 of these cases, only 30% of tumors greater than 2.5 cm in diameter being suitable for a clearly selective approach. Residual pituitary function was preserved in 98% of selective operations, but to a lesser extent with other procedures. In cases followed for more than 1½ years postoperatively, 3 recurrences were noted, all of these being in the group with nonselective removal. In a third series of acromegalics[90] studied 3–12 months following transphenoidal surgery, normal growth hormone levels were found in 9 of 14 patients.

This same study reported that prolactin levels returned to normal postoperatively in 9 of 16 patients with galactorrhea. Normal levels of both hormones were attained within 1–24 hr following ablation. In Hardy's series of 20 patients with galactorrhea[91] (only 4 with radiological evidence of sellar enlargement), galactorrhea disappeared in all postoperatively, and 5 of 18 patients in the premenopausal age group had resumption of menses. Insufficient data were available with regard to any effect on serum prolactin concentrations.

1.5.2.2b. Cushing's Disease. "Cure" was reported[91] in 8 of 10 cases of Cushing's disease treated by transphenoidal hypophysectomy. Of these cases, 4 were associated with radiological evidence of sellar enlargement, 3 of these patients having had bilateral adrenalectomy prior to pituitary surgery. These 3 patients also developed hypopituitarism following surgery. There were no reported endocrine data in this study. There are individual case reports[92–95] concerning an additional 6 patients (4 with radiologically enlarged sellas, 1 demonstrated to be an empty sella; in 2, there was no comment on sellar size). The apparent follow-up period varied from 6 months to 4 years postoperatively. All patients had a return of normal dexamethasone suppressability. The response of plasma corticosteroid levels to insulin-induced hypoglycemia and their circadian periodicity were normal in the 3 patients who were so studied. Function of the other pituitary hormones was also normal postoperatively. It is of interest that 1 case[91] required prolonged corticosteroid maintenance postoperatively (for the 8-month postoperative follow-up period), symptoms of adrenal insufficiency developing when medication was stopped; the author has seen a similar case. This is also similar to the report[96] of transient secondary adrenocortical insufficiency (with no loss of other pituitary hormone function) after α-particle radiation therapy for Cushing's disease, and would suggest temporary feedback suppression of residual ACTH-producing cells in the pituitary as a result of chronic glucocorticoid exposure.

Addendum

A role of somatostatin in the regulation of TSH secretion was further demonstrated by recent studies[97,98] in rats injected with antiserum directed against somatostatin. Basal TSH levels, the response to cold and to injected TRH, and TSH levels in thyroidectomized rats maintained on minimal doses of thyroid hormone were all increased by antisomatostatin treatment. On the basis of these findings, it seems reasonable to suggest that stress induced inhibition of TSH and growth hormone secretion, a characteristic response in this species is due to somatostatin release, and that the prolonged and sometimes abnormally high responses to TRH observed in some patients with hypothalamic hypothyroidism may be due to associated somatostatin deficiency.

References

1. Vanderhaeghen, J. J., Signeau, J. C., and Gepts, W., 1975, New peptide in the vertebrate CNS reacting with antigastrin antibodies, *Nature (London)* **257:**604–605.
2. Said, S. I., and Rosenberg, R. N., 1976, Vasoactive intestinal polypeptide: Abundant immunoreactivity in neural cell lines and normal nervous tissue, *Science* **192:**907–908.
3. Hökfelt, T., Kellerth, J. O., Nilsson, G., and Pernow, B., 1975, Substance P: Localization in the central nervous system and in some primary sensory neurons, *Science* **190:**889–890.
4. Brownstein, M. J., Mroz, E. A., Kizer, J. S., Palkovits, M., and Leeman, S. E., 1976, Regional distribution of Substance P in the brain of the rat, *Brain Res.* **116:**299–305.
5. Carraway, R. E., Demers, L. M., and Leeman, S. E., 1976, Hyperglycemic effect of neurotensin, a hypothalamic peptide, *Endocrinology* **99:**1452–1462.
6. Uhl, G. R., and Snyder, S. H., 1977, Neurotensin receptor binding: Regional and subcellular distributions favor transmitter role, *Eur. J. Pharmacol.* **41:**89–91.
7. Ganten, D., Minnich, J. L., Granger, P., Hayduk, K., Brecht, H. M., Barbeau, A., Boucher, R., and Genest, J., 1971, Angiotensin-forming enzyme in brain tissue, *Science* **173:**64–65.
8. Day, R. P., and Reid, I. A., 1976, Renin activity in dog brain: Enzymological similarity to cathepsin D, *Endocrinology* **99:**93–100.
9. Reid, I. A., and Ramsay, D. J., 1975, The effects of intracerebroventricular administration of renin on drinking and blood pressure, *Endocrinology* **97:**536–542.
10. Krieger, D. T., Liotta, A., and Brownstein, M. J., 1977, Presence of corticotropin in brain of normal and hypophysectomized rats, *Proc. Natl. Acad. Sci. U.S.A.* **74:**648–652.
11. Krieger, D. T., Liotta, A., and Brownstein, M. J., 1977, Presence of corticotropin in limbic system of normal and hypophysectiomized rats, *Brain Res.* **128:**575–579.
12. Oliver, C., Eskay, R. L., Porter, J. C., and Cecil, H., 1976, Distribution in the rat brain of α-MSH and its concentration in hypophysial portal blood, *Proceedings of the 5th International Congress of Endocrinology,* Abstract No. 244.
13. Vaudry, H., Oliver, C., Vaillant, R., and Kraicer, J., 1976, Bioactive and immunoreactive α-MSH in the rat brain, *Proceedings of the 5th International Congress of Endocrinology,* Abstract No. 274.
14. Pacold, S. T., Lawrence, A. M., and Kirsteins, L., 1976, CNS growth hormone: Secretion of GH-like immunoreactivity from monolayer tissue cultures of the amygdala, *Clin. Res.* **24:**563A (abstract).
15. Rudman, D., Del Rio, A. E., Hollins, B. M., Houser, D. H., Keeling, M. E., Sutin, J., Scott, J. W., Sears, R. A., and Rosenberg, M. Z., 1973, Melanotropic–lipolytic peptides in various regions of bovine, simian and human brains and in simian and human cerebrospinal fluids, *Endocrinology* **92:**372–379.

16. Cheung, A. L., and Goldstein, A., 1976, Failure of hypophysectomy to alter brain content of opioid peptides (endorphins), *Life Sci.* **19**:1005–1008.
17. Guillemin, R., 1977, Endorphins, brain peptides that act like opiates, *N. Engl. J. Med.* **296**:226–228.
18. Pearse, A. G. E., 1976, Peptides in brain and intestine, *Nature (London)* **262**:92–94.
19. Snyder, S. H., 1977, Opiate receptors in the brain, *N. Engl. J. Med.* **296**:266–271.
20. Pert, C. B., Kuhar, M. J., and Snyder, S. H., 1976, Opiate receptor: Autoradiographic localization in rat brain, *Proc. Natl. Acad. Sci. U.S.A.* **73**:3729–3733.
21. Lazarus, L. H., Ling, N., and Guillemin, R., 1976, β-Lipotropin as a prohormone for the morphinominetic peptides endorphins and enkephalins, *Proc. Natl. Acad. Sci. U.S.A.* **73**:2156–2159.
22. Rónai, A. Z., Székely, J. I., Graf, L., Dunai-Kovács, Z., and Bajusz, S., 1976, Morphine-like analgesic effect of a pituitary hormone, β-lipotropin, *Life Sci.* **19**:733–738.
23. Bloom, F., Segal, D., Ling, N., and Guillemin, R., 1976, Endorphins: Profound behavioral effects in rats suggest new etiological factors in mental illness, *Science* **194**:630–632.
24. Jacquet, Y. F., and Marks, N., 1976, The C-fragment of β-lipotropin: An endogenous neuroleptic or antipsychotogen?, *Science* **194**:632–635.
25. Graf, L., and Kenessey, A., 1976, Specific cleavage of a single peptide bond (residues 77-78) in β-lipotropin by a pituitary endopeptidase, *FEBS Lett.* **69**:255–260.
26. Bradley, P. B., Briggs, I., Gayton, R. J., and Lambert, L. A., 1976, Effects of microiontophoretically applied methionine-enkephalin on single neurones in rat brainstem, *Nature (London)* **261**:425–426.
27. Gent, J. P., and Wolstencroft, J. H., 1976, Effects of methionine-enkephalin and leucine-enkephalin compared with those of morphine on brainstem neurones in cat, *Nature (London)* **261**:426–427.
28. Guillemin, R., 1976, Somatostatin inhibits the release of acetylcholine induced electrically in the myenteric plexus, *Endocrinology* **99**:1653–1654.
29. De Wied, D., 1977, Peptides and behavior, *Life Sci.* **20**:195–204.
30. Pomeranz, B., and Chiu, D., 1976, Naloxone blockade of acupuncture analgesia: Endorphin implicated, *Life Sci.* **19**:1757–1762.
31. Lampert, A., Nirenberg, M., and Klee, W. A., 1976, Tolerance and dependence evoked by an endogenous opiate peptide, *Proc. Natl. Acad. Sci. U.S.A.* **73**:3165–3167.
32. Tseng, L., Loh, H. H., Li, C. H., 1977, Human β-endorphin: Development of tolerance and behavioral activity in rats, *Biochem. Biophys. Res. Commun.* **74**:390–396.
33. Rivier, C., Vale, W., Ling, N., Brown, M., and Guillemin, R., 1977, Stimulation *in vivo* of the secretion of prolactin and growth hormone by β-endorphin, *Endocrinology* **100**:238–241.
34. Lien, E. L., Fenichel, R. L., Garsky, V., Sarantakis, D., and Grant, N. H., 1976, Enkephalin-stimulated prolactin release, *Life Sci.* **19**:837–840.
35. Ching, M., and Utiger, R. D., 1976, Measurement of thyrotropin releasing hormone (TRH) activity in pituitary portal blood of rats, *Soc. Neurosci.* **2**:648 (abstract).
36. Carmel, P. W., Araki, S., and Ferin, M., 1976, Pituitary stalk portal blood

collection in rhesus monkeys: Evidence for pulsatile release of gonadotrophin-releasing hormone (GnRH), *Endocrinology* **99**:243–248.

37. Zimmerman, E. A., Carmel, P. W., Husain, M. K., Ferin, M., Tannenbaum, M., Frantz, A. G., and Robinson, A. G., 1973, Vasopressin and neurophysin: High concentrations in monkey hypophyseal portal blood, *Science* **182**:925–927.

38. Oliver, C., Mical, R. S., and Porter, J. C., 1977, Hypothalamic–pituitary vasculature: Evidence for retrograde blood flow in the pituitary stalk, *Endocrinology* **101**:598–604.

39. Page, R. B., Munger, B. L., and Bergland, R. M., 1976, Scanning microscopy of pituitary vascular casts, *Am. J. Anat.* **146**:273–302.

40. Raisman, G., and Field, P. M., 1973, Sexual dimorphism in the neuropil of the preoptic area of the rat and its dependence on neonatal androgen, *Brain Res.* **54**:1–29.

41. Dyer, R. G., MacLeod, N. K., and Ellendorff, F., 1976, Electrophysiological evidence for sexual dimorphism and synaptic convergence in the preoptic and anterior hypothalamic areas of the rat, *Proc. R. Soc. London Ser. B* **193**:421–440.

42. Brown-Grant, K., Fink, G., Greig, F., and Murray, M. A. F., 1975, Altered sexual development in male rats after oestrogen administration during the neonatal period, *J. Reprod. Fertil.* **44**:25–42.

43. Araki, S., Toran-Allerand, C. D., Ferin, M., and Wiele, R. L. V., 1975, Immunoreactive gonadotropin-releasing hormone (Gn-RH) during maturation in the rat: Ontogeny of regional hypothalamic differences, *Endocrinology* **97**:693–697.

44. Brown-Grant, K., 1973, Recent studies in the sexual differentiation of the brain, in: *Foetal and Neonatal Physiology* (R. Comline, G. Dawes, and P. W. Nathanielsz, eds.), pp. 527–545, Cambridge University Press, Cambridge.

45. Beach, F. A., and Buehler, M. G., 1977, Male rats with inherited insensitivity to androgen show reduced sexual behavior, *Endocrinology* **100**:197–200.

46. Money, J., and Ehrhardt, A. A., 1972, Gender dimorphic behavior and fetal sex hormones, *Recent Prog. Horm. Res.* **28**:735–763.

47. Goy, R. W., and Resko, J. A., 1972, Gonadal hormones and behavior of normal and pseudohermaphroditic non-human female primates, *Recent Prog. Horm. Res.* **28**:707–733.

48. Witelson, S. F., 1976, Sex and the single hemisphere: Specialization of the right hemisphere for spatial processing, *Science* **193**:425–427.

49. Waber, D. P., 1976, Sex differences in cognition: A function of maturation rate?, *Science* **192**:572–574.

50. Goldman, P. S., Crawford, H. T., Stokes, L. P., Galkin, T. W., and Rosvold, H. E., 1974, Sex-dependent behavioral effects of cerebral cortical lesions in the developing rhesus monkey, *Science* **186**:540–542.

51. Naftolin, F., Ryan, K. J., Davies, I. J., Reddy, V. V., Flores, F., Petro, Z., Kuhn, M., White, R. J., Takaoka, Y., and Wolin, L., 1975, The formation of estrogens by central neuroendocrine tissues, *Recent Prog. Horm. Res.* **31**:295–319.

52. Korach, K. S., and Muldoon, T. G., 1975, Inhibition of anterior pituitary estrogen–receptor complex formation by low-affinity interaction with 5α-dihydrotestosterone, *Endocrinology* **97**:231–236.

53. Gerall, A. A., McMurray, M. M., and Farrell, A., 1975, Suppression of the development of female hamster behaviour by implants of testosterone and

non-aromatizable androgens administered neonatally, *J. Endocrinol.* **67**:439–445.

54. Hayashi, S., 1976, Failure of intrahypothalamic implants of an estrogen antagonist, ethamoxytriphetol (MER-25), to block neonatal androgen-sterilization, *Proc. Soc. Exp. Biol. Med.* **152**:389–392.

55. Arai, Y., and Gorski, R. A., 1968, Critical exposure time for androgenization of the rat hypothalamus determined by antiandrogen injection, *Proc. Soc. Exp. Biol. Med.* **127**:590–593.

56. Schwarzel, W. C., Kruggel, W. G., and Brodie, H., 1973, Studies on the mechanism of estrogen biosynthesis. VIII. The development of inhibitors of the enzyme system in human placenta, *Endocrinology* **92**:866–880.

57. Sar, M., and Stumpf, W. E., 1973, Effects of progesterone or cyproterone acetate on androgen uptake in the brain, pituitary and peripheral tissues, *Proc. Soc. Exp. Biol. Med.* **144**:26–29.

58. Shapiro, B. H., Goldman, A. S., Bongiovanni, A. M., and Marino, J. M., 1976, Neonatal progesterone and feminine sexual development, *Nature (London)* **264**:795–796.

59. Nishizuka, M., 1976, Neuropharmacological study on the induction of hypothalamic masculinization in female mice, *Neuroendocrinology* **20**:157–165.

60. Fox, T. O., 1975, Oestradiol receptor of neonatal mouse brain, *Nature (London)* **258**:441–444.

61. Maclusky, N. J., Chaptal, C., Lieberburg, I., and McEwen, B. S., 1976, Properties and subcellular interrelationships of presumptive estrogen receptor macromolecules in the brains of neonatal and prepubertal female rats, *Brain Res.* **114**:158–165.

62. Attardi, B., and Ohno, S., 1976, Androgen and estrogen receptors in the developing mouse brain, *Endocrinology* **99**:1279–1290.

63. Westley, B. R., and Salaman, D. F., 1976, Role of oestrogen receptor in androgen-induced sexual differentiation of the brain, *Nature (London)* **262**:407–408.

64. Ozaki, Y., Lynch, H. J., and Wurtman, R. J., 1976, Melatonin in rat pineal, plasma and urine: 24-hour rhythmicity and effect of chlorpromazine, *Endocrinology* **98**:1418–1424.

65. Rollag, M. D., and Niswender, G. D., 1976, Radioimmunoassay of serum concentrations of melatonin in sheep exposed to different lighting regimens, *Endocrinology* **98**:482–489.

66. Vaughan, G. M., Pelham, R. W., Pang, S. F., Loughlin, L. L., Wilson, K. M., Sandock, K. L., Vaughan, M. K., Koslow, S. H., and Reiter, R. J., 1976, Nocturnal elevation of plasma melatonin and urinary 5-hydroxyindoleacetic acid in young men: Attempts at modification by brief changes in environmental lighting and sleep and by autonomic drugs, *J. Clin. Endocrinol. Metab.* **42**:752–764.

67. Hedlund, L., Lischko, M. M., Rollag, M. D., and Niswender, G. D., 1977, Melatonin: Daily cycle in plasma and cerebrospinal fluid of calves, *Science* **195**:686–687.

68. Ozaki, Y., and Lynch, H. J., 1976, Presence of melatonin in plasma and urine of pinealectomized rats, *Endocrinology* **99**:641–644.

69. Wetterberg, L., Arendt, J., Paunier, L., Sizonenko, P. C., van Donselaar, W., and Heyden, T., 1976, Human serum melatonin changes during the menstral cycle, *J. Clin. Endocrinol. Metab.* **42**:185–188.

70. Martin, J. E., Engel, J. N., and Klein, D. C., 1977, Inhibition of the *in vitro*

pituitary response to luteinizing hormone-releasing hormone by melatonin, serotonin and 5-methoxytryptamine, *Endocrinology* **100**:675–680.

71. Fideleff, H., Aparicio, N. J., Guitelman, A., Debeljuk, L., Mancini, A., and Cramer, C., 1976, Effect of melatonin on the basal and stimulated gonadotropin levels in normal men and postmenopausal women, *J. Clin. Endocrinol. Metab.* **42**:1014–1017.

72. Jenkins, J. S., Ash, S., and Bloom, H. J. G., 1972, Endocrine function after external pituitary irradiation in patients with secreting and nonsecreting pituitary tumors, *Q. J. Med.* **41**(161):57–69.

73. Waltz, T. A., and Brownell, B., 1966, Sarcoma: A possible late result of effective radiation therapy for pituitary adenoma, *J. Neurosurg.* **24**:901–907.

74. Kelly, K. H., Feldsted, E. T., Brown, R. F., Ortega, P., Bierman, H. R., Low-Beer, B. V. A., and Shimkin, M. B., 1951, Irradiation of the normal human hypophysis in malignancy: Report of three cases receiving 8,100–10,000 r tissue dose to the pituitary gland, *J. Natl. Cancer. Inst.* **11**:967–984.

75. Arnold, A., 1954, Effects of X-irradiation on the hypothalamus: A possible explanation for the therapeutic benefits following X-irradiation of the hypophysial region for pituitary dysfunction, *J. Clin. Endocrinol. Metab.* **14**:859–868.

76. Samaan, N. A., Bakdash, M. M., Caderao, J. B., Cangir, A., Jesse, Jr., R. H., and Ballantyne, A. J., 1975, Hypopituitarism after external irradiation, *Ann. Intern. Med.* **83**:771–777.

77. Perry-Keene, D. A., Connelly, J. F., Young, R. A., Wettenhall, H. N. B., and Martin, F. I. R., 1976, Hypothalamic hypopituitarism following external radiotherapy for tumours distant from the adenohypophysis, *Clin. Endocrinol.* **5**:373–380.

78. Richards, G. E., Wara, W. M., Grumbach, M. M., Kaplan, S. L., Sheline, G. E., and Conte, F. A., 1976, Delayed onset of hypopituitarism: Sequelae of therapeutic irradiation of central nervous system, eye, and middle ear tumors, *J. Pediatr.* **89**:553–559.

79. Shalet, S. M., Beardwell, C. G., Morris Jones, P. H., and Pearson, D., 1976, Growth hormone deficiency after cranial irradiation, *Proceedings of the 5th International Congress of Endocrinology*, Abstract N. 171.

80. Friend, J. N., Judge, D. M., Sherman, B. M., and Santen, R. J., 1976, FSH-secreting pituitary adenomas: Stimulation and suppression studies in two patients, *J. Clin. Endocrinol. Metab.* **43**:650–657.

81. Hamilton, C. R., Jr., and Maloof, F., 1973, Unusual types of hyperthyroidism, *Medicine (Baltimore)* **52**:195–215.

82. Jacobs, H. S., Franks, S., Murray, M. A. F., Hull, G. R., Steele, S. J., and Nabarro, J. D. N., 1976, Clinical and endocrine features of hyperprolactinaemic amenorrhoea, *Clin. Endocrinol.* **5**:439–454.

83. Plotz, C. M., Knowlton, A. I., and Ragan, C., 1952, The natural history of Cushing's syndrome, *Am. J. Med.* **13**:597–614.

84. Ludecke, D., Kautzky, R., Saeger, W., and Schrader, D., 1976, Selective removal of hypersecreting pituitary adenomas?, *Acta Neurochir.* **35**:27–42.

85. Hardy, J., 1975, Trans-sphenoidal microsurgical removal of pituitary microadenoma, in: *Progress in Neurological Surgery*, Vol. 6 (H. Krayenbuhl, P. E. Maspes, and W. H. Sweet, eds.), pp. 200–216, Karger, Basel.

86. Judge, D. M., Kulin, H. E., Page, R., Santen, R., and Trapukdi, S., 1977, Hypothalamic hamartoma: A source of luteinizing-hormone-releasing factor in precocious puberty, *N. Engl. J. Med.* **296**:7–10.

87. Cryer, P. E., and Daughaday, W. H., 1974, Adrenergic modulation of growth hormone secretion in acromegaly: Suppression during phentolamine and phentolamine-isoproterenol administration, *J. Clin. Endocrinol. Metab.* **39:**658–663.
88. Krieger, D. T., 1972, The central nervous system and Cushing's syndrome, *Mt. Sinai J. Med. N. Y.* **39:**416–428.
89. Hardy, J., Somma, M., and Vezina, J. L., 1976, Treatment of acromegaly: Radiation or surgery?, in: *Current Controversies in Neurosurgery* (T. P. Morley, ed.), pp. 377–391, W. B. Saunders, Philadelphia.
90. Jaquet, P., Grisoli, F., Guibout, M., and Lissitzky, J. C., 1976, Résultats de l'exerese chirurgicale par voie trans-sphenoidale dans 30 cas d'adénomes hypophysaires hypersécrétants, *Ann. Endocrinol.* **37:**283–284.
91. Hardy, J., 1973, Transphenoidal surgery of hypersecreting pituitary tumors, in: *Diagnosis and Treatment of Pituitary Tumors* (P. O. Kohler and G. T. Ross, eds.), pp. 179–194, American Elsevier Publishing Co., New York.
92. Lagerquist, L. G., Meikle, A. W., West, C. D., and Tyler, F. H., 1974, Cushing's disease with cure by resection of a pituitary adenoma: Evidence against a primary hypothalamic defect, *Am. J. Med.* **57:**826–830.
93. Muller, O. A., Marguth, F., and Scriba, P. C., 1976, Cushing's disease due to autonomous pituitary ACTH release, *Proceedings of the 5th International Congress of Endocrinology*, Abstract No. 201.
94. Schnall, A. M., Brodkey, J., and Pearson, O. H., 1976, Pituitary function following removal of pituitary microadenomas in Cushing's disease, *Proc. Endocrinol. Soc.* (58th meeting), p. 94.
95. Ganguly, A., Stanchfield, J. B., Roberts, T. S., West, C. D., and Tyler, F. H., 1976, Cushing's syndrome in a patient with an empty sella turcica and a microadenoma of the adenohypophysis, *Am. J. Med.* **60:**306–309.
96. Cook, D. M., Jordan, R. M., Kendall, J. W., and Linfoot, J. A., 1976, Rapid appearance of transient secondary adrenocortical insufficiency after alpha-particle radiation therapy for Cushing's disease, *J. Clin. Endocrinol. Metab.* **43:**295–300.
97. Arimura, A., and Schally, A. V., 1976, Increase in basal and thyrotropin-releasing hormone (TRH)-stimulated secretion of thyrotropin (TSH) by passive immunization with antiserum to somatostatin in rats, *Endocrinology* **98:**1069–1072.
98. Gordin, A., Arimura, A., and Schally, A. V., 1976, Effect of thyroid hormone excess and deficiency on serum thyrotropin in rats immunized passively with antiserum to somatostatin, *Proc. Soc. Exp. Biol. Med.* **153:**319–323.
99. Straus E., Muller, J. E., Choi, H. S., Paronetto, F., and Yalow, R. S., 1977, Immunohistochemical localization in rabbit brain of a peptide resembling the COOH-terminal octapeptide of cholecystokinin, *Proc. Natl. Acad. Sci. U.S.A.* **74:**3033–3034.
100. Krieger, D. T., Liotta, A., Suda, T., Palkovits, M., and Brownstein, G. J., 1977, Presence of immunoassayable β-lipotropin in bovine brain and spinal cord, *Biochem. Biophys. Res. Commun.* **76:**930–936.

Anterior Pituitary

William H. Daughaday

2.1. Introduction

The adenohypophysis, despite its small size, should be considered functionally as at least five different glands, each with separate regulatory mechanisms and with unique disorders. For the purposes of this discussion, we will consider these components in the following order: (1) secretion of corticotropin and related peptides; (2) thyrotropin secretion; (3) gondotropin secretion; (4) prolactin secretion; and (5) somatotropin secretion. This review of contributions during the past year makes no pretense of being comprehensive. The large number of papers and the interests of this author have dictated the selection of papers for consideration.

2.2. Corticotropin-Related Peptides

Pituitary glands contain high-molecular-weight components that react in the radioimmunoassay (RIA) for ACTH. The nature of these

WILLIAM H. DAUGHADAY • Metabolism Division, Department of Medicine, Washington University School of Medicine, St. Louis, Missouri 63110.

components was partially clarified by Eipper *et al.*,[1] who showed by two methods that the big ACTH in mouse pituitaries and pituitary tumors contains carbohydrate substituents. The first experimental approach was to incubate mouse pituitary tumor cells with [³H]glucosamine and [³H]mannose and precipitate products with antibodies against ACTH. Subsequent separation of the ACTH peptides established that 31,000-, 23,000-, and 13,000-dalton molecular forms of "big" ACTH all contained carbohydrate radioactivity.

The second approach was to pass pituitary extracts through a column of concanavalin A linked to agarose. Such a column will retain glycoproteins with terminal mannose substituents; the glycoproteins can subsequently be eluted from the column by α-methyl-D-mannopyranoside. ACTH peptides retained on this column were demonstrated in normal mouse pituitary, neoplastic mouse pituitary cells, and bovine pituitary extracts. Recently, Orth and Nicholson[2] described similar glycoprotein "big" ACTH in human beings. They found that a large fraction of the "big" ACTH in pituitary and ectopic ACTH-producing tumors bound to a concanavalin A–agarose column, suggesting a glycoprotein constituent. Significant but small fractions of "big" ACTH from normal human pituitaries and peripheral plasma were similarly bound.

While these observations have provided new insights into the structure of "big" ACTH, the biological necessity for a pro-ACTH of such large size is not apparent. The observations may help explain, however, the puzzling observation that granules in corticotroph cells stain for carbohydrate with the periodic acid Schiff stain.

It is now evident that the pituitary contains a number of peptides related to ACTH and MSH (see also Chapter 1). These are diagrammatically indicated in Fig. 1. The largest of these peptides is β-lipotropin (β-LPH), which contains 91 amino acids. A cleavage product of 58 amino acids, γ-LPH, has also been isolated. In animals with well-defined intermediate lobes, the LPH molecules are further cleaved at amino acid 41 to yield a 17-amino-acid fragment constituting β-melanocyte stimulating hormone (β-MSH), a major pigmentary hormone of most vertebrates other than man. The amino acid sequences 61–65, 61–76, 61–91, and 61–77 are contained in met-enkephalin and α, β-, and γ-endorphins, respectively.[3] Whether these important peptides, which can react with morphine receptors of the brain, are actually derived *in vivo* from β- or γ-LPH has not been determined.

It is also likely that the molecule of ACTH containing 39 amino acids is cleaved in the intermediate lobe at amino acid 13 to yield α-MSH and at residue 18 to yield a peptide of 21 amino acids, the so-called "CLIP peptide." Because the fetal human pituitary does contain a rudimentary intermediate lobe, Silmen *et al.*[4] compared the corticotropin-related pep-

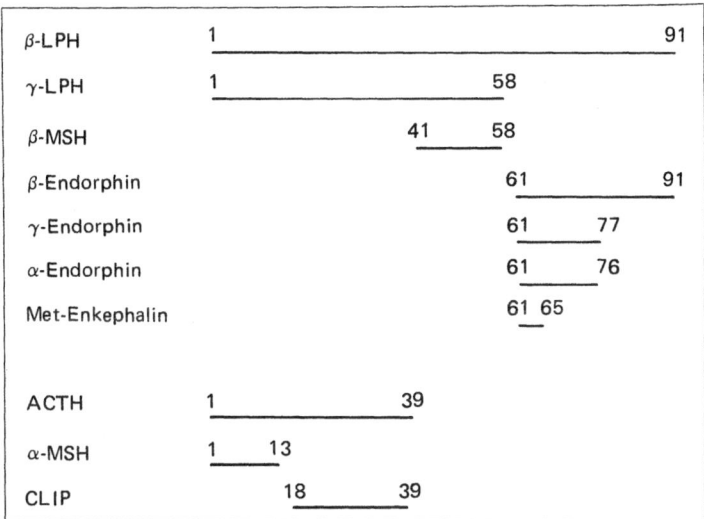

Fig. 1. Diagram indicating relationships among the known corticotropin-related peptides.

tides of fetal pituitaries with those of adult pituitaries. With their separation methods and a RIA for MSH, they found two peaks of material in adult pituitaries corresponding to β- and γ-LPH. Small amounts of the CLIP peptide, but no significant amounts of a MSH, were detected.

Examination of human fetal pituitaries also revealed the presence of β- and λ-LPH, but no detectable β-MSH. Remarkably, these pituitary extracts contained only small amounts of ACTH and relatively larger amounts of CLIP and α-MSH peptides. The predominance of these enzymatic cleavage products of ACTH prompted the authors to speculate that the CLIP and α-MSH might have unique functions in fetal life, such as the stimulation of the fetal cortex of the adrenal gland. With fetal maturity, the cleavage enzymes are less active and intact ACTH becomes the predominant peptide. ACTH acting on the definitive adrenal cortex would thereby provide the potent adrenal steroids required for pulmonary and hepatic maturation in preparation for parturition.

Biological and immunological evidence has established that certain nonpituitary tumors are capable of secretion of β-LPH- and ACTH-like material, but it is not known how closely these peptides resemble those of the normal pituitary. Lowry et al.[5] partially characterized the peptides from a thymic carcinoid tumor associated with the ectopic ACTH syndrome. The purified extracts contained LPH-like peptides and "big" ACTH-like material. On further fractionation, the main ACTH immunoreactive peak contained a minor peak in insufficient quantities for further fractionation and a peak the amino acid composition and end groups of which were established. The amino acid studies indicated that this ectopic ACTH lacked the normal end groups of pituitary ACTH and probably contained the 2–38 amino acid sequence of the native hormone. The authors considered it unlikely that the isolated $ACTH_{2-38}$ peptide was the result of nonspecific exopeptidases, but thought it to be due to cleavage of a "big" ACTH precursor by specific endopeptidase that had different specificities from those in the pituitary gland. It will be of interest to learn how much heterogeneity exists in ectopic ACTH.

Tumors associated with the ectopic ACTH syndrome also produce increased amounts of MSH-active peptides, resulting in hyperpigmentation of affected patients. The question arises whether the peptides produced by these tumors are similar to the active MSH peptides produced by the adenohypophysis. There is now evidence that the human adenohypophysis does not possess the endopeptidases required for the cleavage of the 91-amino-acid peptide β-LPH at positions 41–58 to yield the β-MSH molecule. The β-MSH that had been reported previously in human pituitary extracts may have been the result of nonspecific acid protease activity occurring during the extraction period. Some information concerning the MSH-related peptides of human tumors associated with the ectopic ACTH syndrome was provided by Hirata et al.[6] Peptide extracts were made from 8 such tumors and subjected to gel filtration through Sephadex G-50. In every case, there was detected a high-molecular-weight component the size of β-LPH that possessed a higher MSH bioreactivity in the in vitro frog skin assay that expected from its content of MSH as determined by RIA. Each tumor also contained equal or greater amounts of RIA-reactive material the size of β-MSH, but the authors concluded that this material, not found in the plasma of one subject, was probably formed by acid protease action during extraction. While the evidence for the presence of a β-LPH-like molecule in these tumors producing the ectopic ACTH syndrome seems secure, more evidence is needed before one can state that β-MSH was not also produced in vivo.

There have been attempts to prolong the action of ACTH by modification of the amino acid sequence. One such peptide, D Ser^1-$Lys^{17,18}$-$ACTH_{1-18}$-amide, has about 10 times the potency of an $ACTH_{1-24}$ and a more prolonged action after intramuscular injection. Baumann et al.[7] found that adrenal stimulation lasted for as long as 12 hr following the intranasal insufflation of 1 mg of this analogue, which may be of some practical therapeutic use.

2.2.1. Clinical Abnormalities

The pigmentation that occurs in chronic renal failure is attributable in part to increased levels of β-MSH-related peptides (e.g., LPH). Smith et al.[8] found that β-MSH immunoreactivity increased in uremia in proportion to the creatinine concentration. Dialysis was not effective in clearing the retained β-MSH-like material, but successful renal transplantation lowered β-MSH-like RIA activity to normal. Although little β-MSH-like RIA activity appears in the urine, it is likely that the filtered peptide is reabsorbed and degraded in the renal tubular cell.

Isolated ACTH deficiency remains an infrequently described condition. Limjuco et al.[9] described a case of a 55-year-old man presenting with hypoglycemic coma. In reviewing the literature, they could find only 21 reported cases, of which 15 were male. Eight cases had experienced hypoglycemic episodes. Other symptoms of glucocorticoid deficiency were usually present. The pathological basis of the disease remains unknown, but hypothalamic disease has been suspected. Some cases failing to mobilize ACTH after hypoglycemia or metyrapone will respond to vasopressin, a secretogogue acting directly on the pituitary.[10]

Isolated ACTH deficiency may be difficult to recognize if associated with other conditions. Baba et al.[11] described a patient who had presented with alcohol intoxication and hypoglycemia. Subsequent intensive study, including assessment of the responses to metyrapone and vasopressin administration, failed to demonstrate ACTH secretion. In another report, Yamamoto et al.[12] observed isolated ACTH deficiency associated with hypothyroidism. Thyroid replacement therapy failed to restore ACTH levels as measured by RIA.

2.3. Thyrotropin

2.3.1. Regulation of Secretion

During 1976, there were a number of significant studies of thyrotropin secretion. Parker et al.[13] published a definitive study of the nyctohemeral rhythmicity of plasma thyrotropin. They employed a sensitive TSH RIA capable of detecting as little as 0.2 μU/ml, thereby permitting accurate measurements within the normal range of TSH concentrations. The studies were conducted on 10 normal men in a sleep laboratory with polygraph monitoring. TSH secretion increased during the nighttime hours, the nyctohemeral maximum occurring just before or immediately after the onset of sleep. This peak was not directly related to sleep, because TSH secretion was increased if sleep was delayed or postponed (sleep reversal). In the second 24 hr of sleep reversal, the secretion of TSH was reduced. There was no clear peak at the expected time of 23:00–01:00 hr, but a small peak was noted at about 04:00 hr, suggesting a resetting of the circadian pattern. These studies suggest that TSH secretion is governed by a true circadian rhythm that, unlike that of GH, is not directly linked to sleep.

A similar circadian pattern of TSH secretion was noted in patients with moderate hypothyroidism by Weeke and Laurberg,[14] but the pattern was lost in patients with severe hypothyroidism. Partial treatment of the hypothyroidism with thyroxine restored the circadian pattern.

Inappropriate TSH hypersecretion is usually associated with a demonstrable pituitary tumor, although TSH-induced hyperthyroidism in the absence of a clinically demonstrable pituitary tumor has been recognized. An apparent lack of feedback suppression of TSH by thyroid hormone was described in a woman with Hashimoto's thyroiditis and myxedema.[15] During treatment with 0.15 mg thyroxine and 100 μg triiodothyronine, serum TSH levels initially became unmeasurable. Despite long-term therapy with as much as 0.2 mg T_4, TSH levels rose to as high as 29 ng/ml in the presence of normal serum T_4 and T_3 concentrations. There was no radiological evidence of a pituitary tumor, although a microadenoma could have escaped detection. The authors postulated that the patient had a selective resistence of the pituitary to thyroid hormone that increased the set point required for TSH suppression.

Inappropriately low secretion of TSH may persist after correction of hyperthyroidism. The duration of this dysfunction was carefully studied in 8 patients by Golstein et al.,[16] who used periodic challenges with TRH. Overtreatment with thyroid hormone was avoided by repeated measurements of serum T_4 and T_3. A normal TSH response was observed as early as 11 weeks after treatment was started, but in some patients was delayed beyond 24 weeks after achieving euthyroidism. Physicians should be alert to the unreliability of the TRH test as an indication of normal thyroid status after correction of Graves' disease.

2.3.2. Pituitary Enlargement in Hypothyroidism

In hypothyroidism, major changes occur in pituitary cellular composition and function. There is a great increase in the number, metabolic activity, and secretion of the thyrotroph cells. Somatotroph cells become less numerous, and their secretion decreases. In some instances, lactotroph cells increase their secretory activity. These changes are associated with an increase in the size of the pituitary. McCarten and Kuhns[17] carefully measured lateral sellar area and volume in children of short stature without endocrine disease and compared the findings with those obtained in both primary hypothyroidism and idiopathic hypopituitarism. Pituitary enlargement was demonstrated best in hypothyroidism if the lateral area of the sella was compared to bone age. In some cases, the enlargement of the pituitary was sufficient to suggest pituitary tumor. Clinical findings such as short stature and low urinary corticosteroid secretion might also suggest to the clinician the possibility of primary pituitary disease. Three cases of pituitary enlargement were observed by Leiba et al.[18] in children with congenital defects of thyroid development. Benign hypertrophy of the pituitary in hypothyroidism may be sufficient to cause visual field impairment. In the two adult patients reported by Vagenakis et al.,[19] the pituitary enlargement was attributed to tumor because low serum LH values and impaired serum GH responses to arginine were not corrected by thyroid replacement therapy. In both patients, TSH fell to normal. In the absence of anatomical confirmation of these cases, the diagnosis of the pituitary pathology remains conjectural. In a 24-year-old woman described by Keye et al.,[20] hypothyroidism was associated with pituitary enlargement and amenorrhea. Both TSH and prolactin concentrations were greatly elevated in the serum. Following replacement therapy, menses returned, with eventual pregnancy. Further enlargement of the pituitary did not occur.

These cases confirm that enlargement of the pituitary may occur in hypothyroidism with elevated serum TSH levels, and emphasize the difficulty in distinguishing benign hyperplasia of the pituitary from true neoplasm. Obviously, the physician should treat the hypothyroidism of these patients. In most cases, this will restore hormonal normality and arrest any further pituitary enlargement. If serum TSH levels remain elevated with adequate thyroid hormone replacement or if further enlargement of the pituitary occurs, thyrotroph cell tumor is likely and may require treatment.

2.3.3. TSH Responses to TRH Testing

The thyrotropin response to TRH in normal subjects and in patients with thyroid disease had been established by many investigators prior to 1976, yet interesting observations with this hypophysiotropic hormone continue to be made. The possibility that prostaglandins might be involved in the response to TRH was investigated by Ramey et al.[21] While indomethecin (100 mg/day for 7 days) had no effect on the TSH response to TRH, aspirin (3.6 g/day for 7 days) did lower the TSH response to TRH. Neither agent affected the prolactin response to TRH. Because both agents produced a similar depression of plasma prostaglandin E, it is unlikely that the effects of aspirin were due to inhibition of PGE formation. The dose of aspirin employed did lower total serum T_4 and T_3 concentrations, probably by displacement of bound T_4 and T_3 from thyroxine-binding globulin. The free T_4 and T_3 may have been elevated and thus induced the suppression of TSH response to TRH. Unfortunately, free T_4 and T_3 were not measured, but it is not at all certain that alterations of free T_4 and T_3 induced by displacement from TBG would be sustained for a week.

The response of the human pituitary to an analogue of TRH (pyro-glutamyl-N^{3im}-methyl-histidyl-prolineamide, or methyl-TRH) was measured by Sowers et al.[22,23] Methyl-TRH had previously been shown by Vale et al.[24] to be 8 times more potent than TRH in an in vitro rat pituitary cell assay. In human volunteers, the TSH responses to single intravenous doses of 6.25–500 μg were measured. A dose of 100 μg TRH was required for a maximal response, but a dose as small as 25 μg methyl-TRH sufficed. This would indicate that methyl-TRH is at least 5 times more potent in man than TRH. The absolute rise of TSH, T_3, and T_4 after 100 μg methyl-TRH was considerably greater than that obtained with a maximal dose of TRH (500 μg). Moreover, the duration of stimulation after a single dose was prolonged with methyl-TRH. While it is known that methyl-TRH has a greater affinity for the rat thyrotroph receptor, this cannot explain the difference in response between doses of the two molecules that elicit maximal responses. An additional effect of methyl-TRH on the response mechanism of the cell after binding may be suspected.

The response to TRH was decreased in 13 patients with uremia, all under 20 years of age, undergoing dialysis treatment.[25] No rise in TSH followed TRH administration, but the prolactin response was unimpaired. A significant increase in GH occurred in most patients after TRH. These observations largely confirm earlier studies in adult patients and indicate that significant alterations in pituitary thyrotroph function occur in uremia. No explanation for the impaired TSH response to TRH is evident, because serum T_4 and T_3 levels are generally reduced in uremia.

TRH is useful in differentiating hypothalamic from pituitary causes of secondary hypothyroidism. Earlier workers have established that patients with idiopathic hypopituitarism with dwarfism respond to TRH with a normal or exaggerated rise in TSH. This is evidence for a hypothalamic disturbance. "Isolated" thyrotropin deficiency may exist as a familial disorder recognized in early life or as an acquired condition in later life. In the few cases that have been studied in the past, there has been no detectable rise in thyrotropin after TRH. Boehm et al.[26] evaluated the TSH response to TRH in a 41-year-old man with this condition prior to and after a period of thyroid replacement therapy. Initially, TSH was undetectable in serum both before and after TRH. When the patient was restudied 2 months after discontinuation of thyroid replacement therapy, a rise to 1.8 μU/ml was detected after a single injection of TRH. During a 6-hr TRH infusion (1 μg/min), TSH rose to 1.5 μU/min. At the same time, the secretion of thyroid hormone increased as measured by a double-isotope method. This limited response of TSH to TRH administration that can occur in some patients with isolated TSH deficiency is still consistent with a primary defect in thyrotroph cells, rather than in the hypothalamus.

2.4. Gonadotropins

2.4.1. Heterogeneity and Subunit Characterization

Heterogeneity of molecular sizes of circulating peptide hormones is the rule rather than the exception; in this respect, LH is no exception. When normal human serum was subjected to gel filtration by Graesslin *et al.*,[27] the LH activity detected by RIA, by radioligand receptor assay (RRA), and by an *in vitro* testosterone production assay (TPA) was largely confined to molecular weights of about 30,000 ("little" LH) and about 140,000 ("big" LH). The RRA/RIA of the eluted fractions varied from 1.6 to 8.9; however, the RRA/TPA activities correlated closely. "Big" LH was not converted into "little" LH by 6 M urea, 0.1% mercaptoethanol, or exposure to increased hydrogen ion or salt concentrations. When LRH was administered, the major increment of LH in serum occurred in the "little" component. It could not be determined whether "big" LH was secreted by the pituitary or whether it represented an irreversible aggregation of LH molecules occurring after secretion.

In the studies cited above, the authors noted a small dialyzable component of normal serum that had LH activity in RIA, RRA, and TPA. This latter activity was described in greater detail by Leidenberger *et al.*[28] This component was obtained by dialysis of normal serum against distilled water. The concentrated dialysate contained RIA-measured activity in excess of that in native serum. Heat-labile RRA and TPA activity were also detected in these dialysates. An important finding was that dialysates of serum from hypophysectomized patients contained no activity. When the dialysates were concentrated and gel-filtered through Sephadex G-50, LH activity was associated with a component of molecular weight about 1000. Isoelectric focusing suggested an isoelectric point of 6.2 for the "mini"-LH.

In the interpretation of experiments of this type, the possibility of experimental artifact is difficult to exclude, but it is impressive that three separate detection systems were employed. At this time, it is hard to visualize how a fragment $\frac{1}{30}$ the molecular size of the parent molecule could be cleaved from LH and retain biological and immunological activity. It would be remarkable that an active core could be derived from such large and complex molecules. The small amounts of dialyzable material available for study will make chemical characterization difficult, but clarification of this intriguing observation is needed.

Improvements in the RIA of the gonadotropins continue to be made. The measurement of LH in pregnancy has been difficult because of the nearly complete cross-reactivity of hCG with most antisera against LH. Improved antibody specificity is obtained by using LH-B and hCG-B chains as immunogens. Another approach to this problem was used by Thorell *et al.*[29] Antisera induced in rabbits against human LH were passed through a Sepharose column to which hCG had been coupled. Although 90% of the original LH-binding activity was retained on the column, the remaining antibodies had high specificity for LH, with essentially no cross-reactivity with hCG. With this antiserum, it was possible to show that serum LH during the first trimester fell progressively to below the normal levels for nonpregnant women.

2.4.2. Responses to LHRH

The LH and FSH responses to LHRH continue to be extensively studied in normal and pathological states. Wollensen et al.[30] administered bolus intravenous injections of LRH in doses ranging from 0 to 3000 μg in 16 normal men. The LH response to LHRH was dose-dependent without a maximum effective dose being established. As little as 1–2 μg LHRH produced LH responses that were significantly above base line. About 10 times more LHRH was required to stimulate a significant FSH response. In these subjects, a dose of 100 μg LHRH induced an increase in LH of 400–800% and an increase in FSH of only 100–200%.

Parallel studies of the response to 30, 100, and 300 μg LRH given during the follicular, preovulatory, and luteal phases of the menstrual cycle were carried out in 20 menstruating women by Wollensen et al.[31] Age, body surface area, marital status, or race did not affect the response to LHRH. The absolute rise of LH, as well as the area under the LH response curve, were dose-related, and the integrated response was least during the follicular phase of the cycle and increased progressively during the preovulatory and luteal phases. The same general relationships also held true for the FSH response, but the slope of the dose–response curve was much flatter. The LH responses to LHRH during all phases of the cycle correlated positively with the basal hormone concentration. The authors noted that the FSH/LH ratio in response to LHRH was always less than 1 during all phases of the menstrual cycle, whereas the rise of the FSH/LH ratio that occurred spontaneously during the follicular phase of the spontaneous cycle was usually greater than 1. This led them to speculate that a factor other than LHRH might selectively stimulate FSH secretion during the follicular phase. These studies of LH and FSH responses in men and women are confirmatory of earlier studies, but serve to characterize dose–response characteristics thoroughly and provide a useful base line for comparison of pathological states.

Administration of LHRH as a 2- or 4-hr infusion may have advantages over the bolus method of injection. Koninckx et al.[32] infused LHRH at the rate of 25 μg/hr and observed a diphasic rise in gonadotropin concentration, the dip occurring after 1–2 hr. This pattern of response was interpreted as evidence of a rapidly mobilized pool and a second pool

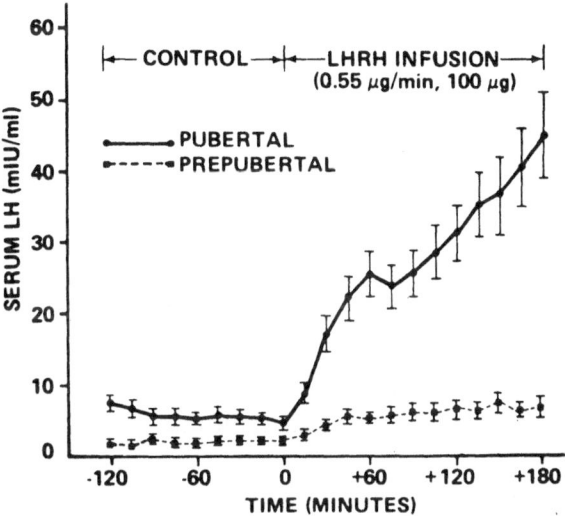

Fig. 2. Serum LH levels (mean ± S.E.) prior to and during 100 μg LHRH infusion in 20 pubertal and 16 prepubertal children depicting the qualitatively different pattern of pituitary LH release. (Reprinted from Reiter *et al.*[34] by permission.)

of stored or newly synthesized gonadotropin. As previously ovserved, the response to LHRH infusion was greater in the luteal than in the follicular phase of the menstrual cycle. Calculations based on a number of reasonable assumptions of the amount of LH released by the pituitary in response to a bolus injection during the follicular and luteal phases were 90 and 141 IU, whereas during the 4-hr infusion, the calculated amount secreted by the pituitary was 336 and 765 IU. FSH response to a bolus LHRH injection in early follicular phase was 7.6 IU and in the luteal phase 7.8 IU/min. The amount released after 4 hr of LHRH in the two phases rose to 52.5 IU and 87.0 IU, respectively.

To describe the response of LH and FSH after the administration of LHRH, multiple blood samples must be drawn. This is expensive, uncomfortable, and inconvenient for ambulatory patients. Beitins *et al.*[33] established that a 3-hr urine collection provided a simple and accurate method for integrating the fluctuating levels of FSH and LH in response to LHRH administration. The correlation between serum and urine measurements was excellent.

The response of children to infusions of LHRH differs in important respects from that of adults. Reiter *et al.*[34] infused 10 and 100 μg LHRH intravenously over a 3-hr period to a group of children. In prepubertal children, there was a single component rise in LH from 2.0±0.4 to 6.2±0.9 mIU/ml (Fig. 2). In the pubertal children, the response was much

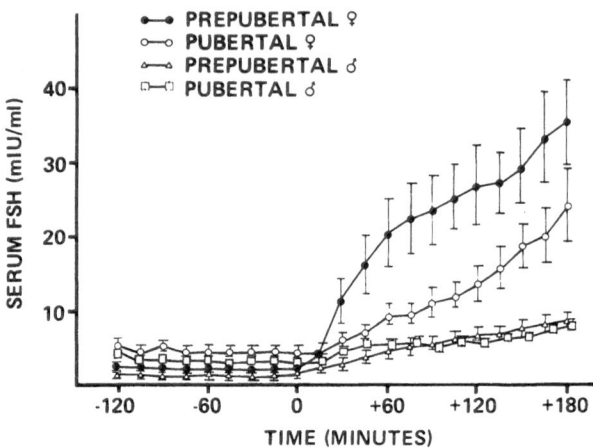

Fig. 3. Serum FSH levels (mean ± S.E.) prior to and during 100 μg LHRH infusion in 8 prepubertal boys, 8 prepubertal girls, 11 pubertal boys, and 9 pubertal girls. The FSH responses were greater in the girls than in the boys in both age groups. (Reprinted from Reiter *et al.*[34] by permission.)

brisker (5.8±0.9 to 28.0±3.6 mIU/ml), and there were two components of response previously described in adult subjects. The base-line values showed pulsatile variation in the pubertal children. Pulsatile release of LH was also evident after LHRH in both prepubertal and pubertal children.

The rise of FSH after LHRH in prepubertal boys was rather small and did not differ significantly from that of pubertal boys (Fig. 3). Prepubertal girls, however, had a brisk rise in FSH (from 2.1±0.4 to a peak of 35.8±6.8 mIU/ml) during LHRH infusion. In pubertal girls, the response was diminished (from 4.6±0.7 to a peak of 25.3±4.6 mIU/ml), but was still greater than that in the pubertal boys.

The response of the fetal pituitary to LHRH is as yet largely undefined. It is known that human fetal pituitary fragments respond to LHRH *in vitro*. Gennser *et al.*[35] attempted to show that human fetuses with a gestational age of 15–22 weeks could respond to LHRH "*in vivo.*" Umbilical vein catheterization was conducted after clamping of the umbilical cord in the course of abortion for "sociomedical reasons," and 10 μg LHRH was injected into the fetus. Blood samples were obtained before and 10 min after LHRH injection. No rise in fetal FSH in either male or female fetuses was noted. There was no rise of LH after LHRH, but the RIA measurement of LH was unreliable because the assay used also cross-reacted with hCG. This study cannot be considered definitive for two reasons: (1) The time of sampling after LHRH was only 10 min; while this is sufficient to document a response in adults, it may not be adequate in fetuses. (2) the fetuses had undergone the stress incident to the hystero-tomy and cord-clamping, with subsequent anoxia. This may have inhib-ited gonadotropin secretion.

The levels of FSH and LH are low in pregnant women, and there is little or no rise in FSH or LH after the administration of LHRH.[36,37] This inhibition of maternal pituitary gonadotropin secretion can be attributed to the high levels of estrogens and progestins that occur in pregnancy. A negative-feedback inhibition of LH secretion by hCG may also be signifi-cant. The recovery of pituitary function in the puerperium of nonnursing mothers was studied by Keye and Jaffee.[38] Baseline FSH and LH rose to levels encountered during the follicular phase of the menstrual cycle by the 3rd week postpartum. After a bolus injection of 100 μg LHRH, a small LH response was observed as early as the 2nd postpartum week, but did not become of normal magnitude until the 4th postpartum week. A period of exaggerated LH response to LHRH was found from the 5th to the 8th week postpartum. The FSH responses to LHRH were similar to those in the follicular phase by the 3rd week and were exaggerated by the 2nd month postpartum.

Andreassen and Tyson[39] compared the response to LHRH in non-nursing and fully nursing women in the puerperium. Between 5 and 12 weeks postpartum, the nursing women had an exaggerated LH and FSH response that exceeded that of nonnursing women. This augmented response may be related to the higher prolactin levels present in the nursing women.

2.4.3. Disorders of Puberty

Patients with idiopathic (true) precocious puberty have normal pub-ertal levels of gonadotropins and a normal pubertal pattern of response to LHRH. This response differs from the prepubertal pattern in that there is an exaggerated response of LH to LHRH with a similar pattern of FSH response.[40] Administration of 50 mg/day of cyproterone acetate, an antiandrogen used extensively in Europe to treat precocious puberty, led to a decrease in the LH response to LHRH. This action of cyproterone acetate cannot be ascribed to its antiandrogen potency, and is probably attributable to the progestagenic action of the drug.

Premature adrenarche of children is characterized by the appearance of pubic hair without accompanying changes of other primary and sec-ondary sex characteristics; it is attributable to an alteration in the secretion of adrenal androgens. Four girls and one boy with this condition, all between 6 and 8 years of age, had base-line levels of FSH and LH and a response to LHRH that were appropriate for prepubertal and not puber-tal children.[41]

2.4.4. Gonadotropin-Secreting Tumors

Gonadotropin-secreting pituitary adenomas are the least commonly recognized secretory pituitary tumors. Some recent observations help to define this condition. Hypogonadism has preceded the development of pituitary tumors in some but not in all cases. Even in the presence of a functioning tumor, plasma levels of FSH and LH may not be much in excess of the levels found in primary gonadal failure. The diagnosis requires demonstration that the pituitary tumor contains gonadotropins either by RIA or immunofluorescent staining or by showing that the tumor can release gonadotropins in tissue culture. In the two cases described by Friend et al.,[42] only one had preceding primary hypogonadism. Elevations of serum hormones were limited to LH, however. In one case, the tumor cells contained LH as well as FSH by immunofluorescent staining. Administration of LHRH resulted in a definite but blunted response of LH, but no response of FSH. Clomiphene was without effect. When testosterone was given, there was a modest fall of both gonadotropins in serum.

Snyder and Sterling[43] described a man who presented with signs of a pituitary tumor and loss of libido and potency. The tumor was removed surgically and postoperative radiation therapy was administered, but the tumor recurred. Libido and potency returned. Endocrine study before the operation showed moderately elevated serum FSH and LH levels and a serum testosterone concentration above normal. Administration of LHRH produced an exaggerated response of LH and a small rise in FSH. An unusual feature of this case was the unequivocal rise in LH and FSH after TRH administration. This response can be compared to the ability of TRH to stimulate GH secretion in acromegaly and connotes an unmasking of potential receptors. This patient also showed a modest elevation of serum prolactin, but this may have been secreted by the compressed normal pituitary tissue, rather than by the neoplasm. Unfortunately, the tumor content of gonadotropins was not directly measured.

These case reports, as well as the few prior descriptions of gonadotropin-secreting tumors, indicate some of the difficulties in recognizing the condition. LH and FSH hypersecretion would be considered physiological in a postmenopausal woman or hypogonadal man. In a man without sexual complaints, it is unlikely that gonadotropins would be measured. Most of the tumors described have led to only moderate elevations of serum FSH. The case described by Snyder and Sterling is an exception in that both gonadotropic hormones were secreted by the tumor. Direct study of the tumor tissue will probably indicate the presence of both hormones in more cases. The clinical significance of gonadotropin-secreting tumors is small, considering the modest level of hypersecretion and the absence of detrimental effects. Further definition of the behavior of these tumors will help us understand the alterations of function that characterize the neoplastic process in the pituitary.

2.4.5. Gonadotropins and Hypothalamic Diseases

Hopes have not been sustained that a single injection of LHRH would permit the physician to distinguish patients whose hypogonadotropism was due to hypothalamic disease from those harboring primary pituitary disease. Mortimer et al.,[44] in an extensive experience with a bolus injection of 100 μg LHRH, found that the response was correlated best with the basal levels of FSH and LH. The test did not distinguish between patients with primary pituitary disease and those with hypothalamic disease. As much information can be obtained by establishment of accurate base-line values of FSH and LH as can be obtained by performing an LHRH test with a single injection. Chronic administration of LHRH probably would be more effective in discriminating different causes of gonadotropin failure.

The value of the base-line levels of LH in predicting the response to LHRH holds true in the polycystic ovary syndrome (PCO) (see also Chapter 8, Section 8.4, for further discussion of this syndrome). In this condition, anovulation is associated with elevated levels of LH and relatively low levels of FSH. An exaggerated and prolonged LH response to LHRH occurs.[45,46] When 17β-estradiol was given intravenously to patients with PCO, there was a fall in LH with little change in FSH. Clomiphene administration also led to increases in FSH and LH. Because these findings suggested integrity of a negative-feedback mechanism, the authors concluded that PCO represents a functional derangement consequent to inappropriate estrogen feedback. The lack of suppression of LH secretion leads to chronic anovulation. Not explained is the apparent dissociation between LH secretion, which is elevated, and FSH secretion, which remains low.

2.5. Prolactin

2.5.1. Normal Physiology

An improved immunohistochemical staining method for localizing prolactin and GH was applied to human pituitaries by Martin-Comin and Robyn.[47] GH-staining cells outnumbered prolactin-staining cells by at least 10 to 1, and there were no cells that contained both GH and prolactin granules. Despite the high levels of prolactin present in fetal plasma, there was no increase in lactotroph cells in the fetal pituitary.

A detailed correlation of serum prolactin levels under basal conditions and after TRH administration as a function of age and sex was performed by Yamaji *et al.*[48] After puberty, prolactin levels were higher in women than in men, confirming earlier studies. Aging *per se* did not affect secretion of this hormone or the response to TRH.

Evidence in lower animals that prolactin regulates certain aspects of salt and water metabolism has prompted clinical investigators to look for similar actions in man. A report by Buckman *et al.*[49] that water loading suppressed plasma prolactin was not confirmed by later studies by Adler *et al.*[50] and others. In a recent paper, Buckman *et al.*[51] reported that 6 patients with pituitary adenomas and hyperprolactinemia had significantly decreased urine volume and solute excretion. The authors attributed the changes to a decrease in osmolar clearance. The difficulty in establishing a control group with exactly comparable fluid and electrolyte intakes makes this conclusion tenuous. The possibility that endogenous prolactin secretion might alter the renal handling of salt and water was also investigated by Baumann and Loriaux.[52] Eight volunteers were studied under metabolic balance conditions while ingesting a 100-mEq-Na diet before and after 10–14 days of fludrocortisone daily. Hyperprolactinemia induced by injection of TRH had no demonstrable effect on renal handling of salt and water or on adrenal steroid levels. These observations fail to confirm earlier studies in sheep in which prolactin administration led to salt and water retension.[53] The difference may reflect species specificity or possibly contamination of administered prolactin with vasopressin.

2.5.2. Pharmacological Modification

The mechanism whereby L-DOPA suppresses prolactin secretion in normal persons, patients with functional hyperprolactinemia, and those with prolactin-secreting tumors has remained moot. That L-DOPA can suppress prolactin secretion in patients with various types of hypothalamic disease associated with hyperprolactinemia suggests that this agent is converted to dopamine within the pituitary and acts directly on the pituitary. Direct experimental proof of this action in rhesus monkeys was provided by Diefenbach *et al.*[54] Stalk sectioning of female monkeys with interposition of a silastic barrier led to a 10-fold rise in serum prolactin. Under these conditions, administration of chlorpromazine, an agent that increases prolactin secretion in normal monkeys, did not increase serum prolactin. In contrast, administration of L-DOPA to stalk-sectioned monkeys still resulted in a profound decrease in serum prolactin concentration. Moreover, the stimulation of prolactin secretion by TRH was blocked in stalk-sectioned monkeys by prior treatment with L-DOPA. These carefully controlled studies resolve some of the confusion that has arisen from conflicting results with different test systems and species, and establish clearly that L-DOPA can act directly on the pituitary. A possible but unlikely explanation of the L-DOPA effect is that the drug acts on the blood vessels to decrease pituitary blood flow, rather than acting via a direct effect on the parenchymal cells. The experiments do not rule out a second effect on the hypothalamus to promote the secretion of a prolactin-inhibiting factor separate from dopamine.

The administration of large doses of estrogens increases serum prolactin levels in both men and women. Because of the possible relationship of prolactin to the development of mammary cancer, Robyn and Mekemans[55] investigated the effects of ethinyl-estradiol in the dose usually prescribed to control menopausal symptoms. Five menopausal women received 25 μg of this estrogen/day for 27 days. Prolactin levels doubled during the first 10 days of treatment and remained elevated throughout the treatment period. Within 2 weeks of discontinuation of treatment, serum prolactin had returned to the original base-line values.

Endogenous estrogen secretion modifies the prolactin response to pharmacological secretagogues. Buckman et al.[56] found that the integrated prolactin response to phenothiazine administration was about 27% greater during the middle of the menstrual cycle than during the early follicular phase.

Estrogens exert a diphasic action on prolactin secretion. Intravenous administration of 17β-estradiol (50 μg/hr for 4 hr) resulted in a significant decrease in prolactin levels.[57] At the conclusion of the infusion, serum prolactin rose to values significantly higher than the original base-line levels. The physiological significance of this observation remains to be determined, but it is obvious that short-term estrogen administration cannot be counted on to stimulate prolactin secretion.

Pharmacological agents that act on the hypothalamus to promote pituitary prolactin secretion are useful diagnostic tools in the evaluation of patients with hypothalamic and pituitary disease. The phenothiazine drugs have been widely utilized for this purpose, but have the disadvantage of inducing hypotension and severe sleepiness, rendering any type of outpatient testing dangerous. Two derivatives of procainamide, sulpiride and metoclopramide, stimulate prolactin secretion. Metoclopramide in particular appears to be a very promising agent. This drug has been extensively employed as an antiemetic and to increase esophageal sphincter pressure and gastric emptying. Sowers et al.[58] observed no adverse side effects of doses of 10 mg orally. Peak serum prolactin levels were reached by 60 min and exceeded those measured after TRH and chlorpromazine. Judd et al.[59] chose to administer metoclopramide intravenously in a dose of 2.5 mg. Prolactin levels rose promptly and reached a peak at 30 min. As with other provocative tests of prolactin secretion, the responses of women were more than twice those observed in men. The failure to observe a rise in serum TSH concentration provides evidence that metoclopramide does not act by stimulating TRH secretion. The site of action of metoclopramide has not been established, but a primary effect on hypothalamic centers is presumed. Two patients with known hypothalamic pathology failed to respond to metoclopramide with a rise in serum prolactin. This provides further support for a hypothalamic site of action.

2.5.3. Hyperprolactinemia Syndromes

A number of reports have appeared describing the clinical features and hormonal measurements in patients with hyperprolactinemia and amenorrhea. Jacobs et al.[60] studied 35 women. Of these patients, 12 had radiological evidence of a pituitary tumor. Despite the hyperprolactinemia, galactorrhea was present in only 12 of the 35 patients. The inconsistent occurrence of galactorrhea in such patients has been commented on by earlier authors. Basal levels of prolactin in the patients with overt tumors were generally above 100 ng/ml. There was a negligible rise in serum prolactin after TRH in patients with pituitary tumors. Base-line gonadotropin levels were usually normal, and LHRH produced a mean response of LH and FSH that was often within the normal range; however, a substantial number of patients had an exaggerated response. In a smaller series of patients, Archer et al.[61] also reported an exaggerated LH and FSH response to LHRH administration. The studies by Bohnet et al.[62] of gonadotropin secretion in patients with hyperprolactinemia are at variance with the preceding findings. Of 127 anovulatory women, 17 were found to be hyperprolactinemic. Galactorrhea had never been present in 8 of the hyperprolactinemic women. Administration of clomiphene did not result in ovulation. Under base-line conditions, the LH levels were low but the FSH levels were similar to those found during the follicular phase of the cycle. The responses to LHRH were variable; in 9 of 17 patients, the LH rise after LHRH was absent; in another 3, the response was subnormal.

At present, therefore, it appears that the defect in gonadotropin secretion in hyperprolactinemia may be in either the hypothalamus or the pituitary. The contradictory reports undoubtedly reflect differences in case selection. None of the authors thus far has specifically studied the factors that control the ovulatory surge of gonadotropins that appear to be most deranged in hyperprolactinemia.

There remains the clinical problem of determining which patients without sellar deformity but with moderate hyperprolactinemia (serum prolactin 30–100 ng/ml) have small pituitary tumors and which patients have only a functional disorder. Of the various provocative and suppression tests that have been proposed, the prolactin response to TRH is most discriminating, as it is impaired in nearly all patients with demonstrable pituitary tumors. In a series of 20 patients with secondary amenorrhea, nearly all patients whose base-line prolactin was greater than 30 failed to respond to TRH with a rise in prolactin. Few endocrinologists would accept, however, the view that all patients with such mild hyperprolactinemia and who are not being medicated have microadenomas. The TRH test may therefore be more a measure of the level of prolactin secretion than of the pituitary pathology. This is an important unresolved question for the clinician.

In the United States, the treatment of hyperprolactinemia with amenorrhea is frustrating because α-bromo ergocryptine, which has been so extensively utilized in other countries, is not yet available here. Obviously, if a pituitary tumor is demonstrable, removal, generally by the transphenoidal approach, is recommended, although heavy-particle irradiation may be equally effective. Administration of pyridoxine in doses of 200–600 ng/day may be effective in some women in lowering prolactin levels and restoring menstruation.[63] It is hypothecated that pyridoxine in the large doses employed increases the concentration of pyridoxal phosphate, a cofactor for the decarboxylase for L-DOPA, and thereby increases hypothalamic and pituitary dopamine.

Hyperprolactinemia has been found in some men with hypogonadism suggesting that there may be a male counterpart to the hyperprolactinemia–amenorrhea syndrome of women. Some new information has been reported on the relationship between prolactin and testosterone secretion. Magrini et al.[64] induced hyperprolactinemia in six men with sulpiride and compared the response to hCG treatment to that found in control subjects. The rise in serum testosterone was no different in the two experimental groups, but the rise of dihydrotestosterone was decreased. An inhibition of 5α-reductase by prolactin was postulated. Using a similar experimental design, Ambrosi et al.[65] found that sulpiride actually increased the testosterone response to hCG. The dopamine antagonist halperidol induced hyperprolactinemia in men, and the changes in serum testosterone were observed by Rubin et al.[66] Instead of the expected fall in testosterone between 10:00 and 18:00 hr, a dose of 0.25 mg halperidol sustained testosterone levels, and 0.5 mg actually caused a rise in serum testosterone. While the authors concluded that "prolactin is another pituitary hormone that stimulates T secretion in adult men," other actions of halperidol may be responsible for the effect. These observations do not suggest that hyperprolactinemia results in decreased gonadal function in the male.

While the findings cited above suggest that prolactin may act in some manner to increase serum testosterone, a similar action in women was not detected by Seppala et al.[67] They measured the serum testosterone by a method that also included dihydrotestosterone, and failed to detect higher levels in women with hyperprolactinemia than in normal women. In addition, when hyperprolactinemia was suppressed by bromocriptine, no change in testosterone levels occurred.

2.5.4. Lactation

Lactation generally suppresses menstruation and decreases fertility, but some women resume regular menstruation. Delvoye et al.[68] measured serum prolactin levels before and 30 min after suckling in 39 women with long-lasting lactation. The menstruating women were found to have lower prolactin levels than the amenorrheic women, suggesting that the level of prolactin secretion might be the determining factor.

Tyson et al.[69] attempted to increase the amount of milk produced by lactating women by stimulating prolactin secretion. Normally lactating women receiving 20 mg TRH orally twice a day did not have higher serum prolactin levels, and no changes in milk composition or infant growth occurred. TSH levels in mothers and infants were not elevated. The results were different when oral TRH was given to women with lactational failure. Four women treated with 5 mg TRH twice daily had a rise in plasma prolactin with improved lactation. In nine women who received 20 mg TRH twice daily, prolactin levels also rose, and increased breast engorgement and milk letdown was noted. They were able to return to full nursing. Two women who received TRH, 40 mg p.o. twice a day, developed clinical and laboratory signs of hyperthyroidism that disappeared when the medication was stopped.

2.5.5. Prolactin Secretion in Nonpituitary Disease

Pseudocyesis is an infrequently encountered psychoendocrine disturbance in which amenorrhea, abdominal distention, and many of the classic features of pregnancy, including galactorrhea, are perceived by the patient. Yen et al.[70] described an interesting case of a 16-year-old girl with pseudocyesis, marked abdominal distention, breast enlargement, and galactorrhea. Repeated samples of serum on the first day of hospitalization established the presence of marked hyperprolactinemia (values in excess of 100 ng/ml) and elevated and irregular hypersecretion of LH. GH, TSH, and FSH secretion were normal. On the second hospital day, the psychological origin of her symptoms was revealed to the patient. Within days, the hormonal abnormalities disappeared, and 2 weeks later the patient menstruated. This case report is of interest in characterizing the pituitary disturbance that can occur in pseudocyesis.

Cushing's disease is characterized by a loss of the normal circadian rhythm of ACTH secretion and the sleep-entrained secretion of growth hormone. It is not surprising to learn that the nocturnal secretion of prolactin was found by Krieger et al.[71] to be suppressed in 6 patients with Cushing's disease (pituitarigenic hyperadrenalcorticism). The abnormality in prolactin secretion was attributed to an underlying disorder of hypothalamic function because it was not observed in 2 patients with adrenal adenoma or in 6 patients receiving long-term high-dose corticosteroid treatment. No defect in lactotroph cell function could be demonstrated in patients with Cushing's disease by TRH testing.

It has long been known that the prolactin response to TRH is suppressed in hyperthyroidism. This suppressed secretory response is not restricted to TRH because the prolactin responses to chlorpromazine[72] and to arginine[73] are similarly depressed.

2.6. Growth Hormone

2.6.1. Molecular Activation

In the past, certain enzymatic treatments of GH have been shown to lead to products of apparent increased hormonal potency. In the case of animal GHs, the objective has been to obtain a modified GH of therapeutic usefulness in man. The latest of these attempts was that carried out by Mills et al.[74] in which porcine GH was treated with human plasmin. Preliminary evidence suggested that the enzyme clipped off a hexapeptide and resulted in a product that was fully potent when injected into hypophysectomized rats. When pGH and the plasmin-treated pGH were given to hypopituitary patients and to patients with myotonic dystrophy, multiple metabolic parameters of GH action failed to show significant response.

Purified plasmin can act on highly purified hGH to yield products, recognized in polyacrylamide electrophorograms by their greater migration, that have greater biological activity in the hypox rat assay. This led Lewis et al.[75] to suggest that the predominant form of GH (hGH-B) in pituitary extracts is in fact a prohormone, and that enzymatic activation is a physiologically significant process required for full hormone action. This hypothesis was examined by Baumann,[76] who incubated [^{131}I]hGH-B and C with human plasma, and with endogenous plasmin in serum and glass-activated serum, for periods up to 24 hr. The formation of GH products of greater electrophoretic migration (hGH-D and E), characteristic of the plasmin-activated GH referred to above, was studied. The labeled hGH-B and C remained remarkably stable in serum and glass-activated serum, and there was no evidence of formation of isohormones hGH-D and E. Even after the removal from serum of natural inhibitors of plasmin action, transformation of hGH to the "activated" forms did not occur. It is therefore unlikely that circulating plasmin has sufficient concentration or activity to convert the intact hGH molecule into cleavage products of greater biological activity.

The possibility that enzymatic activation occurs in peripheral tissues was investigated by Baumann and Hodgen.[77] For these studies, [^{131}I]hGH (either a mixture of hGH-B and C, or hGH-B) was injected into rhesus monkeys, and the hGH isohormones of plasma were determined at intervals up to 90 min. There was no discernible *in vivo* formation of radioactivity with the electrophoretic mobilities of hGH-D and E in serum with either labeled GH preparation. While these studies found no transformation of intact hGH into activated cleavage products (hGH-D and E), they do not rule out the possibility that substantial quantities of the isohormones D and E are secreted by the pituitary. As yet, electrophoretic methods are not sufficiently sensitive to determine the distribution of endogenous GH isohormones in normal human plasma.

2.6.2. Receptors

The study of receptors for hGH in human tissues has been hindered by the lack of availability of an appropriate test system. The binding of hGH by a line of cultured human lymphocytes (IM-9) has been characterized,[78] but the study of hGH receptors in normal human cells has remained difficult. Carr and Friesen[79] succeeded in detecting specific binding of [^{125}I]hGH by microslices of human liver cut on a cryostat and also by hepatic homogenates and crude membrane preparations. Attempts to detect GH receptors in human adrenal, kidney, spleen, and lung were unsuccessful. Specific binding was found in 12 of 15 human livers obtained at autopsy, although nonspecific binding comprised 50–60% of the total counts bound to microslices and homogenates. Scatchard analysis suggested an affinity constant of about 0.8×10^9 liters mol^{-1}, similar to that observed in the IM-9 line of lymphocytes. Studies of the hormonal specificity of binding support the significance of the binding observed. Binding of [^{131}I]hGH to human liver receptors was inhibited by monkey GH, but not by nonprimate growth hormones (beef, ovine, procine, or canine). Purified hPL (placental lactogen) was 0.5% as potent as hGH in this radioreceptor assay, but ovine, bovine, and caprine placental extracts had much higher affinity for the presumed hGH receptor in comparison with their lactogenic activity determined in a prolactin radioreceptor assay. Of interest was the finding that culture media preincubated with spargana of *Spirometra mansonoides* (which possess GH-like activity in hypophysectomized rats) reacted with GH receptors in rabbit liver membranes, but did not compete with [^{125}I]hGH in human liver preparations.

This demonstration of specific GH binding by human liver is convincing, but the investigative potential of this approach is less promising. The degree of binding observed was variable and possibly subject to artifacts due to occupancy of receptors by endogenous GH. Moreover, ethical considerations make the study of GH receptors in liver obtained by needle biopsy of patients unjustifiable. A more accessible GH receptor system is needed for clinical research.

2.6.3. Placental Growth-Hormone-Like Peptides

Human placental lactogen (mammosomatotropin) resembles hGH in structure. It has strong lactogenic potency, but only weak somatotrophic action. Little had been known about the biological properties of placental peptides related to GH in other species until information concerning receptor reactivity was provided by Kelly et al.[80] The potency of serum from pregnant animals and placental extracts was tested in a radioreceptor assay (RRA) for lactogenic activity (membranes from rabbit mammary gland and [125I]-labeled ovine prolactin) and a RRA for GH-related activity (membranes from pregnant rabbit liver and [125I]hGH). During pregnancy, all species except the cow had a marked increase in serum lactogenic activity detected by the prolactin RRA. This was usually evident by midgestation and continued to term (in goat, sheep, and monkey, as well as in man). In hamster and guinea pig, levels fell after a midgestational peak. A well-defined double peak was evident during gestation. The concentration of GH-like activity detected by the GH RRA also rose in guinea pig, goat, and monkey to the same extent as the prolactinlike activity. The apparent rise in human and sheep was less than that observed in the other species. Measurement of GH-like activity by RRA was not possible in mouse, rat, and hamster because the sera of these species appeared to bind the [125I]hGH tracer in the RRA.

Studies were also carried out on the placentas of a number of species. Human and sheep placentas contained the highest concentration of peptide reactive in the RRA. The relative lactogenic (L) and GH-like (G) activities as revealed by the respective RRAs was determined. Human placental extracts had a G/L ratio of 40, while those of sheep and the other species had G/L ratios of near unity. The high GH-like activity demonstrated in this study in the pregnant rabbit placental membrane was also noted in the human liver [125I]hGH-binding system.[79] These fascinating observations suggest that the sheep placental peptide might be as potent as a GH substitute in man. If the sheep peptide should prove to have low immunogenic activity in man, it might have potential therapeutic usefulness in the treatment of pituitary dwarfism.

The effects of secretion of hPL on pituitary function in pregnancy are also of interest. During pregnancy, the absolute plasma levels of pituitary GH are difficult to measure because of the small reactivity of most anti-GH antibodies with the massive amounts of hPL that are present. With the most specific RIAs, basal serum GH levels are low and the responses to most GH secretagogues are markedly blunted. Support for the possible role of hPL in inhibiting GH secretion is provided by observations made on women with hydatidiform moles. This abnormal trophoblastic tissue secretes chorionic gonadotropin in large amounts, but there is generally little elevation of hPL in serum. Mochizuki et al.[81] administered arginine to 20 women with molar pregnancies of between 13 and 19 gestational weeks and compared the GH and Prl responses to those of both normal nonpregnant women and pregnant women of the same gestational duration. The GH responses of the women with molar pregnancy equaled that of normal women, whereas the pregnant women had the blunted responses observed by others. Basal prolactin levels in the women with molar pregnancy were elevated more than in normal pregnancy, and the response to arginine was exaggerated. These findings are consistent with the following conclusions: (1) hCG has no significant inhibitory effect on GH and Prl secretion by the pituitary; (2) in normal pregnancy, the pituitary secretion of Prl is partially inhibited by the lactogenic potency of hPL, and the secretion of GH is nearly totally inhibited by the somatotrophic actions of hPL; (3) the low levels of hPL that occur in molar pregnancy are insufficient to inhibit GH and Prl; (4) the plasma estrogen levels are sufficiently elevated in molar pregnancy to raise basal Prl levels and increase the Prl response to arginine.

2.6.4. Growth Hormone Effects

It has been difficult to establish a role for the normal concentrations of GH in the regulation of carbohydrate and lipid metabolism because compensatory alterations in the various agonist and antagonist hormones concerned with control of metabolism adjust for the effect of GH. Somatostatin provides the investigator with the ability to suppress the secretion of GH, insulin, and glucagon simultaneously. Gerich et al.[82] infused somatostatin intravenously and separately replaced GH, glucagon, and insulin intravenously at a rate that restored peripheral venous concentrations of the respective hormones to normal. When glucagon was added to an insulin infusion, mean plasma glucose rose from 94 to 126 mg/dl, without changes in β-hydroxybutyrate, free fatty acids, or glycerol. Withdrawal of insulin led to a further rise in plasma glucose, with a rise in β-hydroxybutyrate, free fatty acids, and glycerol. When similar experiments were carried out with GH and insulin, no apparent changes were seen in plasma glucose or in the parameters of lipolysis. When insulin was stopped and GH infusion continued, there was a rise in β-hydroxybutyrate, glycerol, and free fatty acids, but no change in plasma glucose. These observations suggest that basal glucagon secretion exerts an antiinsulin action in respect to carbohydrate metabolism, whereas basal GH secretion stimulates lipolysis.

2.6.5. Pharmacological Modification of Growth Hormone Secretion

Intravenous administration of arginine is a routine provocative stimulus for GH secretion. The mechanism of the stimulation is unknown and the response is often delayed for 60–90 min, suggesting that the action of arginine may be indirect. Chambers and Brown[83] suggest that volume expansion from the administered saline solution may be important in stimulating GH secretion. In experiments in monkeys, saline or dextran solutions alone proved to be as effective as arginine plus saline in stimulating GH secretion. Moreover, it was hypothesized that volume expansion activates somatostatin secretion. Delayed GH secretion was attributed to rebound following cessation of secretion of endogenous somatostatin. These are challenging ideas, but control mechanisms in monkeys may not be identical to those in man.

The effects of serotonin on GH secretion remain undefined, with considerable conflicting evidence concerning the effects of activation of serotoninergic pathways in man. Pontiroli et al.[84] provided new information on this topic. They gave normal adult subjects a 3-day period of treatment with metergoline (12 mg/day), a serotonin inhibitor. Arginine infusions performed at the completion of the medication resulted in higher GH peaks than occurred prior to metergoline. When the same protocol was used to study the response to L-DOPA, metergoline had no significant effect on the GH response. These results suggest that serotoninergic pathways are selectively inhibitory to the GH response to arginine, but not to L-DOPA. Administration of another agent, p-chlorophenylalanine, is at variance with this conclusion. This agent, a tryptophan hydroxylase inhibitor, depletes serotonin stores and lowers the excretion of 5-hydroxyindolacetic acid. When p-chlorophenylalanine was given to patients with Duchenne's muscular dystrophy as a therapeutic trial, there was no alteration of the circadian pattern of GH and prolactin secretion.[85] Obviously, further work in this field is needed before a clear picture of the significance of serotoninergic pathways in the CNS regulation of GH secretion will emerge.

Ritalin (methylphenidate) is believed to stimulate dopamine release from nerve endings and to act directly on dopamine receptor sites. It is also a potent stimulator of GH secretion in young men in a dose of 20 mg orally.[86] The failure of cortisol to rise after this dose argues against a nonspecific stress response.

The function of the adenohypophysis is modified in anorexia nervosa. The secretion of gonadotropins is reduced and basal levels of GH are occasionally elevated but more often normal. An abnormality in the GH response to TRH is frequently present. In the studies of Maeda *et al.*,[87] 9 of 11 patients given an intravenous dose of 500 μg TRH had a rise in their plasma GH levels. Peak levels were noted as late as 60–90 min postinjection. Interaction between TRH and hypothalamic adrenergic pathways was suspected as the cause of this response, but the explanation remains speculative.

2.6.6. Hypopituitarism

The availability of TRH and LHRH has permitted the recognition that Sheehan's syndrome is not solely the result of destruction of adenohypophysial tissue, but can also result from hypothalamic damage or disturbed portal circulation. In a remarkable case described by Herbai and Werner,[88] a 25-year-old diabetic woman developed toxemia and delivered prematurely. Postdelivery, she incurred frequent insulin reactions and evidenced the classic manifestations of hypopituitarism. Endocrine studies established the presence of hypoadrenalcorticism, hypothyroidism, and low basal GH levels. Following TRH administration, there was a normal rise in TSH. LHRH stimulated a rise in LH from 0.7 to 2.9 ng/ml, and vasopressin increased plasma cortisol to as high as 27.8 μg/dl. These findings are evidence that functional pituitary tissue was not receiving hypothalamic stimulation.

The endocrine consequences of suprasellar tumors were reported in detail by two groups. Korsgaard *et al.*[89] studied 35 patients with a variety of suprasellar tumors. Craniopharyngiomas and hypothalamic gliomas were generally associated with severe pituitary secretory deficiencies. Milder hormonal disturbances were generally found in patients with simple suprasellar cysts, meningiomas, and optic nerve gliomas.

Jenkins *et al.*[90] evaluated pituitary function in 20 patients with craniopharyngiomas. GH and gonadotropin secretion was decreased in nearly all patients. ACTH secretion, as judged from cortisol responses to hypoglycemia, was abnormal in half the patients. Of 14 patients, 6 had subnormal TSH responses to TSH, whereas 12 of 20 had low serum thyroxine. Only half the patients studied exhibited a modest elevation of serum prolactin; the highest value was 42 ng/ml. The latter finding suggests that isolation of pituitary tissue from hypothalamic control is rarely complete. Low gonadotropins were the rule, but injection of a single dose of LHRH rarely stimulated a normal rise in gonadotropin secretion. More prolonged LHRH administration might have stimulated gonadotropin secretion.

Hypoglycemia is encountered in about 10% of patients with pituitary dwarfism. Haymond et al.[91] clarified the mechanism of production of this complication. Under controlled conditions, mild hypoglycemia was induced by fasting in five panhypopituitary children. Plasma alanine and glutamine fell during fasting to values significantly less than those found in normal fasting children. Infusion with alanine restored plasma glucose, providing further evidence of deficiency of gluconeogenic substrates. The hypoglycemia was corrected by cortisone and GH treatment.

Laron dwarfism is a condition of GH refractoriness characterized phenotypically by severe growth impairment and by signs of GH deficiency despite elevated levles of plasma GH. The plasma GH of these patients is immunologically normal, and Jacobs et al.[92] found that plasma of 7 patients with Laron dwarfism reacted normally in a GH RRA utilizing pregnant rabbit liver receptors. Thes observations suggest, but do not prove, that the circulating hormone in these patients is biologically active. The failure of GH treatment in patients with this condition is therefore probably attributable to a defect in cellular response.

Clemons et al.[93] studied a 13½-year-old boy with Laron drawfism. Low somatomedin levels did not rise after GH treatment, but the patient grew at an accelerated rate. This growth cannot be ascribed to the GH therapy, however, because puberty ensued with a rise in plasma testosterone from 85 to 748 ng/dl during the period of growth. An interesting observation was the increase in insulin secretion during this period of growth. Possibly the insulinotropic action of GH was retained in this patient. The possible modifying effect of the puberty on pancreatic function should also be considered.

Hemochromatosis is often accompanied by signs of hypogonadism, a condition that has been variously attributed either to the accompanying cirrhosis or to hemosiderosis of the pituitary. That the latter pathogenetic mechanism is unusual follows from the studies of Walsh et al.[94] These workers studied 12 men with hemosiderosis and found clinical manifestations of hypogonadism in 9. Serum testosterone levels were subnormal in only 2 patients, and the rise in gonadotropins after LHRH was subnormal in only 2 patients. In general, other pituitary functions were well maintained. The authors suggested that hemosiderosis per se was not a frequent cause of hypogonadism in the absence of alcoholism or diabetes.

2.6.7. Growth Hormone Treatment

The limited availability of hGH has restrained investigators from evaluating the full range of dosage of hGH in the treatment of pituitary dwarfism; doses of 5–7 mg a week are commonly used. There are indications that higher doses of hGH might be more effective than these customary doses.[95] In 38 patients treated with either 10 or 20 IU hGH/ week, the height velocity was 1.3 times greater during the first year of treatment with the higher dose of GH. At the end of 3 years, the authors predicted that the net increase in height would have been 3.4 cm. The increased height velocity was achieved without a proportionate increase in bone age. Unfortunately, the limited supply of GH for treatment makes this study of little practical importance at present.

To conserve GH supplies, intermittent GH therapy has been undertaken in an attempt to prolong the period of "catch-up" growth. On the basis of observations made in a series of patients with pituitary deficiency over a period of 3–7 years, Pertzelan et al.[96] claimed that intermittent treatment was not associated with a progressive decline in growth velocity. The study was uncontrolled, however, the therapeutic program was not uniform, and no patients received continuous therapy.

Both GH and testosterone are potent "growth hormones" in hypopituitary children. The characteristics of the growth produced by each hormone and their interaction have been investigated. Aynsley-Green et al.[97] measured the growth of a large number of hypogonadal pubertal aged boys with and without GH deficiency and compared the effect of various therapies on growth velocity with that expected in normal adolescent boys. With hypogonadism uncomplicated by GH deficiency, testosterone therapy induced normal or greater than normal pubertal increases in growth velocity. When testosterone was administered to GH-deficient hypogonadal boys, a lesser stimulation of growth occurred. When testosterone was administered to such patients during GH therapy, however, growth velocities reached the expected normal levels. For maximum effectiveness, GH should be continued during testosterone administration or spontaneous puberty.

The pattern of growth induced by sex steroids during puberty differs from that induced by GH. Tanner et al.[98] carefully measured pituitary dwarfs who were observed during alternate 3-month period with and without hGH treatment. The patients included 6 boys and 4 girls with isolated GH deficiency who entered spontaneous puberty and 7 boys with gonadotropin as well as GH deficiency who received androgen therapy. During the "off-GH" periods, growth continued at about two-thirds the expected rate in the adolescent boys. The retardation of growth was not uniformly observed in all bones, because increase in leg length virtually ceased, while growth in sitting height continued. This phenomenon was not evident in girls. Muscle thickness, determined radiographically, also appeared to be GH-dependent, and most boys lost muscle mass during the "off-GH" periods. Bone age progressed during the "off-GH" periods.

These studies showed somewhat better growth with endogenous or exogenous androgens in the absence of GH than that observed byAynsley-Green *et al.*,[97] but the authors are in agreement that GH treatment should be continued throughout puberty to achieve normal growth.

2.6.8. Acromegaly

GH and prolactin evolved from a common peptide primitive hormone closer to prolactin than to GH in its biological attributes. It is understandable, therefore, that some patients with acromegaly should hypersecrete prolactin as well as GH. This was noted in 7 of 26 patients by Franks *et al.*,[99] and prolactin hypersecretion had no apparent relationship to the level of GH secretion. Corenblum *et al.*[100] asked the question whether the same cell could secrete both hormones. In pituitary adenomas of 6 acromegalic patients with hyperprolactinemia, two well-defined cell types with characteristic granule morphology were identified by electron microscopy. Two cell populations were also recognized by immunoperoxidase staining; some cells stained with anti-GH serum and others with antiprolactin serum. No cells contained both types of granules. No intermediate forms that would suggest the transformation of one cell type into the other were seen. Unresolved is the question whether or not the two cell types arose from a common precursor stem cell.

Patients with somatotroph adenomas frequently respond to TRH and LHRH with a prompt increase in the secretion of GH. This has been interpreted as reflecting the acquisition of normally suppressed receptors for these hypophysiotrophic hormones. It is not unexpected to learn that LHRH administration can also stimulate prolactin secretion in some acromegalic patients.[101]

A fascinating disorder of GH secretion exists in some patients with carcinoid tumors. Acromegaly has been noted in the past in patients with carcinoid tumors, and has generally been attributed to a pluriglandular syndrome with a separate pituitary tumor. Evidence that ectopic production of GH-like peptides by carcinoid tumors can occur was provided by Dabek.[102] Another source of GH was suggested by the case reported by Sönksen *et al.*[103] The patient, a woman 60 years of age, had clinical acromegaly with carpal tunnel syndrome. The sella turcica was enlarged (18×20 mm), and plasma GH concentrations varied from 156 to 260 mU/liter. 5-Hydroxyindoleacetic acid secretion was normal. The patient had a bronchial adenoma with collapse of the right lower lobe, which was removed surgically. A remarkable finding was that plasma GH fell promptly postoperatively to near normal, and there was a remission of the acromegaly. The tumor contained typical secretory granules of a carcinoid. 5-Hydroxytryptamine and dopamine were demonstrated in tumor extracts, but GH was not. The tumor was successfully grown in cell culture, and no significant amounts of GH could be detected in the culture medium. Although the culture medium of the tumor cells failed to stimulate GH secretion in a dog, the authors still postulated that this tumor was secreting a GH-releasing substance. A possible, but unlikely, explanation is that the patient did have a somatotroph tumor that infarcted, resulting in a self-cure of GH hypersecretion. Clinicians should be on the alert for this interesting endocrine situation.

The molecular size and receptor activity of the circulating GH of acromegalic patients may be different from those of normal persons. Gorden et al.[104] found that the acromegalic patients had relatively more "little" GH, corresponding in size to GH monomer, and relatively less "big" and "pre-big" fractions of immunoreactve GH. In addition, when the amount of "little" GH was measured in a RRA and expressed as a ratio of RRA/RIA, the "little" GH in acromegaly was more potent than "little" GH from normal subjects. The authors speculated that the alteration of GH receptor activity could explain the presence in some patients of active acromegaly with relatively low radioimmunoreactive GH.

An interrelationship between serotoninergic pathways and dopaminergic pathways in the regulation of GH secretion in acromegaly has been proposed. Two groups of clinical investigators have found that metergoline, a serotonin antagonist, can lower GH secretion in acromegaly. The degree of suppression was similar to that induced by the dopaminergic agents L-DOPA and 2-Br-α-ergocryptine. While Delitala et al.[105] attributed the changes in GH secretion after metergoline to interference with serotoninergic pathways, Chiodini et al.[106] found that 4 patients who responded to metergoline did not respond to another potent serotonin inhibitor, cyproheptadine. They suggested that metergoline might directly stimulate dopaminergic pathways in a manner unrelated to its antiserotoninergic effects.

Further observations on serotonin antagonists in acromegaly were reported by Feldman el al.[107] Cyprohepatidine given for 2 days lowered basal GH levels in 4 of 6 patients, and the "paradoxical" rise in GH that followed glucose ingestion was abolished in 1. Methysergide administration for 2 days lowered GH secretion in only 1 of 4 acromegalic patients, however. From this, we may conclude that serotonin antagonists are relatively weak and inconstant inhibitors of GH secretion in acromegaly.

The site of action of administered dopamine on GH secretion could be either on the hypothalamus or directly on the pituitary. In normal persons, dopamine infusion does not stimulate GH secretion, whereas L-DOPA, a precursor of dopamine that has access to the hypothalamus, stimulates GH secretion. Because dopamine infusions can suppress GH levels in acromegaly, Verde et al.[108] reasoned that dopaminergic suppression of GH release in acromegaly involves receptors present on adenomatous somatotroph cells.

Most acromegalic patients with goiter are euthyroid. In a large series of acromegalic patients,[109] 9% were hyperthyroid. In many other patients, the TSH response to TRH was definitely subnormal. This could be taken as evidence that subclinical hyperthyroidism commonly may exist in acromegalic patients.

A follow-up of an unusual case of hyperthyroidism and acromegaly has appeared.[110] As originally reported by Hamilton and Maloof,[111] this patient had clinical hyperthyroidism with exophthalmos, together with elevated TSH with thyroid hormone concentrations in the blood. The pituitary was treated with proton-beam therapy, with remission of the acromegaly and hyperthyroidism. Three years later, the patient was again hyperthyroid. TSH during this period was repeatedly undetectable in serum. Treatment with ^{131}I corrected the hyperthyroidism, but TSH levels remained low. It is difficult to decide whether this patient initially had pituitary hyperthyroidism and subsequently had Graves' disease or whether the entire disease was Graves' disease and the initial high thyrotropin values were in error or represented immunoreactive, but biologically inactive, TSH. A dissociation between immunoreactive and biologically active TSH occurs in some cases of pituitary hypothyroidism.

Despite the presence of enlarged muscles, weakness is a common complaint in patients with long-established acromegaly. Muscle biopsies obtained in 18 patients most commonly showed hypertrophy of the type 1 fibers and atrophy of the type 2 fibers.[112]

2.7. Somatomedins

The somatomedins consist of a number of peptide substances in plasma the concentration of which is GH-dependent. Somatomedins stimulate growth-related processes in cartilage, and possibly in other tissues, *in vitro*. It is widely accepted, but as yet unproved, that GH stimulates skeletal growth *in vivo* indirectly by regulating the level of somatomedins. The past work in this field was extensively reviewed in a *Nobel Symposium*.[113]

The recognized somatomedins present in human serum include: (1) somatomedin A (present as two closely related peptides), (2) somatomedin C, and (3) NSILA-s (which also exists as two separate peptides). All are small peptides with molecular masses less than 10,000 daltons. They circulate in plasma complexed to specific binding proteins. The partial amino acid sequences of NSILA-s I and II have revealed that these two peptides have very similar structures.[114] Of the first 31 residues from the amino terminal end, 22 were identical. Of great interest was the finding that 47% of the amino acid residues of NSILA-s I and 51% of NSILA-s II were identical to those on the insulin β-chain (Fig. 4). On the basis of this finding, the authors proposed that NSILA-s be renamed *insulinlike growth factor.*

Schlumph *et al.*[115] developed a simple method for quantitating growth factors in serum. The bound factors were dissociated from their binding protein in 1 M acetic acid and separated from the higher-molecular-weight proteins by gel filtration. The fraction that the authors call NSILA-s undoubtedly contains somatomedins A and C also. The fraction had insulinlike effects in adipose tissue and promoted sulfate uptake in cartilage. The effect of whole serum on adipocytes did not appear to be GH-dependent, whereas the cartilage stimulation induced by serum was GH-dependent. This suggests a greater specificity of cartilage than of adipose tissue in response to the somatomedin-related peptides in whole serum.

Franklin *et al.*[116] described an adipocyte assay for somatomedinlike peptides (NSILA-s) in which an acid ethanol extract of plasma is added to isolated adipocytes, with subsequent measurement of the stimulation of incorporation of radioactivity from $[U^{14}C]$glucose into lipid. Despite the laborious preparation of extracts, which involved considerable loss of activity, the assay statistics were impressive and provided a clean separation of activity in normal serum from that in the serum of hypopituitary and acromegaly patients.

Garland *et al.*[117] measured the response of isolated chick embryo chondrocytes to serum growth factors. The uptake of thymidine by these cells was stimulated in a dose-dependent manner by normal human serum; greater stimulation occurred on addition of serum from acromegalic patients and less stimulation on addition of serum from hypopituitary subjects. The different groups, however, were not as well separated as has been observed with other assay systems, suggesting that these collagenase-treated cells were responding nonspecifically to nonhormonal serum components. Exposure to dilutions of serum for only 15 min was sufficient to stimulate leucine and thymidine uptake for the next 24–25 hr.[118] This suggests that rapid, virtually irreversible binding of somatomedin peptides to receptors in chondrocyte membrane occurs. The residual serum after exposure to chondrocytes was depleted of the stimulating activity.

The measurement of somatomedin by bioassay has the virtue of providing an index of the net stimulating effects of all somatomedins, but is quite impractical for routine clinical studies. Newer procedures depend on the availability of highly purified peptides for radioactive labeling. Takano *et al.*[119] employed a RRA for somatomedin A in patients with

		% Homology (residues 1–30) to:	
		NSILA I	NSILA II
NSILA I			73.3
NSILA II		73.3	
Insulin B chain Man		46.7	40.0
Tuna II		56.7	50.0
Coypu		43.3	50.0

```
                 -2 -1 1  2  3  4  5            10              15          20            25              30
NSILA I              G  P  E  T  L  C  G  A  E  L  V  D  A  L  Q  F  V  C  G  D  R  G  F  Y  F  N  K  P  T  G  Y
NSILA II          A  Y  R  P  S  E  T  L  C  G  G  E  L  V  D  T  L  Q  F  V  C  G  D  R  G  F  Y  F  S  R  E
Insulin B chain
Man                  F  V  N  Q  H  L  C  G  S  H  L  V  E  A  L  Y  L  V  C  G  E  R  G  F  F  Y  T  P  K  T
Tuna II           V  A  P  P  Q  H  L  C  G  S  H  L  V  D  A  L  Y  L  V  C  G  D  R  G  F  F  Y  N  P  K
Coypu             Y  V  S  Q  R  L  C  G  S  Q  L  V  D  T  L  Y  S  V  C  R  H  R  G  F  Y  R  P  N  D
```

Fig. 4. Alignments of amino acid sequences of NSILA I, NSILA II, and insulin β-chains from man, tuna fish, and coypu. The one-letter symbols for amino acid residues recommended by the *Journal of Biological Chemistry* are used. The numbering of residues of NSILA was chosen to correspond to conventional numbering of insulin β-chains. Dashed-line boxes indicate residues identical in NSILA I and II; Solid-line boxes indicate residues identical in NSILA and insulin β-chains. (Reprinted from Rinderknecht and Humbel,[114] with permission.)

disorders of growth. This assay measures the binding of [^{125}I]somatomedin A by a membrane preparation derived from human placentas. In general, the somatomedin levels correlated with plasma GH measurements. An unexpected finding was an increase in somatomedin A levels in patients with uremia.

A very important development was the preliminary report by Furlanetto et al.[120] of a RIA for somatomedin C. Antibodies were raised in rabbits to a somatomedin C–ovalbumin complex. The binding of [^{125}I]somatomedin C by antibody was highly specific and was not inhibited by pituitary peptides. Somatomedin A and NSILA-s cross-reacted to an extent of only 1–2%. Serum from a number of animal species appeared to cross-react. Initial results of measurements in human serum with this assay correlated with the GH status of the patients from whom serum was obtained. If these promising results can be confirmed, investigators and clinicians will have a simpler and more accurate method for measuring somatomedin in patients.

Another approach to the measurement of growth factors was utilized by Heinrich et al.[121] They measured the competitive displacement of [^{125}I]NSILA-s from its plasma binding protein. NSILA-s from serum was separated from its plasma binding protein by acid dissociation and gel filtration before introduction into the binding system. The results correlated with the GH secretion of the patients.

These promising results with competitive protein binding assay are welcomed by all workers in the field. Unresolved is the question whether the binding proteins in plasma for these tissue growth factors present obstacles to direct assay. Another important question is the relative contribution of the separate somatomedin peptides to the total biological activity of plasma. Until this question is resolved, a competitive binding assay that has a high specificity for only one somatomedin peptide may not properly reflect the total growth-promoting activity of plasma.

The plasma binding protein for somatomedin may itself be GH-dependent. Cohen and Nissley[122] measured the disappearance of somatomedin activity as measured by a chick fibroblast assay after injection of serum into hypophysectomized rats. The half-life of disappearance of somatomedin from normal serum was about 3 hr, but the disappearance of activity after injection of serum from operated rats briefly treated with GH was only 8 min. More prolonged GH treatment of hypophysectomized rats yielded serum the somatomedin activity of which disappeared with a half-life of about 4 hr. The shorter half-life of somatomedin in these GH-treated rats was attributed to less binding by plasma.

There has been considerable interest in the subject of somatomedin and fetal growth. D'Ercole et al.[123] detected specific binding of human somatomedin C by a number of tissues of fetal pig at all stages of gestation. Moreover, fetal pig serum contained detectable somatomedin by bioassay. These observations support the possibility that somatomedin might be importantly related to fetal growth. The authors also found that human cord serum contained low but detectable levels of somatomedin. The cord blood of both small-for-gestational date and postmature infants appeared to have lower somatomedin content.

A more comprehensive study of human cord blood, in which somatomedin was measured by a porcine cartilage bioassay, was reported by Gluckman and Brinsmead.[124] The mean cord blood somatomedin activity was 0.65 ± 0.21 U/ml, but the variability between samples was large. Somatomedin concentration correlated positively with gestational age, birth weight, and other parameters of fetal size. Plasma somatomedin levels in newborn infants, as reported by Giordano et al.,[125] were similar to those found in cord blood.

Amniotic fluid obtained at parturition has low somatomedin activity,[126] but expressed per milligrams of protein, it is comparable to that of plasma. Most of the bioassayable activity is complexed to high-molecular-weight proteins and can be dissociated by acid to yield a biologically active function of smaller size. In these properties, amniotic fluid resembles plasma somatomedin.

Application of a somatomedin C RRA to amniotic fluid demonstrated a reactive material that was detectable at 12 weeks of gestation, but reached a peak at 20 weeks of gestation.[127] Thereafter, there was a progressive decline in the amount of material detected until term, when only small amounts of material were detected. The reactive material in midterm amniotic fluid is not somatomedin C, but a 30,000-molecular-weight protein with specific somatomedin-C-binding activity and no cartilage-stimulating activity.[128] Whether this material represents a monomer of the normal plasma binding protein or a special fetal binding protein remains to be determined.

Somatomedin activity in the serum of 100 children of various ages was measured by the chick embryo cartilage bioassay.[129] These studies confirmed the lower levels of activity during the first few years of life that had been observed previously. Growth at this age may be less dependent on somatomedin than is the case later, or else somatomedin in the plasma of infants may be more available because of reduced protein binding. Tissue sensitivity to somatomedin may also be increased so that less is required.

There are a number of interesting exceptions to the correlation between GH and somatomedin levels. The condition that has attracted the greatest attention is so-called *growth-hormone-independent growth*. This situation is encountered in children with hypothalamic tumors who on presentation are short, but grow at a normal or accelerated rate after operative intervention. During this period of growth, serum GH levels are low, but somatomedin levels are normal. Prolactin levels are occasionally elevated, but elevated prolactin levels are probably not required to maintain somatomedin in such patients, because in one case complete suppression of prolactin to undetectable levels by bromocryptine administration did not affect somatomedin levels.[130] Costin *et al.*[131] studied 8 patients with this paradoxical postoperative growth. All had GH deficiency, but the mean somatomedin level was within the normal range. Prolactin levels were all normal. The insulin responses to oral glucose and intravenous tolbutamide were significantly greater than those observed in hypopituitary children who were not growing. The improved insulin response, perhaps related to improved nutrition, may have been important in maintaining somatomedin levels.

While GH, prolactin, and insulin may be capable of increasing somatomedin levels under certain circumstances, supraphysiological amounts of estrogen can lower somatomedin levels. This has been shown previously in acromegalic patients and in hypopituitary patients treated with GH.[132] The same suppressive effect is evident in men without pituitary disease receiving ethinyl estradiol, 0.5 mg/day for 7–70 days.[133] A fall of 40–62% in serum somatomedin activity occurred. Intravenous administratin of 25 mg of conjugated estrogens (Premarin[R]) also led to a prompt fall in somatomedin activity to from 40 to 80% of its initial level. The apparent half-time of disappearance was only 2 hr. In both situations, estrogens raised plasma GH, a result that the authors suggested might be secondary to a decreased negative feedback exerted by somatomedin. Ethinyl estradiol in a dose of 0.25 mg/day was also effective in producing a significant decrease in somatomedin activity in patients with Turner's syndrome, although the magnitude of response was less than the responses reported to occur in men given 0.5 mg/day.[134]

References

1. Eipper, B. A., Mains, R. E., and Guenzi, D., 1976, High molecular weight forms of adrenocorticotropic hormone are glycoproteins, *J. Biol. Chem.* **251**:4121–4126.
2. Orth, D. N., and Nicholson, W. E., 1977, High molecular weight forms of human ACTH are glycoproteins, *J. Clin. Endocrinol. Metab.* **44**:214–217.
3. Guillemin, R., 1976, Physiological and clinical signifcance of hypothalamic and extrahypothalamic brain peptides, *Triangle (Engl. Ed.)* **15**:1–7.
4. Silman, R. E., Chard, T., Lowry, P. J., Smith, I., and Young, I. M., 1976, Human foetal pituitary peptides and parturition, *Nature (London)* **260**:716–718.
5. Lowry, P. J., Rees, L. H., Tomlin, S., Gillies, G., and Landon, J., 1976,

Chemical characterization of ectopic ACTH purified from a malignant thymic carcinoid tumor, *J. Clin. Endocrinol. Metab.* **43**:831–835.

6. Hirata, Y., Matsukura, S., Imura, H., Nakamura, M., and Tanaka, A., 1976, Size heterogeneity of β-MSH in ectopic ACTH-producing tumors: Presence of β-LPH-like peptide, *J. Clin. Endocrinol. Metab.* **42**:33–40.

7. Baumann, G., Walser, A., Desaulles, P. A., Paesi, F. J. A., and Geller, L., 1976, Corticotropic action of an intra-nasally applied synthetic ACTH derivative, *J. Clin. Endocrinol. Metab.* **42**:60–63.

8. Smith, A. G., Shuster, S., Thody, A. J., Alvarez-ude, F., and Kerr, D. N., 1976, Role of the kidney in regulating plasma immunoreactive beta-melanocyte-stimulating hormone, *Br. Med. J.* **1**:874–876.

9. Limjuco, R. A., Sherman, L., and Kolodny, H. D., 1976, Isolated ACTH deficiency, *N. Y. State J. Med.* **76**:439–444.

10. Laron, Z., Karp, M., Pertzelan, A., and Frankel, J., 1970, ACTH deficiency in children and adolescents (clinical and psychological aspects), *Prog. Brain Res.* **32**:305–315.

11. Baba, S., Takase, S., Uenoyama, R., Morita, S., Mizoi, S., and Hishida, S., 1976, Isolated corticotrophin-deficiency found through alcohol-induced hypoglycemic coma, *Horm. Metab. Res.* **8**:274–278.

12. Yamamoto, T., Ogihara, T., Miyai, K., Kumahara, Y., and Hirata, Y., 1976, Co-existent primary hypothyroidism and isolated ACTH deficiency, *Acta Endocrinol.* **82**:467–474.

13. Parker, D. C., Pekary, A. E., and Hershman, J. M., 1976, Effect of normal and reversed sleep–wake cycles upon nyctohemeral rhythmicity of plasma thyrotropin: Evidence suggestive of an inhibitory influence in sleep, *J. Clin. Endocrinol. Metab.* **43**:318–329.

14. Weeke, J., and Laurberg, P., 1976, Diurnal TSH variations in hypothyroidism, *J. Clin. Endocrinol. Metab.* **43**:32–37.

15. Hood, S., Vaughan-Jackson, J. D., and Farid, N. R., 1976, Inappropriate TSH secretion. Paradoxical rise in serum TSH in response to thyroxine therapy, *J. Clin. Endocrinol. Metab.* **43**:1360–1364.

16. Golstein, J., Vanhaelst, L., Camus, M., and Glinoer, D., 1976, Paradoxical modulation of thyrotrope responsiveness to TRH during the treatment of thyrotoxic patients. Apparent absence of feed-back regulation, *Horm. Metab. Res.* **8**:128–31.

17. McCarten, K. M., and Kuhns, L. R., 1976, The area and volume of the sella turcica in childhood primary hypothyroidism, *Radiology* **119**:645–650.

18. Leiba, S., Shani, M., Zahavi, I., Samuel, R., Borohowsky, S., and Ber, A., 1976, Secondary pituitary insufficiency; Report of three cases of ectopia or hemiagenesis of the thyroid gland, *Arch. Intern Med.* **136**:1010–1015.

19. Vagenakis, A. G., Dole, K., and Braverman, L. E., 1976, Pituitary enlargement, pituitary failure, and primary hypothyroidism, *Ann. Intern. Med.* **85**:195–198.

20. Keye, W. R., Jr., Yuen, B. H., Knopf, R. F., and Jaffe, R. B., 1976, Amenorrhea, hyperprolactinemia and pituitary enlargement secondary to primary hypothyroidism. Successful treatment with thyroid replacement, *Obstet. Gynecol.* **48**:697–702.

21. Ramey, J. N., Burrow, G. N., Spaulding, S. W., Donabedian, R. K., Speroff, L., and Frantz, A. G., 1976, The effect of aspirin and indomethacin on the TRH response in man, *J. Clin. Endocrinol. Metab.* **43**:107–114.

22. Sowers, J. R., Hershman, J. M., Pekary, A. E., Nair, M. G., and Baugh, C. M., 1976, Effect of N^{3im}-methyl-thyrotropin releasing hormone on the human pituitary–thyroid axis, *J. Clin. Endocrinol. Metab.* **43:**741–748.
23. Sowers, J. R., Hershman, J. M., Carlson, H. E., Pekary, A. E., Reed, A. W., Nair, M. G., and Baugh, C. M., 1976, Dose-response of prolactin and thyrotropin to N^{3im}-methyl-thyrotropin releasing hormone in euthyroid men, *J. Clin. Endocrinol. Metab.* **43:**856–860.
24. Vale, W., Rivier, J., and Burgus, R., 1971, Synthetic TRF (thyrotropin releasing factor) analogues: II. pGlu-N^{3im}me-His-Pro-NH_2: A synthetic analogue with specific activity greater than that of TRF, *Endocrinology* **89:**1485–1488.
25. Czernichow, P., Dauzet, M. C., Broyer, M., and Rappaport, R., 1976, Abnormal TSH, PRL and GH response to TSH releasing factor in chronic renal failure, *J. Clin. Endocrinol. Metab.* **43:**630–637.
26. Boehm, T. M., Dimond, R. C., and Wartofsky, L., 1976, Isolated thyrotropin deficiency with thyrotropin-releasing-hormone induced TSH secretion and thyroidal release, *J. Clin. Endocrinol. Metab.* **43:**1041–1046.
27. Graesslin, D., Leidenberger, F. A., Lichtenberg, V., Glismann, D., Hess, N., Czygan, P. J., and Bettendorf, G., 1976, Existence of big and little forms of luteinizing hormone in human serum, *Acta Endocrinol.* **83:**466–482.
28. Leidenberger, F. A., Graesslin, D., Scheel, H. J., Hess, N., Lichtenberg, V., and Bettendorf, G., 1976, A low molecular weight substance obtained from serum which has luteinizing hormone like activity ("mini LH"), *J. Clin. Endocrinol. Metab.* **43:**1410–1413.
29. Thorell, J. I., Jeppsson, S., and Holmström, B., 1976, Production of specific antisera for radioimmunoassay of human luteinizing hormone (LH) in the presence of human chorionic gonadotropin (hCG), *J. Clin. Endocrinol. Metab.* **43:**708–711.
30. Wollensen, F., Swerdloff, R. S., and Odell, W. D., 1976, LH and FSH responses to luteinizing-releasing hormone in normal human males, *Metabolism* **25:**845–863.
31. Wollensen, F., Swerdloff, R. S., and Odell, W. D., 1976, LH and FSH responses to luteinizing releasing hormone in normal fertile women, *Metabolism* **25:**1275–1285.
32. Koninckx, P., De Hertogh, R., Heyns, W., Meulepas, E., Brosens, I., and De Moor, P., 1976, Secretion rates of LH and FSH during infusion of LH-FSH/RH in normal women and in patients with secondary amenorrhea: Suggestive evidence for two pools of LH and FSH, *J. Clin. Endocrinol. Metab.* **43:**159–167.
33. Beitins, I. Z., O'Loughlin, K., Ostrea, T., and McArthur, J. W., 1976, Gonadotropin determinations in timed 3-hour urine collections during the menstrual cycle and LHRH testing, *J. Clin. Endocrinol. Metab.* **43:**46–55.
34. Reiter, E. O., Root, A. W., and Duckett, G. E., 1976, The response of pituitary gonadotropes to a constant infusion of luteinizing hormone-releasing hormone (LHRH) in normal prepubertal and pubertal children and in children with abnormalities of sexual development, *J. Clin. Endocrinol. Metab.* **43:**400–411.
35. Gennser, G., Liedholm, P., and Thorell, J., 1976, Pituitary hormone levels in plasma of the human fetus after administration of LRH, *J. Clin. Endocrinol. Metab.* **43:**470–473.

36. Jeppsson, S., and Rannevik, G., 1976, Studies on the gonadotropin response after administration of LH-FSH-releasing hormone (LRH) during pregnancy and after therapeutic abortion in the second trimester, *Am. J. Obstet. Gynecol.* **125**:484–490.
37. Reyes, F. I., Winter, J. S. D., and Faiman, C., 1976, Pituitary gonadotropin function during human pregnancy: Serum FSH and LH levels before and after LHRH administration, *J. Clin. Endocrinol. Metab.* **42**:590–592.
38. Keye, W. R., Jr., and Jaffe, R. B., 1976, Changing patterns of FSH and LH response to gonadotropin-releasing hormone in the puerperium, *J. Clin. Endocrinol. Metab.* **42**:1133–1138.
39. Andreassen, B., and Tyson, J. F., 1976, Role of the hypothalamic–pituitary–ovarian axis in puerperal infertility, *J. Clin. Endocrinol. Metab.* **42**:1114–1122.
40. Angeli, A., Boccuzzi, G., Fonzo, D. B. D., Frajria, R., De Sanctis, C., and Ceresa, F., 1976, Effect of cyproterone acetate therapy on gonadotropin response to synthetic luteinizing hormone-releasing hormone (LRH) in girls with idiopathic precocious puberty, *J. Clin. Endocrinol. Metab.* **42**:551–560.
41. Lee, P. A., and Gareis, F. J., 1976, Gonadtropin and sex steroid response to lutenizing hormone-releasing hormone in patients with premature adrenarche, *J. Clin. Endocrinol. Metab.* **43**:195–197.
42. Friend, J. N., Judge, D. M., Sherman, B. M., and Santen, R. J., 1976, FSH-secreting pituitary adenomas: Stimulation and suppression studies in two patients, *J. Clin. Endocrinol. Metab.* **43**:650–657.
43. Snyder, P. J., and Sterling, F. H., 1976, Hypersecretion of LH and FSH by a pituitary adenoma, *J. Clin. Endocrinol. Metab.* **42**:544–550.
44. Mortimer, R. H., Fleischer, N., Lev-Gur, M., and Freeman, R. G., 1976, Correlation between integrated LH and FSH levels and the response to luteinizing hormone releasing factor (LRF), *J. Clin. Endocrinol. Metab.* **43**:1240–1249.
45. Katz, M., Pimstone, B. L., Carr, P. J., and Hendricks, S., 1976, Plasma gonadotropin and gonadotropin-releasing hormone levels after intranasal administration of gonadotropin releasing hormone, *J. Clin. Endocrinol. Metab.* **43**:215–221.
46. Rebar, R., Judd, H. L., Yen, S. S. C., Rakoff, J., Vandenberg, G., and Naftolin, F., 1976, Characterization of the inappropriate gonadotropin secretion in polycystic ovary syndrome, *J. Clin. Invest.* **57**:1320–1329.
47. Martin-Comin, J., and Robyn, C., 1976, Comparative immunoenzymatic localization of prolactin and growth hormone in human and rat pituitaries, *J. Histochem. Cytochem.* **24**:1012–1016.
48. Yamaji, T., Shimamoto, K., Ishibashi, M., Kosaka, K., and Orimo, H., 1976, Effect of age and sex on circulating and pituitary prolactin levels in human, *Acta Endocrinol. (Copenhagen)* **83**:711–719.
49. Buckman, M. T., Kaminsky, N., Conway, M., and Peake, G. T., 1973, Utility of L-dopa and water loading in evaluation of hyperprolactinemia, *J. Clin. Endocrinol. Metab.* **36**:911–919.
50. Adler, R. A., Noel, G. L., Wartofsky, L., and Frantz, A. G., 1975, Failure of oral water loading and intravenous hypotonic saline to suppress plasma prolactin in men, *J. Clin. Endocrinol. Metab.* **41**:383–389.
51. Buckman, M. T., Peake, G. T., and Robertson, G., 1976, Hyperprolactinemia influences renal function in man, *Metabolism* **25**:509–516.

52. Baumann, G., and Loriaux, D. L., 1976, Failure of endogenous prolactin to alter renal salt and water excretion and adrenal function in man, *J. Clin. Endocrinol. Metab.* **43**:643–649.
53. Horrobin, D. F., Manku, M. S., and Robertshaw, D., 1973, Water-losing action of antidiuretic hormone in the presence of excess cortisol: Restoration of normal action by prolactin or by oxytocin, *J. Endocrinol.* **58**:135–136.
54. Diefenbach, W. P., Carmel, P. W., Frantz, A. G., and Ferin, M., 1976, Suppression of prolactin secretion by L-Dopa in the stalk-sectioned rhesus monkey, *J. Clin. Endocrinol. Metab.* **43**:638–642.
55. Robyn, C., and Vekemans, M., 1976, Influence of low dose oestrogen on circulation prolactin, LH and FSH levels in post-menopausal women, *Acta Endocrinol.* **83**:9–14.
56. Buckman, M. T., Peake, G. T., and Srivastava, L. S., 1976, Endogenous estrogen modulates phenothiazine stimulated prolactin secretion, *J. Clin. Endocrinol. Metab.* **43**:901–906.
57. Ehara, Y., Siler, T. M., and Yen, S. S. C., 1976, Effects of large doses of estrogen on prolactin and growth hormone release, *Am. J. Obstet. Gynecol.* **125**: 455–458.
58. Sowers, J. R., McCallum, R. W., Hershman, J. M., Carlson, H. E., Sturdevant, R. A. L., and Meyer, N., 1976, Comparison of metoclopramide with other dynamic tests of prolactin secretion, *J. Clin. Endocrinol. Metab.* **43**:679–681.
59. Judd, S. J., Lazarus, L., and Smythe, G., 1976, Prolactin secretion by metoclopramide in man, *J. Clin Endocrinol. Metab.* **43**:313–317.
60. Jacobs, H. S., Franks, S., Murray, M. A. F., Hull, M. G. R., Steele, S. J., and Nabarro, J. D. V., 1976, Clinical and endocrine features of hyperprolactinaemic amenorrhoea, *Clin. Endocrinol. (Oxford)* **5**:439–454.
61. Archer, D. F., Sprong, J. W., Nankin, H. R., and Josimovich, J. B., 1976, Pituitary gonadotropin response in women with idiopathic hyperprolactinemia, *Fertil. Steril.* **27**:1158–1164.
62. Bohnet, H. G., Dahlén, H. G., Wuttke, W., and Schneider, H. P. G., 1976, Hyperprolactinemic anovulatory syndrome, *J. Clin. Endocrinol. Metab.* **42**:132–143.
63. McIntosh, E. N., 1976, Treatment of women with the galactorrhea–amenorrhea syndrome with pyridoxine (vitamin B_6), *J. Clin. Endocrinol. Metab.* **42**:1192–1195.
64. Magrini, G., Ebiner, J. R., Burckhardt, P., and Felber, J. P., 1976, Study on the relationship between plasma prolactin levels and androgen metabolism in man, *J. Clin. Endocrinol. Metab.* **43**:944–947.
65. Ambrosi, B., Travaglini, P., Beck-Peccoz, P., Bara, R., Elli, R., Paracchi, A., and Faglia, G., 1976, Effect of sulphiride-induced hyperprolactinemia on serum testosterone response to HCG in normal men, *J. Clin. Endocrinol. Metab.* **43**:700–703.
66. Rubin, R. T., Poland, R. E., and Tower, B. B., 1976, Prolactin-related testosterone secretion in normal adult men, *J. Clin. Endocrinol. Metab.* **42**:112–116.
67. Seppälä, M., Hirvonen, E., Unnérus, H. A., Ranta, T., and Laatikainen, T., 1976, Prolactin and testosterone: Independent circulating levels in hyperprolactinemic and normoprolactinemic amenorrhea. The effect of prolactin suppression by bromocriptine, *J. Clin. Endocrinol. Metab.* **43**:198–200.
68. Delvoye, P., Delogne-Desnoeck, J., and Robyn, C., 1976, Serum-prolactin in long-lasting lactation amenorrhoea, *Lancet* **2**:288–289.

69. Tyson, J. E., Perez, A., and Zanartu, J., 1976, Human lactational response to oral thyrotropin releasing hormone, *J. Clin. Endocrinol. Metab.* **43**:760–768.
70. Yen, S. S. C., Rebar, R. W., and Quesenberry, W., 1976, Pituitary function in pseudocyesis, *J. Clin. Endocrinol. Metab.* **43**:132–136.
71. Krieger, D. T., Howantiz, P. J., and Frantz, A. G., 1976, Absence of nocturnal elevation of plasma prolactin concentrations in Cushing's disease, *J. Clin. Endocrinol. Metab.* **42**:260–272.
72. Onishi, T., Miyai, K., Izumi, K., Nakanishi, H., and Kumahara, Y., 1975, Prolactin response to chlorpromazine and thyrotropin-releasing hormone in hyperthyroidism, *J. Clin. Endocrinol. Metab.* **40**:30–32.
73. Onishi, T., Itoh, K. F., Miyai, K., Izumi, K., Shima, K., and Kumahara, Y., 1976, Prolactin response to arginine in normal subjects and in patients with hyperthyroidism, *J. Clin. Endocrinol. Metab.* **42**:148–151.
74. Mills, J. B., Zeringue, M., Harris, R., Wilhelmi, A. E., and Rudman, D., 1976, Assay of pig growth hormone preparations for metabolic activities in the rat and in man, *J. Clin. Endocrinol. Metab.* **42**:1127–1132.
75. Lewis, U. J., Pence, S. J., Singh, R. N. P., and VanderLaan, W. P., 1975, Enhancement of the growth promoting activity of human growth hormone, *Biochem. Biophys. Res. Commun.* **67**:617–624.
76. Baumann, G., 1976, Failure of endogenous plasmin to convert human growth hormone to its "activated" isohormones, *J. Clin Endocrinol. Metab.* **43**:222–225.
77. Baumann, G., and Hodgen, G., 1976, Lack of *in vivo* transformation of human growth hormone to its "activated" isohormones in peripheral tissues of the rhesus monkey, *J. Clin. Endocrinol. Metab.* **43**:1009–1014.
78. Lesniak, M. A., Gorden, P., Roth, J., and Gavin, J. R., III, 1974, Binding of ^{125}I-human growth hormone to specific receptors in human cultured lymphocytes, *J. Biol. Chem.* **249**:1661–1667.
79. Carr, D., and Friesen, H. G., 1976, Growth hormone and insulin binding to human liver, *J. Clin. Endocrinol. Metab.* **42**:484–493.
80. Kelly, P. A., Tsushima, T., Shiu, R. P. C., and Friesen, H. G., 1976, Lactogenic and growth hormone-like activities in pregnancy determined by radioreceptor assay, *Endocrinology* **99**:765–774.
81. Mochizuki, M., Morikawa, H., Kawaguchi, K., and Tojo, S., 1976, Growth hormone, prolactin and chorionic somatomammotropin in normal and molar pregnancy, *J. Clin. Endocrinol. Metab.* **43**:614–621.
82. Gerich, J. E., Lorenzi, M., Bier, D. M., Tsalikian, E., Schneider, V., Karam, J. H., and Forsham, P. H., 1976, Effects of physiologic levels of glucagon and growth hormone on human carbohydrate and lipid metabolism. Studies involving administration of exogenous hormone during suppression of endogenous hormone secretion with somatostatin, *J. Clin. Invest.* **57**:875–884.
83. Chambers, J. W., and Brown, G. M., 1976, Stimulation of rhesus monkey GH release: Arginine vs. plasma volume expansion, *J. Clin. Endocrinol Metab.* **42**:169–172.
84. Pontiroli, A. E., Viberti, G. C., Tognetti, A., and Pozza, G., 1976, Effect of metergoline, a specific serotonin antagonist, on human growth hormone response to arginine and L-Dopa, *Horm. Metab. Res.* **8**:106–108.
85. Malarkey, W. B., and Mendell, J. R., 1976, Failure of serotonin inhibitor to effect nocturnal GH and prolactin secretion in patients with Duchenne muscular dystrophy, *J. Clin. Endocrinol. Metab.* **43**:889–892.
86. Brown, W. A., and Williams, B. W., 1976, Methylphenidate increases serum growth hormone concentrations, *J. Clin. Endocrinol. Metab.* **43**:937–939.

87. Maeda, K., Kato, Y., Yamaguchi, N., Chihara, K., Ohgo, S., Iwasaki, Y., Yoshimoto, Y., Moridera, K., Kuromaru, S., and Imura, H., 1976, Growth hormone release following thyrotropin-releasing hormone injection into patients with anorexia nervosa, *Acta Endocrinol. (Copenhagen)* **81:**1–8.
88. Herbai, G., and Werner, I., 1976, Sheehan's syndrome of hypothalamic origin in a woman with juvenile diabetes mellitus, *Acta Med. Scand.* **199:**539–541.
89. Korsgaard, O., Lindholm, J., and Rasmussen, P., 1976, Endocrine function in patients with suprasellar and hypothalamic tumours, *Acta Endocrinol. (Copenhagen)* **83:**1–8.
90. Jenkins, J. S., Gilbert, C. J., and Ang, V., 1976, Hypothalamic–pituitary function in patients with cranio pharyngiomas, *J. Clin. Endocrinol. Metab.* **43:**394–399.
91. Haymond, M. W., Karl, I., Weldon, V. V., and Pagliara, A. S., 1976, The role of growth hormone and cortisone on glucose and gluconeogenic substrate regulation in fasted hypopituitary children, *J. Clin. Endocrinol. Metab.* **42:**846–856.
92. Jacobs, L. S., Sneid, D. S., Garland, J. T., Laron, Z., and Daughaday, W. H., 1976, Receptor-active growth hormone in Laron dwarfism, *J. Clin. Endocrinol. Metab.* **42:**403–406.
93. Clemons, R. D., Costin, G., and Kogut, M. D., 1976, Laron dwarfism: Growth and immunoreactive insulin following treatment with human growth hormone, *J. Pediatr.* **88:**427–433.
94. Walsh, C. H., Wright, A. D., Williams, J. W., and Holder, G., 1976, A study of pituitary function in patients with idiopathic hemochromatosis, *J. Clin. Endocrinol. Metab.* **43:**866–872.
95. Preece, M. A., Tanner, J. M., Whitehouse, R. H., and Cameron, N., 1976, Dose dependence of growth response to human growth hormone in growth hormone deficiency, *J. Clin. Endocrinol. Metab.* **42:**477–483.
96. Pertzelan, A., Kauli, R., Assa, S., Greenberg, D., and Laron, Z., 1976, Intermittent treatment with human growth hormone (GH) in isolated GH deficiency and in multiple pituitary hormone deficiencies, *Clin. Endocrinol. (Oxford)* **5:**15–24.
97. Aynsley-Green, A., Zachmann, M., and Prader, A., 1976, Interrelation of the therapeutic effects of growth hormone and testosterone on growth in hypopituitarism, *J. Pediatr.* **89:**992–999.
98. Tanner, J. M., Whitehouse, R. H., Hughes, P. C. R., and Carter, B. S., 1976, Relative importance of growth hormone and sex steroids for the growth at puberty of trunk length, limb length, and muscle width in growth hormone-deficient children, *J. Pediatr.* **89:**1000–1008.
99. Franks, S., Jacobs, H. S., and Nabarro, J. D., 1976, Prolactin concentrations in patients with acromegaly—clinical significance and response to surgery, *Clin. Endocrinol. (Oxford)* **5:**63–69.
100. Corenblum, B., Sirek, A. M. T., Horvath, E., Kovacs, K., and Ezrin, C., 1976, Human mixed somatotrophic and lactotrophic pituitary adenomas, *J. Clin. Endocrinol. Metab.* **42:**857–863.
101. Catania, A., Catalamessa, L. and Reschini, E., 1976, Plasma prolactin response to luteinizing hormone releasing hormone in acromegalic patients, *J. Clin. Endocrinol. Metab.* **43:**689–691.

102. Debek, J. T., 1974, Bronchial carcinoid tumor with acromegaly in two patients, *J. Clin. Endocrinol. Metab.* **38:**329–333.
103. Sönksen, P. H., Ayres, A. B., Braimbridge, M., Corrin, B., Davies, D. R., Jeremiah, G. M., Oaten, S. W., Lowy, C., and West, T. E. T., 1976, Acromegaly caused by pulmonary carcinoid tumours, *Clin. Endocrinol. (Oxford)* **5:**503–13.
104. Gorden, P., Lesniak, M. A., Eastman, R., Hendricks, C. M., and Roth, J., 1976, Evidence for higher proportion of "little" growth hormone with increased radioreceptor activity in acromegalic plasma, *J. Clin. Endocrinol. Metab.* **43:**364–373.
105. Delitala, G., Masala, A., Alagna, S., Devilla, L., and Lotti, G., 1976, Growth hormone and prolactin release in acromegalic patients following metergoline administration, *J. Clin. Endocrinol. Metab.* **43:**1382–1386.
106. Chiodini, P. G., Liuzzi, A., Muller, E. E., Botalla, L., Cremascoli, G., Oppizzi, G., Verde, G., and Silvestrini, F., 1976, Inhibitory effect of an ergoline derivative, metergoline, on growth hormone and prolactin levels in acromegalic patients, *J. Clin. Endocrinol. Metab.* **43:**356–363.
107. Feldman, J. M., Plonk, J. W., and Bivens, C. H., 1976, Inhibitory effect of serotonin antagonists on growth hormone release in acromegalic patients, *Clin. Endocrinol. (Oxford)* **5:**71–78.
108. Verde, G., Oppizzi, G., Colussi, G., Cremascoli, G., Botalla, L., Muller, E. E., Silverstrini, F., Chiodini, P. G., and Liuzzi, A., 1976, Effect of dopamine infusion on plasma levels of growth hormone in normal subjects and in agromegalic patients, *Clin. Endocrinol. (Oxford)* **5:**419–423.
109. Lamberg, B. A., Pelkonen, R., Aro, A., and Grahne, B., 1976, Thyroid function in acromegaly before and after transsphenoidal hypophysectomy followed by cryoapplication, *Acta Endocrinol.* **82:**254–266.
110. Sandler, R., 1976, Recurrent hyperthyroidism in an acromegalic patient previously treated with proton beam irradiation: Graves' disease as probable etiology based on follow-up observations, *J. Clin. Endocrinol. Metab.* **42:**163–168.
111. Hamilton, C. R., Jr., and Maloof, F., 1972, Acromegaly and toxic goiter. Cure of the hyperthyroidism and acromegaly by proton-beam partial hypophysectomy, *J. Clin. Endocrinol. Metab.* **35:**659–664.
112. Nagulesparen, M., Trickey, R., Davies, M J., and Jenkins, J. S., 1976, Muscle changes in acromegaly, *Br. Med. J.* **2:**914–915.
113. Luft, R., and Hall, K. (eds.), 1975, Somatomedin and some other growth factors, in: *Advances in Metabolic Disorders*, Vol. 8, Academic Press, New York.
114. Rinderknecht, E., and Humbel, R. E., 1976, Amino-terminal sequences of two polypeptides from human serum with nonsuppressible insulin-like and cell-growth-promoting activities: Evidence for structural homology with insulin B chain, *Proc. Natl. Acad. Sci. U.S.A.* **73:**4379–4381.
115. Schlumpf, U., Heimann, R., Zapf, J., and Froesch, E. R., 1976, Non-suppressible insulin-like activity and sulphation activity in serum extracts of normal subjects, acromegalics and pituitary dwarfs, *Acta Endocrinol.* **81:**28–42.
116. Franklin, R. C., Rennie, G. C., Burger, H. G., and Cameron, D. P., 1976, A bioassay for NSILA-S in individual serum samples and its relationship to somatotropin, *J. Clin. Endocrinol. Metab.* **43:**1164–1169.
117. Garland, J. T., Jennings, J., Levtsky, L. I., and Buchanan, F., 1976, Stimula-

tion of DNA synthesis in isolated chrondrocytes by somatomedin. II. Validation of the assay for clinical use and comparison with the stimulation of protein synthesis, *J. Clin. Endocrinol. Metab.* **43**:847–851.

118. Garland, J. T., and Buchanan, F., 1976, Stimulation of RNA and protein synthesis in isolated chondrocytes by human serum, *J. Clin. Endocrinol. Metab.* **43**:842–846.

119. Takano, K., Hall, K., Ritzén, M., Iselius, L., and Sievertsson, H., 1976, Somatomedin A in human serum, determined by radioreceptor assay, *Acta Endocrinol.* **82**:449–459.

120. Furlanetto, R. W., D'Ercole, A. J., Underwood, L. E., and Van Wyk, J. J., 1976, A radioimmunoassay for somatomedin-C: Development, specificity and results, 5th International Congress of Endocrinology, Hamburg, Brühlsche Universitätsdruckerei, Giessen, Abstract No. 392.

121. Heinrich, U. E., Schalch, D. S., Koch, J. G., and Johnson, C. J., 1976, Nonsuppressible insulin-like activity (NSILA-s): Plasma levels and their relationship to growth hormone and NSILA-s carrier protein concentration, 5th International Congress of Endocrinology, Hamburg, Brühlsche Universitätsdruckerei, Giessen, Abstract No. 398.

122. Cohen, K. L., and Nissley, S. P., 1976, The serum half-life of somatomedin activity: Evidence for growth hormone dependence, *Acta Endocrinol.* **83**:243–58.

123. D'Ercole, A. J., Foushee, D. B., and Underwood, L. E., 1976, Somatomedin-C receptor ontogeny and levels in porcine fetal and human cord serum, *J. Clin. Endocrinol. Metab.* **43**:1069–1077.

124. Gluckman, P. D., and Brinsmead, M. W., 1976, Somatomedin in cord blood: Relationship to gestational age and birth size, *J. Clin. Endocrinol. Metab.* **43**:1378–1381.

125. Giordano, G., Foppiani, E., Minuto, F., and Perroni, D., 1976, Growth hormone and somatomedin behaviour in the newborn, *Acta Endocrinol.* **81**:449–454.

126. Bala, R. M., and Smith, G. R., 1976, Partial characterization of somatomedin bioactivity in term human amniotic fluid, *J. Clin. Endocrinol. Metab.* **43**:907–912.

127. Chochinov, R. H., Ketupanya, A., Mariz, I. K., Underwood, L. E., and Daughaday, W. H., 1976, Amniotic fluid reactivity detected by somatomedin C radioreceptor assay correlation with growth hormone, prolactin and fetal renal maturation, *J. Clin. Endocrinol. Metab.* **42**:983–986.

128. Chochinov, R. H., Mariz, I. K., Hajek, A. S., and Daughaday, W. H., 1977, Characterization of a protein in mid-term human amniotic fluid which reacts in the somatomedin-C radioreceptor assay, *J. Clin. Endocrinol. Metab.* **44**:902–908.

129. Pierson, M., Grignon, G., Malaprade, D., and Hartemann, P., 1976, L àctivité somatomédine du sérum au cours de lènfance chez le sujet normal et dans les retards de croissance, *Ann. Biol. Clin.* **34**:11–18.

130. Gluckman, P. D., and Holdaway, I. M., 1976, Prolactin and somatomedin studies in the syndrome of growth hormone-independent growth, *Clin. Endocrinol. (Oxford)* **5**:545–549.

131. Costin, G., Kogut, M. D., Phillips, L. S., and Daughaday, W. H., 1976, Craniopharyngioma: The role of insulin in promoting postoperative growth, *J. Clin. Endocrinol. Metab.* **42**:370–379.

132. Wiedemann, E., and Schwartz, E., 1972, Suppression of growth hormone-dependent human serum sulfation factor by estrogen, *J. Clin. Endocrinol. Metab.* **34:**51–58.
133. Wiedemann, E., Schwartz, E., and Frantz, A. G., 1976, Acute and chronic estrogen effects upon serum somatomedin activity, growth hormone, and prolactin in man, *J. Clin. Endocrinol. Metab.* **42:**942–952.
134. Saenger, P., Schwartz, E., Wiedemann, E., Levine, L. S., Tsai, M., and New, M. I., 1976, The interaction of growth hormone, somatomedin and oestrogen in patients with Turner's syndrome, *Acta Endocrinol.* **81:**9–18.

The Thyroid

Kenneth A. Woeber and Lewis E. Braverman

3.1. Introduction

This chapter will focus on those advances relating to the thyroid that have been reported during 1976 and early 1977 and that have particular impact with respect to human physiology and disease. We elected to retain the organizational format that we employed last year in the hope that over time it will readily permit a longitudinal review of a given general area.

3.2. Hypothalamic–Pituitary–Thyroid Interrelationships

During the past year, elucidation of the factors that regulate the secretion of thyrotropin (TSH) has been given added impetus through the development of exquisitely sensitive radioimmunoassays for TSH. Many laboratories are now able to conduct assays that attain sensitivities of the order of 0.2 μU/ml. While earlier work utilizing less sensitive radioimmunoassay methodology was contradictory as to whether TSH in plasma underwent a circadian variation, recent studies have indicated quite convincingly that TSH is subject to both briefly episodic and circadian varia-

KENNETH A. WOEBER • Department of Medicine, Mt. Zion Hospital and Medical Center, and University of California, San Francisco, California. LEWIS E. BRAVERMAN • Department of Medicine, University of Massachusetts Medical School, Worcester, Massachusetts.

tions. The latter variation is characterized by a nocturnal surge or nycto-hemeral maximum that appears not to be determined by the circadian rhythm of cortisol secretion or by fluctuations in thyroxine (T_4) or $3,5,3^1$-triiodothyronine (T_3) concentrations.

Parker et al.[1] undertook a major study in healthy men to define the time of occurrence of the nocturnal surge of TSH in relation to poly-graphically monitored sleep in both normal and acutely reversed sleep–wake cycles. As has been shown to be the case for other hormones, plasma TSH concentrations were found to fluctuate at 1 to 2 hr intervals, suggest-ing a briefly episodic release pattern. Superimposed on this pattern was a larger peak the onset of which always anteceded lights-off or onset of sleep and the maximum of which frequently anteceded onset of sleep. This nocturnal surge of TSH occurred at about 11:00 PM when sleep onset began between 11:00 PM and midnight. When sleep onset was delayed or sleep postponed to the next day, the TSH surge was accen-tuated and prolonged. Conversely, early onset of sleep resulted in a nocturnal surge that was of lesser magnitude and of shorter duration. The foregoing observations indicate that TSH secretion, unlike that of growth hormone or prolactin or that of luteinizing hormone during puberty, is not augmented by sleep. Rather, sleep appears to be accompa-nied by inhibitory influences that modulate the expression of a funda-mental circadian rhythmicity of TSH. A pattern of TSH secretion that is virtually identical from a qualitative standpoint to that seen in normal men has been reported to occur in both men and women with mild primary hypothyroidism. On the other hand, in patients with severe hypothyroid-ism and very high serum TSH concentrations, the circadian variation may be lost, but is restored when serum TSH concentrations are reduced by thyroid replacement therapy.[2]

Although the existence of a specific thyrotropin-release-inhibiting factor has not been identified, evidence is mounting to suggest that somatostatin (growth hormone-release-inhibiting factor, GRIF) may fulfill this function. Earlier work had demonstrated that the infusion of soma-tostatin suppresses basal plasma TSH concentration, the nocturnal surge of TSH, and the responsiveness of TSH to thyrotropin-releasing hor-mone (TRH). Nevertheless, the physiological significance of these find-ings was open to question in view of the doses of somatostatin that were required to elicit an effect. To circumvent this problem, a different approach was employed by Gordin et al.[3] and by Arimura and Schally.[4] These investigators passively immunized rats with antisomatostatin anti-serum to neutralize endogenous somatostatin. This maneuver resulted in increases in basal plasma TSH concentration and enhanced responsive-ness to TRH. This finding supports the view that somatostatin may indeed modulate TSH secretion under physiological circumstances. The mechanism through which somatostatin elicits this effect and the manner in which it interacts with TRH and thyroid hormones in regulating TSH secretion are, however, unclear.

The role that other factors play in regulating TSH secretion has also been given some emphasis during the past year. Re et al.[5] demonstrated that the administration of metyrapone is accompanied by an increase in basal plasma TSH concentration, suggesting that physiological quantities of glucocorticoid may modulate TSH secretion. It is uncertain whether the effect of physiological perturbations of glucocorticoid is mediated through a direct action on the pituitary or through inhibition of endogenous TRH elaboration.

To assess whether prostaglandins play a role in the response of TSH to TRH, Raney et al.[6] administered either indomethacin or aspirin to men for 1 week. Although both agents led to decreases in serum prostaglandins E and F, only salicylate was accompanied by suppression of the TSH response to TRH, an effect that may be due to the known ability of salicylate to displace thyroid hormones from binding proteins in plasma. Thus, this study does not support a role for prostaglandins in mediating the TSH response to TRH in man.

The relative importance of T_4 and T_3 as determinants of basal plasma TSH concentration and its responsiveness to TRH was examined,[7] and a possible influence of reverse T_3 in this regard was also assessed.[8] In hypothyroid patients replaced with T_4 alone, normal basal TSH values and normal TSH responses to TRH required restoration to normal of both T_4 and T_3, rather than of T_4 alone. Administration of $3,3',5'$-triiodothyronine (reverse T_3, rT_3) to normal men was shown not to affect serum T_4, T_3, or TSH concentrations or TSH responsiveness to TRH. This is an important observation in view of the earlier findings that rT_3 is capable of inhibiting the conversion of T_4 to T_3 in tissue preparations in vitro, though very high concentrations are required. These findings indicate that rT_3 in vivo does not affect TSH secretion, either directly or indirectly through inhibition of peripheral T_3 generation from T_4.

Further elucidation of the factors that regulate TSH secretion has been hampered by the lack of a reliable assay method for TRH measurement. This is largely owing to rapid degradation of TRH in plasma. A noteworthy finding, however, is that degradative activity is increased in plasma from hyperthyroid and decreased in plasma from hypothyroid rats and man relative to normal.[9-11] Degradative activity is absent in the plasma of neonatal rats, but develops with maturation.[12] These findings have led to the suggestion that thyroid-hormone-dependent TRH degradation in plasma may represent still another level of regulatory control of thyroid hormone economy.

Recent work has demonstrated that degradation of immunoreactive

TRH in serum does not occur in the presence of 8-hydroxyquinoline sulfate and Tween 20, and this observation has been exploited in developing a satisfactory radioimmunoassay for TRH.[13] With this assay, TRH was found to be detectable in normal serum, to be below the limit of detectability in serum from hyperthyroid patients or from patients with hypothalamic hypothyroidism, and to be increased in the serum of patients with primary or pituitary hypothyroidism. In the patients with primary hypothyroidism, serum TRH returned toward normal during thyroid hormone administration, and in most of the patients with hyperthyroidism became detectable during antithyroid drug treatment. These findings provide a hint of the potential value of a workable radioimmunoassay in elucidating hypothalamic–pituitary–thyroid relationships.

The availability of synthetic TRH has led to further exploration of its effects *in vivo*. Studies undertaken in the pregnant rhesus monkey demonstrated convincingly that TRH can cross the primate placenta in both directions.[14] What role, if any, such transplacental passage of TRH plays in initiating neuroendocrine stimulation of thyroid function in the fetus remains to be determined, however.

In view of its ability to provoke prolactin secretion, the influence of TRH on lactation was examined both in normal lactating women and in women with defective lactation.[15,16] In the former group, the oral administration of TRH did not augment milk production, despite inducing increases in basal prolactin and its responsiveness to suckling. In contrast, in some mothers with defective lactation, the oral administration of TRH led to increases in basal prolactin and in milk production with full restoration of nursing. Thus, TRH may have clinical utility in the management of some cases of defective lactation. It is noteworthy, however, that in two women who were given large doses of TRH, hyperthyroidism ensued, though it disappeared after TRH was withdrawn.

3.3. Thyroid Hormones

3.3.1. Synthesis and Secretion

This general area has received considerable emphasis during the past year, and several aspects that are judged to be particularly important will be considered in some detail.

Last year, mention was made of a "short-loop" feedback mechanism whereby T_4 and T_3 act directly on the thyroid to impair its responsiveness to TSH. Further studies on this phenomenon include the findings that prior administration of thyroid hormones to the rat and mouse inhibits the TSH-induced increase in thyroid ornithine decarboxylase (ODC) activity and thyroid secretion of T_4 and T_3.[17] Other data suggest that there exists in the rat an intrathyroid autoregulatory mechanism that prevents excessive concentrations of thyroid hormones in the serum following large doses of bTSH.[18] This "short-loop" regulatory mechanism probably exists in man, since exogenous bTSH and endogenous TSH did not induce ^{131}I uptake in the suppressed lobe of a patient with an autonomous "hot" thyroid nodule.[19] In addition to this mechanism for modulating TSH action, development of relative refractoriness to TSH with resultant dampening of its stimulatory effects was recently shown to occur. Bovine thyroid slices that had previously been exposed to TSH displayed blunted responses of cAMP, protein kinase activity, glucose oxidation, and phospholipid synthesis to subsequent TSH stimulation, but displayed no decrease in the binding of ^{125}I-labeled TSH.[20,21] This phenomenon of relative refractoriness to TSH was also observed in dog thyroid cells in tissue culture.[22] Since thyroid responsiveness to TSH is also depressed by inhibitors of prostaglandin synthesis, it is possible that prostaglandins play a role in modulating the effects of TSH.[23] It has also been suggested that refractoriness to TSH depends on new protein synthesis.[24]

A number of studies have dealt with the impact of TSH stimulation on thyroid intermediary metabolism and hormone secretion. The observation that TSH stimulates ODC activity and polyamine synthesis and that polyamines increase RNA polymerase activity suggests a possible mechanism for the long-term effects of TSH on RNA synthesis.[25] Nonetheless, the principal mechanism for the increase in RNA and protein synthesis that TSH induces is probably one mediated through increased generation of cAMP. Both cAMP and cGMP increase thyroid RNA synthesis, while cytidine monophosphate decreases RNA synthesis and blunts the stimulatory effects of cAMP and cGMP.[26]

The biogenic amines, especially histamine and norephinephrine, have thyroid receptors different from those of TSH and prostaglandin E_2 (PGE_2) in human and mouse thyroid tissue, and, in the case of histamine, it is a histamine$_2$-receptor.[27,28] Like TSH, these biogenic amines also stimulate the AC–cAMP system and probably exert their stimulatory effect through this system. Although PGE_1 and TSH stimulate cAMP synthesis in normal and thyrotoxic human thyroids *in vitro*, differences in cAMP responses to these agents in normal and toxic glands, the failure of thyroid hormones to suppress the PGE_1 response, and additive effects of both hormones strongly suggest the possibility of different membrane receptors and/or mode of action of these two stimulators.[29] Propranolol inhibits the TSH stimulation of cAMP production and enhances the binding of TSH to human thyroid membranes, leading to the suggestion that this β-blocker reduces the efficiency of the receptor–AC coupling system.[30]

It has been suggested that prolonged TSH stimulation of the thyroid results in a disproportionate increase in the secretion of T_3 relative to T_4. Recent studies of TSH-perfused canine thyroids isolated *in situ* demonstrated, however, that this is only a transient phenomenon that abates during prolonged TSH stimulation.[31] Moreover, significant changes in serum T_3 concentration were not observed following small increases in serum TSH for a prolonged period after hemithyroidectomy in the rat, even though compensatory hypertrophy of the residual lobe occurred.[32]

Although the mechanisms underlying the inhibitory effects of iodide on various aspects of thyroid function remain elusive, recent studies may serve to provide some clarification. The administration of iodide to iodine-deficient mice and rats was shown to inhibit the generation of thyroid cAMP that is induced by TSH and other thyroid stimulators; this appears to be due to the formation of an unknown organic form of iodine, since the concurrent administration of methimazole (MMI) prevents the inhibitory effects of iodide.[33,34] The iodide-induced inhibitor of cAMP was neither soluble nor freely diffusible.[35] Excess iodide was also shown to inhibit RNA and protein synthesis; again, the inhibitory effect is apparently due to an organic form of iodine.[36,37] Although both inhibition and stimulation of thyroid proteolytic activity have been reported to follow large doses of iodide, a recent study employing cultured thyroid glands demonstrated inhibition of thyroglobulin (Tg) hydrolysis following the addition of iodide; again, the formation of an organic form of iodide appears to be necessary for this inhibition.[38] In contrast to these inhibitory effects, administration of iodide to hypophysectomized rats or to thyroid-hormone-treated intact rats stimulated thyroid secretion by increasing intrathyroidal cAMP in the absence of TSH.[39] Since MMI blocked this response, formation of an organic form of iodine appears to be required for this stimulatory effect.

A study of the sequential alterations of serum T_4, T_3, and TSH was carried out in the rat during the ingestion of a low-iodine diet.[40] Serum T_4 concentration decreased rapidly within days, accompanied by only a small increase in serum TSH until 15 days, when TSH rose abruptly. Serum T_3 concentration remained essentially unchanged for 26 days, but decreased to about 50% of the control values in more prolonged experiments. Despite the availability of T_3, though not T_4, long-term iodine-deficient rats were hypothyroid since they did not survive exposure to a cold environment. The formation of labeled 3,3'-diiodothyronine (3,3'-T_2) was significant only in iodine-deficient thyroids, and the greatest quantities were observed in the most severely iodine-deficient glands, presumably due to the increased probability of coupling of two molecules of monoiodotyrosine (MIT). The formation of rT_3 was similar in iodine-deficient and iodine-sufficient thyroids. Studies of thyroglobulin iodinated *in vitro* gave similar results.[41]

In view of great variation in the iodine content of different low-iodine diets and the postulated presence of a goitrogen in some low-iodine diets, a careful study was undertaken to assess the effects of various low-iodine diets on goiter formation and thyroid function in the rat.[42] The results suggest that iodine deficiency alone is sufficient to account for the goiter formation and abnormalities of thyroid function observed, and that the degree of abnormality was directly related to the degree of iodine deficiency. Indeed, an inverse relationship was found to exist between thyroid iodine content and thyroid peroxidase (TPO) activity.[43] The clinical manifestations of excess iodine administration were recently reviewed,[44] and either hypothyroidism or hyperthyroidism may occur, depending on the underlying thyroid disorder and the iodine intake. Administration of iodized oil to Nepalese living in a severely iodine-deficient area resulted in a decrease in serum T_3 and increase in serum TSH in subjects with small goiters or normal thyroids, suggesting an acute inhibitory effect of iodine, and in a marked increase in serum T_4 and T_3 and a decrease in serum TSH in subjects with large multinodular goiters and elevated basal serum TSH concentrations, suggesting the induction of the Jodbasedow phenomenon.[45] Finally, small doses of iodide (10 mg/day) given to normal subjects resulted in small but significant increases in serum TSH,[46] as has previously been reported with larger doses.

During the past year, several studies bearing on intrathyroid thyroglobulin (Tg) have appeared. In support of earlier observations, conformation of Tg is important for TPO-catalyzed coupling.[47] An *in vitro* system provided direct evidence for the formation of phagolysosomes by the fusion of lysosomes with Tg-containing endocytic vesicles.[48] Indirect evidence suggesting that apical vesicles are involved in the transport of Tg and that colloid droplets, the formation of which is induced by TSH, do contain Tg was directly confirmed by electron-microscopic immunohistochemical localization.[49]

The mechanism of action of the thionamide drugs, propylthiouracil (PTU) and MMI, has been studied in some detail. Taurog believes that these drugs act primarily to inhibit the formation of "activated iodine" and the subsequent iodination of tyrosyl residues, and that this inhibition is antagonized by iodide (Fig. 1).[50] Nagasaka and Hidaka[51] presented evidence to indicate that PTU interacts with the product of TPO action (oxidized iodide) without affecting TPO activity, and the inhibitory effect is removed by dialysis; MMI, in contrast, inhibits enzyme activity directly and the inhibition is not removed by dialysis. These findings may explain why MMI is a more potent inhibitor of iodination than PTU.

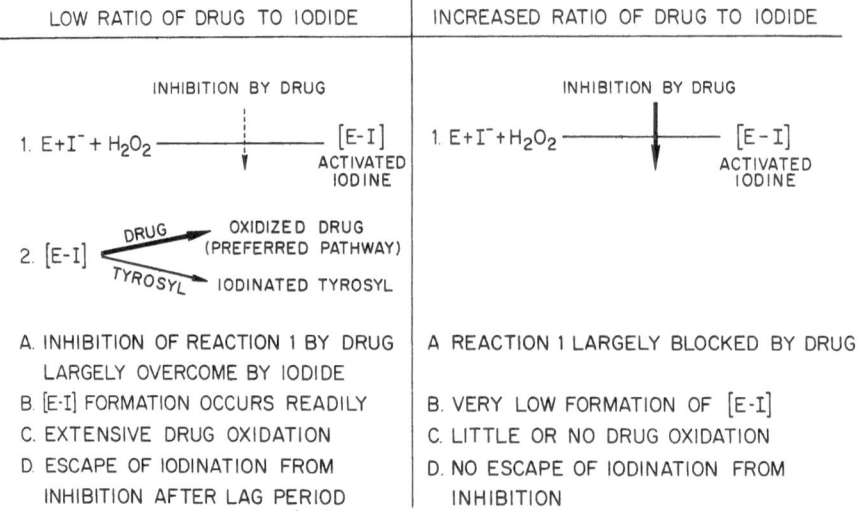

Fig. 1. Proposed scheme for the mechanism of inhibition by thionamide drugs of TPO-catalyzed iodination.

Functioning microtubules are essential for the stimulation of thyroid hormone secretion by TSH and cAMP. Drugs such as colchicine and vinblastine that disrupt microtubules inhibit endocytosis of colloid and decrease hormone secretion *in vivo* and *in vitro*.[52] It is uncertain, however, whether drugs such as colchicine will affect thyroid function in man.

Iodotyrosine dehalogenase deficiency is a rare hereditary disorder associated with decreased thyroid iodothyronine content. This syndrome was reproduced in the iodine-deficient rat by administering 3-nitro-L-tyrosine (MNT), an inhibitor of iodotyrosine dehalogenase,[53] and was reversed by either administration of iodide or removal of the MNT. Other defects in hormone synthesis that result in goiter with or without hypothyroidism have been described in man. Pommier *et al.*[54] carefully analyzed the thyroids from two goitrous patients. One lacked peroxidase activity, and the other had a marked decrease in iodinated Tg.

3.3.2. Peripheral Metabolism

It has been 60 years since Kendall crystallized and identified T_4; 25 years since Gross and Pitt-Rivers first identified T_3 in human serum; approximately 10 years since the concentration of T_3 was first accurately measured in serum; 7 years since the first conclusive demonstration that in man T_4 is peripherally deiodinated in its outer ring and converted to T_3 and that the alanine side chain of T_4 is deaminated and decarboxylated to form tetraiodothyroacetic acid (tetrac); 3 years since rT_3, the product of the inner-ring deiodination of T_4, was measured in the serum of man; and about 1 year since further deiodinated products of T_3 and rT_3 metabolism were identified in the serum.

There is now general agreement that in normal subjects, the thyroid gland is a minor source of T_3 production, the bulk of T_3 ($\approx 80\%$) being produced through 5′-monodeiodination of T_4 in peripheral tissues. A greater proportion of the circulating T_3 derives from thyroid secretion in the hyperfunctioning gland in hyperthyroidism, the TSH-stimulated failing thyroid, and the thyroid gland in iodine deficiency. As discussed last year, impairment of the peripheral conversion of T_4 to T_3 has been invoked as the mechanism for the decreased serum T_3 concentrations that occur in a variety of physiological and pathological states, such as early neonatal life and old age, starvation, protein–caloric malnutrition, anorexia nervosa, severe systemic illness, the postoperative state, and during the administration of PTU or dexamethasone. In these circumstances, total and free T_4 concentrations in serum are normal or marginally increased, while total and free T_3 concentrations are subnormal. During the past year, impaired conversion of T_4 to T_3 has also been invoked as the cause of subnormal T_3 concentrations in other clinical states, including cord blood from newborn infants with the respiratory distress syndrome,[55] patients with acute illnesses[56] or in diabetic coma,[57] and during surgery and epidural analgesia.[58] The administration of amiodarone, an iodine-containing drug used in Europe for the treatment of arrhythmias and angina pectoris, results in decreased serum T_3 concentration and an enhanced TSH response to TRH.[59] The radiographic contrast agent sodium iopanoate (Telepaque®) also decreases serum T_3 concentration, but increases serum T_4 concentration. The latter finding may be due to enhanced thyroid secretion of T_4 secondary to the observed rise in serum TSH concentration,[60] although an effect of Telepaque on the metabolic clearance rate of T_4 has not been ruled out. Previous studies have not demonstrated any significant decrease in serum T_3 concentration in animals or man receiving propranolol or other β-adrenergic antagonists. A recent report[61] suggests, however, that propranolol does impair peripheral conversion of T_4 to T_3 and that some of the clinical improvement seen in thyrotoxic patients treated with β-blockers might result from a decrease in T_3 generation.

In view of the marked decrease in serum T_3 concentration observed during various states of starvation or caloric deprivation, several studies have been carried out to determine the factor(s) responsible for the impaired generation of T_3 from T_4. It seems probable that carbohydrate is a major modulator of the hepatic conversion of T_4 to T_3, since low or normal caloric, carbohydrate-free diets result in a decreased serum T_3 concentration,[62,63] and carbohydrate, but not lipid, overfeeding increases serum T_3 concentration.[62] Essentially similar findings were reported in the rat; here, the ability of liver homogenates from starved rats to generate T_3 from T_4 added *in vitro* is impaired and is partly restored by the oral[64] or intravenous[65] infusion of glucose. Infusion of isocaloric quantities of amino acids, but not lipid, also partly restores T_3 generation from T_4.[65] Finally, serum T_3 concentration is positively and significantly correlated with body weight.[66]

In view of the frequency of the low-T_3 syndrome, a major unresolved question is whether patients with impaired peripheral generation of T_3 are hypothyroid at the tissue level. Although basal serum TSH concentrations and TSH responsiveness to TRH are occasionally increased, serum TSH concentration is usually normal, indicating both the presence of a euthyroid state and a regulatory effect of T_4 on pituitary TSH secretion. Growth hormone (GH) concentrations in both the pituitary and the plasma after barbiturate stimulation are lower in hypothyroid rats receiving T_4 plus PTU than T_4, alone. Since PTU is known to inhibit generation of T_3 from T_4, this suggests that conversion of T_4 to T_3 *in vivo* plays an important role in the expression of T_4 action on GH secretion.[67] In contrast, others have reported that the thyrotroph can respond acutely to both increases and decreases in either T_4 or T_3, but that the hepatocyte responds primarily to T_3, as assessed from mitochondrial α-glycerophosphate dehydrogenase activity.[68] The lack of sensitive metabolic indices by which to assess mild hypothyroidism in man is a major problem in determining whether patients with the low-T_3 syndrome are clinically and biochemically hypothyroid. Recent studies in patients with anorexia nervosa and low T_3 and normal T_4 concentrations in serum have suggested that these patients display several abnormalities found in hypothyroidism. These include a decreased basal metabolic rate,[69] an increased plasma cortisol concentration with a prolonged half-life, increased urinary tetrahydrocortisol/tetrahydrocortisone ratios,[70] and decreased urinary androsterone/etiocholanolone ratios.[71] These abnormalities were corrected by the administration of T_3. Further studies are obviously required to assess the metabolic significance of the low-serum-T_3 syndrome.

Monodeiodination of the inner ring of T_4, yielding rT_3, is the other major pathway of T_4 deiodination. Although the major source of rT_3 production was demonstrated by indirect methods to be T_4,[72,73] direct evidence of a small thyroid contribution to rT_3 production in man has now been obtained.[74] Comparison of direct analyses of T_4, T_3, and rT_3 concentrations in thyroid and peripheral venous blood has revealed calculated relative secretion rates of $T_4/T_3/rT_3$ to be 85:9:1, indicating that almost all of rT_3 and most of T_3 is produced by extrathyroidal conversion of T_4, not thyroid secretion.[74] In virtually all situations in which T_4 conversion to T_3 is impaired, serum rT_3 concentration is increased. Accordingly, it was suggested that T_4 deiodination has been shifted from the 5' to the 5 position.[75] Recent observations have questioned this hypothesis, however, since the clearance rate of rT_3 in clinical situations such as cirrhosis and starvation, in which T_3 production and serum concentration are strikingly reduced, is decreased, and this could account for most of the increase in serum rT_3 concentration observed.[72,76,77] If the mechanism of the low-T_3 syndrome is solely an inhibition of 5'-deiodination, further deiodination of rT_3 would also be impaired and could account for the decreased clearance and subsequent increase in serum rT_3 concentration.

Recent studies of the peripheral metabolism of rT_3 in normal subjects have revealed metabolic clearance rates (MCR) ranging from 77 to 138 liters/day (82–108 liters/70 kg per day) and absolute disposal (or production) rates ranging from 31 to 63 μg/day (21–50 μg/70 kg per day).[72,76–79] The wide variability in the normal mean serum rT_3 concentration reported from many laboratories (17–60 ng/dl),[72–74,76–82] as well as the variability in the reported values for MCR, will obviously result in discrepancies in calculated rT_3 production rates. It should be pointed out, however, that a recent comparative study[83] of serum T_3 concentrations from various laboratories also revealed wide variations, and that seasonal variations in serum T_4 and T_3 concentrations have also been reported,[84] with the lowest values occurring in the summer.

Pharmacological quantities of rT_3 added *in vitro* were reported to enhance GH release and oxygen consumption in cultured pituitary cells,[85] to inhibit the conversion of T_4 to T_3 by rat liver homogenates,[86] and to decrease TSH release from incubated rat pituitaries.[87] Physiological doses of rT_3 administered to the rat *in vivo* increase hepatic L-triiodothyronine aminotransferase activity similar to that induced by T_3.[88] Relatively large physiological amounts of rT_3 administered to normal man, however, do not affect serum T_4, T_3, and TSH concentrations or the TSH response to TRH,[8] confirming previous work indicating that rT_3 has little if any metabolic activity. The entire question of the direct metabolic effect of rT_3 or its role in regulating T_4 metabolism remains unclear, especially since the cellular rate of rT_3 production and degradation is extremely rapid, and plasma concentrations may therefore not accurately reflect cellular action. The rT_3 concentration is greatly increased in amniotic fluid and cord blood as a result of both increased hepatic conversion of T_4 and decreased metabolic clearance of rT_3. Accordingly, it has been suggested that prenatal and neonatal screening for hypothyroidism be carried out by measurement of rT_3.[89] Preliminary data suggest, however, that rT_3 screening is not as accurate as T_4 or TSH in detecting neonatal hypothyroidism.

During the past year, the further metabolic fate of T_3 and rT_3 has been studied (Fig. 2). Rudolph *et al.*[90] identified labeled 3,3'-T_2 and 3'-T_1 in serum following the intravenous administration of ^{125}I-labeled T_3 or ^{125}I-labeled rT_3 and labeled 3',5'-T_2 after administration of ^{125}I-labeled rT_3, as well as the sulfo- and glucuronoconjugates of both T_2's and T_1. The acetic acid derivatives of T_3 and rT_3 were not found, perhaps due to their extremely rapid clearance rate. The fates of inner-ring-labeled T_3 and rT_3 have not been studied. A radioimmunoassay for 3,3'-T_2 has now been described, and T_2 has been found in amniotic fluid, cord blood, and serum from normal subjects.[91-93] T_2 is derived almost entirely from the peripheral deiodination of T_3 and rT_3. Its metabolic activity, if any, remains to be determined.

The initial enthusiasm for the possibility that elevated serum Tg concentrations might prove to be a clinically useful marker in the detection of thyroid carcinoma *in situ* has waned with the observation that serum Tg concentration is often elevated in states of thyroid gland stimulation in rat and man[94] and with the finding that serum Tg concentrations in patients with a history of head and neck radiation did not correlate with the presence of thyroid cancer.[95] A new radiometric assay for the presence of Tg–antiTg immune complexes in human serum has been described.[96] These complexes were not found in the sera of normal subjects, but were detected in the sera of 24% of patients with Graves' disease.

A radioimmunoassay (RIA) for thyroxine-binding globulin (TBG) has been available for the past several years. Serum TBG concentration in normal subjects has now been reported to be 1.5 ± 0.5 μg/dl.[97] A comparison of the values for TBG (RIA) and for the maximum T_4-binding capacity of TBG yielded a molar ratio of 1:1 for T_4 and TBG. The increase in serum TBG concentration during estrogen administration is due to stimulation of hepatic synthesis of TBG. This was demonstrated both *in vivo* in the monkey and *in vitro* with hepatocytes isolated from monkeys treated with estradiol.[98,99] Finally, *in vivo* studies of the kinetics of labeled TBG metabolism in patients with an X-chromosome-linked increase or decrease in serum TBG concentration revealed that the abnormalities were due to alterations in TBG synthesis, while abnormalities of TBG degradation or rate of synthesis or both were found in clinical conditions associated with acquired abnormalities of serum TBG concentration.[100]

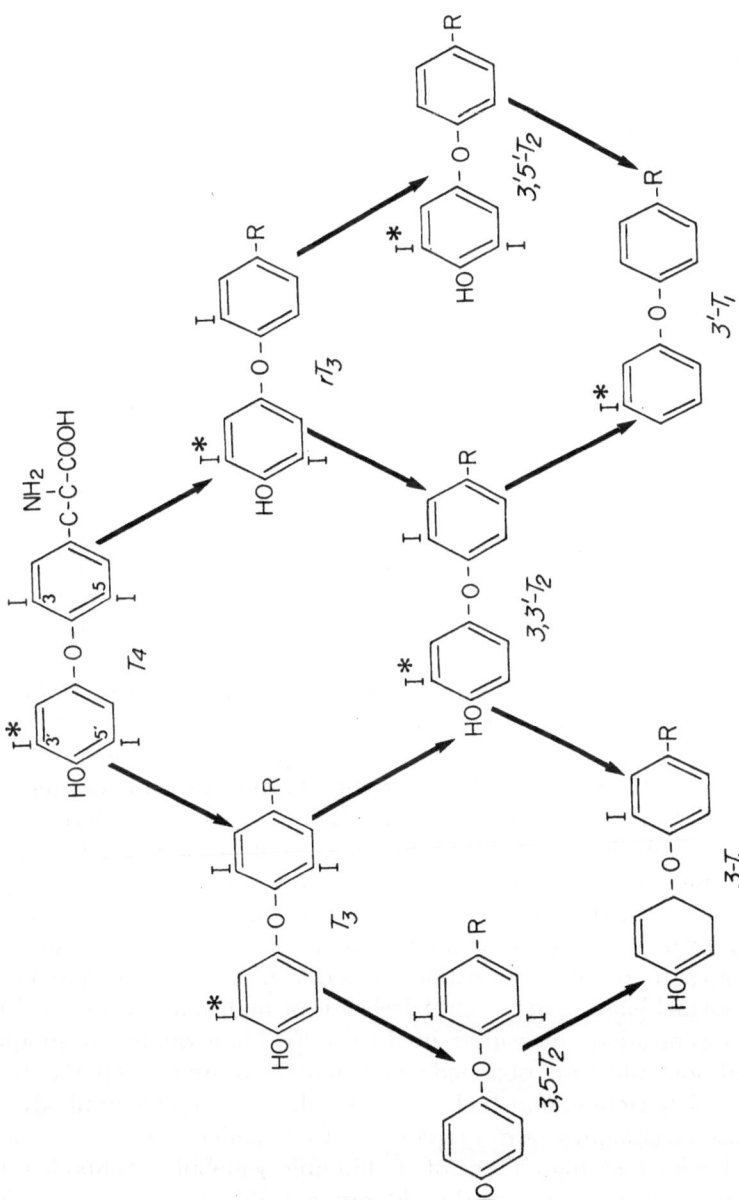

Fig. 2. Sequential deiodination of thyroxine and identification of the resulting iodinated thyronines. (*) Site of the ^{125}I label.

Studies on the cellular distribution and metabolism of the thyroid hormones have continued to appear. The role of the human polymorpho-nuclear leukocyte (PMN) in T_4 and T_3 deiodination was further explored. The bulk of deiodinative activity has been shown to reside in the granule fraction, and the stimulation of activity that phagocytosis induces appears not to depend upon the generation of either hydrogen peroxide or the superoxide radical.[101,102] In addition, the human PMN has been shown to possess saturable nuclear binding sites for T_3 that bind T_3 without the intermediation of a cytosol receptor.[103] In rat muscle and liver homoge-nates, T_3 and T_4 share cellular sites, and in muscle, which constitutes over half the rat body weight, T_4 is preferentially deiodinated.[104] The major role of the liver in thyroid hormone economy has been reemphasized by the findings that pregnenolone-16α-carbonitrile (PCN) enhanced biliary excretion of T_4, resulting in a goiter and increased TSH secretion as a compensatory response to maintain a euthyroid state,[105] and that partial hepatectomy resulted in a rapid, progressive fall in serum T_4 and T_3 concentrations due, at least in part, to increased utilization and turnover of thyroid hormones by the regenerating liver remnant.[106] Langer *et al.*[107] concluded from studies of the acute redistribution of T_4 after the adminis-tration of various drugs, including salicylate and barbituate, that there are two different effects of drugs on plasma T_4 concentration: an immediate effect due to decreased plasma protein binding and a prolonged effect due to increased hormone turnover by peripheral tissues. Extrathyroid iodoprotein concentrations correlate inversely with thyroid state, being decreased in hyperthyroidism and increased in hypothyroidism as a result of alterations in the degradation of these compounds.[108] Finally, Oppen-heimer and colleagues reported that the shorter duration of nuclear occupancy of triac noted last year can be attributed to a more rapid fractional metabolism, and this finding may explain the lesser hormone action of this compound in spite of significant nuclear binding.[109]

Abnormal binding of thyroid hormones to γ-globulins has been observed over the past 20 years in patients with thyroid carcinoma, Hashimoto's thyroiditis, idiopathic myxedema, and hyperthyroidism. Such abnormal binding may yield falsely low or high values for serum T_4 or T_3 concentrations measured by RIA depending on the technique employed; low values are obtained when charcoal is used to separate free from bound hormone, and high values result when double-antibody or solid-phase techniques are employed. Two patients were recently described who had high titers of T_3-binding γ-globulin antibodies in serum; one of the two was hypothyroid, probably due to the large quantity of antibody in the serum.[110] Kinetic studies in the euthyroid patient revealed a slow T_3 clearance rate resulting in a slightly elevated serum T_3 concentration measured in ethanol extracts of serum and a normal T_3 production rate.[111] Although thyroid hormone antibodies are not common, they should be considered in patients in whom values for serum T_4 and T_3 concentrations are discordant with the clinical state.

3.4. Mechanisms of Thyroid Hormone Action

Within the cell, thyroid hormones bind to several subcellular constituents. Saturable nuclear binding sites have been demonstrated in several tissues, and a good correlation has been shown to exist between the relative affinities of thyroid hormone analogues for such sites and their relative biological potencies. There is now nearly general agreement that these nuclear binding sites serve as receptors for thyroid hormones in the cell, and that occupancy of these sites is a prerequisite for induction of at least some aspects of hormone action. Evidence in support of this view was recently provided by Samuels and his associates,[112,113] who examined the relationship between the occupancy by T_3 of nuclear binding sites and the rate of *de novo* synthesis of GH in a GH-producing rat pituitary tumor cell line (GH cell line). They found that the dose–response curve for GH synthesis after 24 hr of incubation with T_3 was displaced to the left of the dose-dependent nuclear-binding curve obtained after 4 hr of incubation, but coincided more closely with the nuclear-binding curve obtained after 24 hr of incubation. This time-dependent shift of the nuclear-binding curve could not be attributed to decreased cell permeability to T_3 or to T_3 degradation, and was interpreted as reflecting receptor depletion. Receptor depletion with time was shown to be T_3-concentration-dependent, and derivation of the receptor-depletion curve resulted in virtually complete superimposition on the dose–response curve for GH synthesis. This latter observation suggests that the unoccupied T_3 receptor might act as a repressor of mRNA synthesis that is rate-limiting for GH synthesis, and that T_3 elicits its action through induction of receptor depletion. This apparent T_3-mediated modulation of nuclear receptor concentration *in vitro* is difficult to reconcile, however, with earlier work demonstrating that T_3 binding by rat liver nuclei was independent of the thyroid state of the animals from which the liver had been obtained. Additional studies are therefore required to determine whether receptor modulation by T_3 occurs *in vivo* and with tissues other than GH_1 cells *in vitro*.

High-affinity, saturable binding sites for thyroid hormones have also been demonstrated in the mitochondrial fraction of certain rat tissues by

Sterling and his associates. These putative mitochondrial receptors are found in those tissues that have classically been considered to be thyroid-hormone-responsive in displaying a calorigenic response to thyroid hormones, but are lacking in nonresponsive tissues, such as adult brain, spleen, and testis. The receptor has been localized to the inner mitochondrial membrane. Preliminary work by these investigators suggests that T_3 binding to the receptor is accompanied by increased O_2 consumption and ATP formation in the isolated mitochondrial vesicles.[114] In the view of Sterling, the mitochondrial receptor is responsible for mediating the early effects of thyroid hormones on cell energy metabolism, while the nuclear receptor mediates the later and more sustained effects of thyroid hormones on protein synthesis. Nonetheless, the latter nuclear action is in all likelihood responsible for the enhancement of Na^+-dependent energy expenditure that thyroid hormones induce. Edelman and his co-workers[115] recently provided evidence suggesting that T_3 elicits an increase in the total number of Na^+, K^+-ATPase sites in rat skeletal muscle. The increased ADP so generated would drive mitochondrial oxidative activity, resulting in a sustained effect on energy metabolism.

The existence of binding proteins in the cytosol of the cell is now firmly established. Recent work with human liver has provided evidence for three distinct binding proteins for T_4 and two for T_3.[116] The function of these cytosol binding proteins has not been defined. Unlike the case with steroid hormones, they are not required for the transport of thyroid hormones to nuclear sites. Rather, they may have a function analogous to that of the binding proteins in plasma in maintaining a readily available intracellular pool of hormone in a dissociable complex.

3.5. Clinical Thyroidology

3.5.1. Hyperthyroidism

A variety of clinical studies concerned with various aspects of hyperthyroidism appeared during the past year. The availability of a number of review articles dealing with the pathogenesis of Graves' disease[117,118] and the diagnosis and treatment of thyrotoxicosis[119] obviate a comprehensive review of these areas, but recent reports pertaining to some of these aspects will be discussed.

At the outset, it would seem appropriate to review briefly the various assays that have been developed to detect the thyroid stimulators found in the immunoglobulin fraction of plasma from patients with Graves' disease. These include: release of radioiodine from prelabeled mouse thyroid (long-acting thyroid stimulator, LATS); prevention of neutralization of LATS activity in thyroid gland extracts (LATS protector, LATS-P); colloid droplet formation and cAMP generation in human thyroid slices (human thyroid stimulator, HTS); adenylyl cyclase stimulation and cAMP generation in human thyroid membranes (human thyroid adenylyl cyclase stimulator, H-TACS[120]; and displacement of labeled TSH in a receptor assay using thyroid membranes (thyroid-stimulating immunoglobulins, TSI). Although the stimulators detected in the different assay systems were initially believed to represent distinct entities, McKenzie and Zakarija[121] recently proposed the theory that a TSI is probably present in all patients with Graves' disease, that the antibody is polyclonal, and is directed against a single human thyroid antigen with variable cross-reactivity in other species. The receptor assay for detection of TSI is currently the one that is most commonly employed. Recent observations suggested that the TSI activity of γ-globulin is not confined to the IgG fraction,[122] and that activation of thyroid AC in bovine plasma membranes can be produced by antisera and antisera IgG from rabbits immunized against bovine thyroid plasma membranes, suggesting that such antibodies manifest properties similar to those of the abnormal thyroid stimulators of Graves' disease.[123]

TSIs have now been detected in the serum of the vast majority of patients with Graves' disease. Previous attempts to correlate the presence of abnormal thyroid stimulators with escape from normal regulatory control of thyroid function have generally been unsuccessful. Clague *et al.*,[124] however, recently noted a positive correlation between the presence of TSI, as assessed by receptor assay, and the absence of TSH control of thyroid function, as assessed by T_3-suppression and TRH-stimulation tests in 48 of 50 hyperthyroid or euthyroid patients, most of whom had Graves' disease. In 2 patients, TSI was present, but T_3 suppression and TRH-stimulation tests were normal.

The presence of ophthalmopathy in euthyroid patients strongly suggests underlying Graves' disease. LATS-P was found, however, in only 9 of 17 patients with euthyroid Graves' ophthalmopathy. Of these 9 patients, 6 had thyroid nonsuppressibility, goiters, and high thyroid antibody titers, suggesting the presence of thyroid autoimmunity, and 3 had suppressible thyroid function. These 3 patients, and 3 patients without LATS-P, but without normal thyroid suppressibility, could not be classified. The 5 remaining patients had neither LATS-P nor goiter and were normally suppressible; they were designated as having "isolated" Graves' ophthalmopathy.[125] Ophthalmopathy may also occur in hypothyroid patients without a previous history of thyroid disease. Either LATS or thyroid autonomy is present, and this aspect of the Graves' disease spectrum has been termed *hypothyroid Graves' disease*.[126] A mechanism for the development of Graves' ophthalmopathy has been proposed based on the identification of Tg or a derivative of Tg in normal human orbital tissue. T lymphocytes obtained from patients with Graves' disease and ophthalmopathy elaborate migration-inhibitory factor (MIF) when exposed to orbital tissues.[127]

Lymphocytes cultured from patients with Graves' disease and exposed to thyroid antigen and phytohemagglutinin have now been shown to produce TSI, as assessed by cAMP stimulation in human thyroid slices.[128,129] Antithyroid antibodies and serum immunoglobulins often decrease during pregnancy and increase postpartum in patients with autoimmune thyroid disease. It is therefore not surprising that active Graves' disease may transiently recur after delivery in patients whose disease has been inactive during pregnancy.[130] These observations further emphasize the importance of immune mechanisms in the etiology of Graves' disease.

A major problem in the management of hyperthyroid Graves' disease with antithyroid drugs is to determine the appropriate time for withdrawal of drug therapy. Thyroid suppression and TRH tests have not proved to be of great help in this regard. It has therefore been suggested that antithyroid drugs be discontinued approximately 3–6 months after euthyroidism has been achieved.[131] The remission rate in patients treated in this way is similar to that obtained after more prolonged therapy. The high recurrance rate of hyperthyroidism following drug therapy has been attributed to the increasing dietary iodine intake. This suggestion has not been confirmed in a study[132] from Denmark, however, where a high relapse rate (approximately 70%) occurred following long-term treatment in an area with a relatively low iodine intake. It is not surprising that thyrotoxicosis recurs so often after antithyroid drug therapy, since abnormal responses to TRH and thyroid suppression occur frequently during the early[133] and late[134] periods following withdrawal of the drugs.

Painful, subacute thyroiditis continues to be a relatively common disorder, and a careful study of 11 biopsy-proved patients revealed the classic three phases of the disorder: hyperthyroidism, hypothyroidism, and recovery to euthyroidism, although 2 patients may have remained permanently hypothyroid.[135] The syndrome of painless thyroiditis is characterized by a nontender goiter, or normal-sized gland, hyperthyroidism, low thyroid radioiodine uptake, and recovery within a few weeks.[136,137] The persistence of anti-Tg antibody titers in some patients for many months raises the possibility that this syndrome is a variant of Hashimoto's thyroiditis. It is evident, however, that needle biopsies of the thyroid must be carried out more frequently before the etiology of this disease can be determined. Since painless thyroiditis is a self-limited disorder and may be difficult to differentiate from Graves' disease on clinical grounds, thyroid ^{123}I uptakes should be carried out more frequently.

Multinodular goiters are more common in the elderly, and the diagnosis of hyperthyroidism is often difficult because serum T_4 and T_3 concentrations may be within the normal range or only marginally increased. Since mild hyperthyroidism is more devastating in elderly patients, and iodide-induced hyperthyroidism may occur in these patients during the administration of iodine-containing medications, physiological hyperthyroidism should be diagnosed early. In two large series of patients with multinodular goiters and normal serum T_4 and T_3 concentrations, serum TSH concentrations were lower than in normal subjects or in patients with diffuse nontoxic goiter,[138] and unresponsiveness to TRH[139] was common, suggesting preclinical hyperthyroidism due to autonomously functioning nodular tissue.

A series of papers that describe in great detail thyroid function in patients with molar pregnancy or choriocarcinoma appeared this year.[140–142] Again, the clinical hyperthyroidism is generally mild in these disorders, despite greatly increased serum T_4 and T_3 concentrations. Absence of frank thyrotoxicosis might be due to the relatively low T_3/T_4 ratios as compared to patients with classic diffuse or nodular toxic goiter, to the often normal proportion of free hormone in serum, and to the limited duration of the disease. As expected, TRH unresponsiveness is usually found, and returns to normal after removal of the trophoblastic tissue. The presence of very high concentrations of hCG, a weak thyroid stimulator, is the probable cause of the thyroid hyperfunction.

Thyrotoxicosis secondary to TSH-secreting pituitary adenomas is rare, but three additional patients were recently reported,[143–145] one with accompanying galactorrhea, amenorrhea, and hyperprolactinemia.[145] The occurrence of frank Graves' disease in one patient previously reported to have had hyperthyroidism on the basis of a TSH-secreting pituitary tumor justifies caution in interpreting the etiology of the hyperthyroidism in these patients.[146] Finally, hyperthyroid Graves' disease may occur in patients with a hereditary decrease in serum TBG concentration.[147,148] These patients have normal serum T_4 and normal or increased serum T_3 concentrations, but free T_4 and T_3 concentrations are increased. This association should be considered in all patients with clinical hyperthyroidism and normal total serum hormone concentrations.

A few unusual clinical and chemical abnormalities associated with hyperthyroidism were noted during the past year. A patient with thyrotoxic, normokalemic periodic paralysis, with unusual manifestations of the disease consisting of main d'accoucheur, diplopia, and lid lag, was reported,[149] and complete quadriplegia was induced by glucose and insulin infusions in patients with thyrotoxic periodic paralysis.[150] Thyrotoxicosis occurred in three patients with myotonic dystrophy, and marked clinical improvement in muscle weakness resulted when the patients became euthyroid.[151] Hyperthyroidism has been reported to be associated with a decrease in the content of zinc and carbonic-anhydrase I and an increase in sodium concentrations in erythrocytes, suggesting that these measurements might prove useful in the diagnosis of hyperthyroidism.[152,153]

The effect of hyperthyroidism on other endocrine systems has received some emphasis in the past. Nonetheless, a few recent observations are noteworthy. In hyperthyroidism, pancreatic alpha and beta cells display decreased functional responses to l-arginine, but not to insulin-induced hypoglycemia.[154,155] The prolactin response to TRH may be blunted in hyperthyroidism, but a normal or exaggerated response occurs in euthyroid patients previously treated for thyrotoxicosis with ^{131}I or antithyroid drugs, despite a blunted or absent TSH response.[156] The prolactin response to l-arginine is diminished[157] in hyperthyroid patients. In contrast to these blunted hormone responses, fasting plasma gastrin levels are increased,[158] plasma catecholamine concentrations[159] and epinephrine secretion rates[160] are normal, and absolute urine cAMP excretion is greater in ambulant patients with thyrotoxicosis than in normals.[161]

Long-standing hyperthyroidism may be associated with negative calcium balance and osteoporosis or osteomalacia. A direct effect of thyroid hormone in stimulating bone resorption *in vitro* was reported.[162] However, a recent study of bone biopsies from 27 hyperthyroid patients revealed a normal degree of bone mineralization as assessed by the phosphorus/hydroxyproline ratio.[163] In a large series of hyperthyroid patients, total and ionized serum calcium were frequently elevated, without an elevation in serum parathyroid hormone concentration.[164] The hypercalcemia induced by hyperthyroidism was invoked as the precipitating cause of acute pancreatitis and renal tubular acidosis observed in one patient.[165] Since hepatic microsomal enzyme activity is enhanced in hyperthyroidism, plasma 25-OH vitamin D concentrations were measured in thyrotoxic patients;[166] subnormal concentrations were noted, and this finding might contribute to the osteomalacia reported to occur in some cases.

Several useful innovations have appeared with respect to drug treatment of hyperthyroidism. The addition of small quantities of iodide (1 mg/day) to PTU therapy results in a more rapid fall in serum hormone concentrations during the early phase of treatment relative to that which occurs with PTU alone.[167] Lithium was reported to be a useful agent in the treatment of severe thyrotoxicosis, potentiating the effects of carbimazole[168] and iodides.[169] It should be emphasized, however, that iodide administration to euthyroid subjects receiving lithium may induce either hypo- or hyperthyroidism.[170] Like iodide, lithium may also induce hypothyroidism in euthyroid patients previously treated for Graves' disease.[171]

Propranolol alleviates many of the signs and symptoms of hyperthyroidism and has been recommended as the sole therapeutic agent in the chronic treatment of thyrotoxic Graves' disease or in the preparation of patients for surgery.[172] Continuous cardiac monitoring indicates that 40 mg propranolol every 6 hr for 3 or 4 days is sufficient preoperative preparation,[173] Propranolol alone, however, may not improve the adverse metabolic effects of hyperthyroidism, such as weight loss, carbohydrate intolerance, and elevated plasma free fatty acid concentrations.[174] Furthermore, in a recent case report, propranolol alone did not prevent thyroid storm, although this might have been due to the relatively low doses that were employed.[175]

Earlier suggestions that ^{125}I might be preferable to ^{131}I in the treatment of hyperthyroidism have not been borne out by recent data. The incidence of hypothyroidism following ^{125}I therapy is similar to that observed after ^{131}I therapy and consequently ^{125}I offers no advantage and should be abandoned.[176,177] The occurrence of hypothyroidism during the first 2 years following ^{131}I therapy depends on the radiation dose administered, while that occurring in later years does not appear to be dose-dependent.[178] Although serum T_4 and T_3 concentrations may increase following ^{131}I therapy of hyperthyroidism, this is not commonly seen. In a recent series, however, 7% of patients with severe thyrotoxicosis became clinically and chemically more toxic after treatment with ^{131}I, irrespective of the dose employed.[179] Thus, it seems advisable to treat elderly hyperthyroid patients or severely thyrotoxic younger patients with antithyroid drugs prior to therapy with ^{131}I. Inadvertent ^{131}I therapy for hyperthyroidism during the first and second trimesters of pregnancy resulted in congenital hypothyroidism in six infants.[180] Pregnancy tests should be carried out in all women in the child-bearing age prior to ^{131}I therapy to avoid this unfortunate complication.

Surgical therapy for thyrotoxicosis also results in hypothyroidism. It has been suggested that temporary hypothyroidism is often present during the first few months following subtotal thyroidectomy, but that normal thyroid function may return by 6 months.[181] It is not necessary to treat this transient hypothyroidism, and long-term replacement therapy should be deferred for approximately 6 months, at which time hypothyroidism, if present, is probably permanent. Postoperative transient hypocalcemia is common following subtotal thyroidectomy for toxic or nontoxic goiters and has been attributed to release of thyrocalcitonin rather than the presence of thyrotoxic osteodystrophy or parathyroid gland damage, although the latter mechanism was not definitely excluded.[182]

3.5.2. Hypothyroidism

During the past year, several reports appeared concerning the patho-physiological abnormalities that are the consequence of the hypothyroid state. Some of this work has important implications with respect to diagnosis and management, and accordingly merits discussion.

The exquisite sensitivity of the myocardium to alterations in hormone availability supports a major role for thyroid hormones in sustaining optimum ventricular performance. In the hypothyroid state, myocardial contractility, as reflected in both the rate of tension development and the peak tension attained, is depressed. In addition, systolic time intervals are altered. For example, the pre-ejection period (PEP), representing electro-mechanical delay and isovolumic contraction, is distinctly prolonged in hypothyroidism and shortened in thyrotoxicosis. A recent study by Crowley et al.[183] examined the serial changes in systolic time intervals in hypothyroidism in response to gradual T_4 replacement and sought a correlation with changes in serum T_4, and TSH concentrations. Systolic time intervals were obtained noninvasively by simultaneous recording of the ECG, phonocardiogram, and carotid-pulse tracing in 15 patients with primary hypothyroidism. Consonant with earlier work, PEP was found to be prolonged and the ratio of PEP to left ventricular ejection time (PEP/LVET) increased in the untreated hypothyroid state. With progressive increments in the dosage of thyroxine replacement, there was a progressive shortening of PEP and decrease in PEP/LVET. In addition, these systolic indices displayed a significant inverse correlation with serum T_4 over a wide range of concentrations and varied directly with serum TSH concentration. With a daily levothyroxine dose of 100 μg, systolic indices and serum T_4 concentration were normal, but serum TSH concentration was still increased. Increasing the dose to 150 μg resulted in restoration to normally detectable values of serum TSH with retention of normal systolic time intervals and serum T_4 concentration. When thyroxine replacement was increased to 200 and 300 μg daily, TSH became undetectable in serum, and the systolic indices declined further. This work suggests that systolic time intervals assessed by noninvasive techniques are a sensitive index of the metabolic impact of the thyroid hormones. Accordingly, they may serve as a useful means for monitoring the response to replacement therapy in the elderly patient or in the patient with coexisting cardiac disease in whom even slight excess of thyroid hormone would be undesirable.

It has long been recognized that enlargement of the sella turcica accompanies hypothyroidism dating from infancy or childhood. This phenomenon has been ascribed to hypertrophy and hyperplasia of the thyrotrophs in response to long-standing deficiency of thyroid hormone. Recently, Yamada *et al.*[184] provided evidence that enlargement of the sella is a frequent accompaniment of adult hypothyroidism. They assessed the volume of the sella by a three-dimensional radiologic technique in 26 patients with primary hypothyroidism. In 21 of the 26 patients, the volume exceeded the maximum value in normal subjects. In these patients, sellar volume correlated directly with serum TSH concentration and inversely with serum thyroid hormone concentrations, indicating that it was a reflection of pituitary enlargement. Rarely, hypertrophy and hyperplasia of the thyrotrophs in long-standing primary hypothyroidism may occur to such a degree that function of other pituitary cells is compromised, resulting in pituitary insufficiency.[185]

3.5.3. Thyroid Cancer

The increased risk of papillary carcinoma of the thyroid and parotid tumors following low-dose therapeutic radiation to the head and neck in early life and adolescence is now well recognized, and the risk of radiation-induced malignant and benign goiter persists for at least 35 years following exposure.[186,187] In the most recent large series of patients, palpable nodular disease was found in 16% and nonpalpable lesions were detected by thyroid imaging in an additional 11%. Thyroid cancer was found in one-third of the patients operated on for nodular disease. The American Thyroid Association has published guidelines for the management of patients at risk.[188] The major controversies concern (1) the advisability of scanning patients at risk who do not have palpable tissue and (2) whether surgery should be done if cold areas are detected, especially since focal carcinoma is often found in areas other than those observed on scan. Until a well-controlled study is carried out, the correct approach to these patients remains uncertain. In our clinic, all patients at risk are scanned, and those with palpable cold nodules are subjected to surgery. Patients with cold areas on scan that are not palpable or patients with enlarged glands without cold areas are placed on long-term thyroid suppression. There is general agreement that all surgically treated patients should be on permanent thyroid suppressive therapy whether the lesions are benign or malignant. The initial enthusiasm for measuring plasma Tg concentration as a screening test for the initial detection of thyroid carcinoma has not proved to be warranted.[95] However, a rise in Tg concentrations following surgery for thyroid carcinoma might indicate recurrent disease. In addition, the presence of Tg in serum after surgery indicates residual, nonsuppressed malignant or benign thyroid tissue, and may indicate the need for a higher dose of thyroid hormone as well as more careful follow-up observation. Measurement of serum TSH concentration and the TSH response to TRH are useful guides to the optimum replacement dose of thyroid hormone in postoperative patients with thyroid carcinoma.[189] The effective dose is that which suppresses both the basal and TRH-stimulated TSH concentrations.

The use of postoperative ablative doses of ^{131}I in patients with carcinoma localized to the thyroid and adjacent nodes is open to debate. If such therapy is used, however, low doses (30 mCi) appear to be as efficacious as the usual higher doses (80–100 mCi) in maintaining patients disease-free.[190] Finally, an excellent review of the results of therapy of 576 patients with papillary carcinoma of the thyroid was recently published.[191]

3.5.4. Miscellaneous

A thorough study of the epidermis in patients with thyroid disease revealed that epidermal thickness was reduced in hypothyroidism, and that epidermal cell division and anabolic activity measured in skin biopsies were increased in hyperthyroidism and reduced in hypothyroidism.[192] Antibodies to *Yersinia enterocolitica* were found more frequently in patients with thyroid disease, especially the autoimmune disorders, both in New York and Denmark, and an association between this infection and thyroid disorders has been suggested.[193,194] The TRH test is normal in patients with a hereditary decrease in TBG despite a low serum free T_4 concentration, suggesting that the normal free T_3 concentration often observed in these patients maintains normal pituitary TSH function.[195] Antimicrosomal thyroid antibodies detected by tanned red cell agglutination are almost always present in high titer in the serum from patients with Hashimoto's thyroiditis and Graves' disease, in contrast to the rather low prevalence of antiTg antibodies measured by this technique.[196] TSH receptors have been found in human thyroid carcinomas for the first time, suggesting that these tumors may be TSH-dependent.[197] Finally, another study of thyroid dysfunction in uremia was carried out, and it suggests that patients treated with chronic hemodialysis often have goiter and low mean serum T_4 and T_3 concentrations, while the serum T_4 is normal and serum T_3 decreased in nondialyzed patients with chronic renal failure. Both groups of uremic patients appear to have both intrathyroid and hypophyseal defects, since the T_4 response to exogenous TSH and the TSH response to exogenous TRH were decreased.[198]

ACKNOWLEDGMENT

The authors' research was supported in part by grants AM19081 and AM18919 from the National Institutes of Health.

References

1. Parker, D. C., Pekary, A. E., and Hershman, J. M., 1976, Effect of normal and reversed sleep–wake cycles upon nyctohermeral rhythmicity of plasma thyrotropin: Evidence suggestive of an inhibitory influence in sleep, *J. Clin. Endocrinol. Metab.* **43**:318–329.
2. Weeke, J., and Laurberg, P., 1976, Diurnal TSH variations in hypothyroidism, *J. Clin. Endocrinol. Metab.* **43**:32–37.
3. Gordin, A., Arimura, A., and Schally, A. V., 1976, Effect of thyroid hormone excess and deficiency on serum thyrotropin in rats immunized passively with antiserum to somatostatin, *Proc. Soc. Exp. Biol. Med.* **153**:319–323.
4. Arimura, A., and Schally, A. V., 1976, Increase in basal and thyrotropin-releasing hormone (TRH)-stimulated secretion of thyrotropin (TSH) by passive immunization with antiserum to somatostatin in rats, *Endocrinology* **98**:1069–1072.
5. Re, R. N., Kourides, I. A., Ridgway, E. C., Weintraub, B. D., and Maloof, F., 1976, The effect of glucocorticoid administration on human pituitary secretion of thyrotropin and prolactin, *J. Clin. Endocrinol. Metab.* **43**:338–346.
6. Ramey, J. N., Burrow, G. N., Spaulding, S. W., Donabedian, R. K., Speroff, L., and Frantz, A. G., 1976, The effect of aspirin and indomethacin on the TRH response in man, *J. Clin. Endocrinol. Metab.* **43**:107–114.
7. Maeda, M., Kuzuya, N., Masuyama, Y., Imai, Y., Ikeda, H., Uchimura, H., Matsuzaki, F., Kumagai, L. F., and Nagataki, S., 1976, Changes in serum triiodothyronine, thyroxine, and thyrotropin during treatment with thyroxine in severe primary hypothyroidism, *J. Clin. Endocrinol. Metab.* **43**:10–17.
8. Nicod, P., Burger, A., Strauch, G., Vagenakis, A. G., and Braverman, L. E., 1976, The failure of physiologic doses of reverse T_3 to affect thyroid-pituitary function in man, *J. Clin. Endocrinol. Metab.* **43**:478–481.
9. White, N., Jeffcoate, S. L., Griffiths, E. C., and Hooper, K. C., 1976, Effect of thyroid status on the thyrotrophin-releasing hormone-degrading activity of rat serum, *J. Endocrinol.* **71**:13–19.
10. Bauer, K., 1976, Regulation of degradation of thyrotropin-releasing hormone by thyroid hormones, *Nature (London)* **259**:591–593.
11. Dupont, A., Labrie, F., Levasseur, L., Dussault, J.-H., and Schally, A. V., 1976, Effect of thyroxine on the inactivation of thyrotropin-releasing hormone by rat and human plasma, *Clin. Endocrinol.* **5**:323–330.
12. Neary, J. T., Kieffer, J. D., Federico, P., Mover, H., Maloof, F., and Soodak, M., 1976, Thyrotropin releasing hormone: Development of inactivation system during maturation of the rat, *Science* **193**:403–405.
13. Mitsuma, T., Hirooka, Y., and Nihei, N., 1976, Radioimmunoassay of thyrotropin releasing hormone in human serum and its clinical application, *Acta Endocrinol.* **83**:225–235.
14. Azukizawa, M., Murata, Y., Ikenoue, T., Martin, C. B., and Hershman, J. M., 1976, Effect of thyrotropin-releasing hormone on secretion of thyrotropin, prolactin, thyroxine, and triiodothyronine in pregnant and fetal rhesus monkeys, *J. Clin. Endocrinol. Metab.* **43**:1020–1028.
15. Zarate, A., Villalobos, H., Canales, E. S., Soria, J., Arcovedo, F., and MacGregor, C., 1976, The effect of oral administration of thyrotropin-releasing hormone on lactation, *J. Clin. Endocrinol. Metal.* **43**:301–305.
16. Tyson, J. E., Perez, A., and Zanartu, J., 1976, Human lactational response to oral thyrotropin releasing hormone, *J. Clin. Endocrinol. Metab.* **43**:760–768.

17. Yu, S., Friedman, Y., Richman, R., and Burke, G., 1976, Altered thyroidal responsivity to thyrotropin induced by circulating thyroid hormones: A "short-loop" regulatory mechanism?, *J. Clin. Invest.* **57**:745–755.
18. Gafni, M., Saddok, C., Sirkis, N., and Gross, J., 1977, The mechanism of damping of the serum thyroxine and triiodothyronine levels caused by increasing thyrotropin dosage in mice, *Endocrinology* **100**:1186–1191.
19. Gluzman, B. E., Varela, A. S., and Niepomniszeze, H., 1976, Altered thyroidal responsivity to TSH: Probable clinical example of a newly proposed "short-loop" regulatory mechanism, *Rev. Biol. Med. Nucl.* **8**:75–78.
20. Shuman, S. J., Zor, U., Chayoth, R., and Field, J. B., 1976, Exposure of thyroid slices to thyroid-stimulating hormone induces refractoriness of the cyclic AMP system to subsequent hormone stimulation, *J. Clin. Invest.* **57**:1132–1141.
21. Field, J. B., Bloom, G., Chou, C.-Y., and Kerins, M. E., 1977, Inhibition of thyroid-stimulating hormone stimulation of protein kinase, glucose oxidation, and phospholipid synthesis in thyroid slices previously exposed to the hormone, *J. Clin. Invest.* **59**: 659–665.
22. Rapoport, B., 1976, Dog thyroid cells in monolayer tissue culture: Adenosine 3′,5′-cyclic monophosphate response to thyrotropic hormone, *Endocrinology* **98**:1189–1197.
23. Thompson, M. E., Orczyk, G. P., and Hedge, G. A., 1972, *In vivo* inhibition of thyroid secretion by indomethacin, *Endocrinology* **100**:1060–1067.
24. Rapoport, B., and Adams, R. J., 1976, Induction of refractoriness to thyrotropin stimulation in cultured thyroid cells: Dependence on new protein synthesis, *J. Biol. Chem.* **251**:6653–6661.
25. Spaulding, S. W., 1977, Effect of thyrotropin on ornithine decarboxylase and of polyamines on RNA polymerase in the thyroid, *Endocrinology* **100**:1039–1946.
26. Pisarev, M. A., and Kleiman de Pisarev, D. L., 1977, Action of cyclic nucleotides on protein and RNA synthesis in the thyroid, *Acta Endocrinol.* **84**:297–302.
27. Sato, A., Hashizume, K., Onaya, T., Miyakawa, M., Makiuchi, M., and Furihata, R., 1976, Effects of biogenic amines on the formation of adenosine 3′,5′-monophosphate in human thyroid slices, *Endocrinol. Jpn.* **23**:319–325.
28. Onaya, T., Hashizume, K., Sato, A., Takazawa, K., Akasu, F., and Endo, W., 1977, Evidence for the existence of a histamine H_2-receptor in the mouse thyroid, *Endocrinology* **100**:61–66.
29. Takasu, N., Sato, S., Tsukui, T., Yamada, T., Miyakawa, M., Makiuchi, M., and Furihata, R., 1976, Comparison of prostaglandin E_1 and TSH stimulation of cyclic AMP synthesis in thyroid tissues from euthyroid subjects and thyrotoxic patients, *J. Clin. Endocrinol. Metab.* **43**:69–79.
30. Davies, T. F., McLachlan, S. M., Povey, P. M., Smith, B. R., and Hall, R., 1977, The influence of propranolol on the thyrotropin receptor, *Endocrinology* **100**:974–979.
31. Laurberg, P., 1977, The relative contribution of thyroxine and triiodothyronine to the hormone secretion from the perfused canine thyroid during various degrees of stimulation, *Endocrinology* **100**:656–662.
32. Clark, O. H., Lambert, W. R., Cavalieri, R. R., Rapoport, B., Hammond, M. E., and Ingbar, S. H., 1976, Compensatory thyroid hypertrophy after hemithyroidectomy in rats, *Endocrinology* **99**:988–995.

33. Hashizume, K., Akasu, F., Takazawa, K., Endo, W., and Onaya, T., 1976, The inhibitory effect of acute administration of excess iodide on the formation of adenosine 3′,5′-monophosphate induced by thyrotropin in mouse thyroid lobes, *Endocrinology* **99**:1463–1468.
34. Rapoport, B., West, M. N., and Ingbar, S. H., 1976, On the mechanism of inhibition by iodine of the thyroid adenylate cyclase response to thyrotropic hormone, *Endocrinology* **99**:11–22.
35. Rapoport, B., Adams, R. J., and Rose, M., 1977, Cultured thyroid cell adenosine 3′,5′-cyclic monophosphate response to thyrotropin: Loss and restoration of sensitivity to iodide inhibition, *Endocrinology* **100**:755–764.
36. Pisarev, M. A., Aiello, L. O., and Kleiman de Pisarev, D. L., 1976, Action of KI, thyroxine and cyclic AMP on [^{3}H]uridine incorporation into the RNA of thyroid slices, *Acta Endocrinol.* **83**:313–320.
37. Pisarev, M. A., and Aiello, L. O., 1976, Studies on the mechanism of action of potassium iodide on thyroid protein biosynthesis, *Acta Endocrinol.* **82**:298–305.
38. Bagchi, N., Brown, T., Shivers, B., and Mack, R. E., 1977, Effect of inorganic iodide on thyroglobulin hydrolysis in cultured thyroid glands, *Endocrinology* **100**:1002–1007.
39. Yukimura, Y., Ikejiri, K., Kojima, A., and Yamada, T., 1976, Effect of excess iodide and other anions on thyroid hormone secretion in normal or hypophysectomized rats treated with graded doses of thyroid hormone, *Endocrinology* **99**:541–548.
40. Riesco, G., Taurog, A., Larsen, P. R., and Krulich, L., 1977, Acute and chronic responses to iodine deficiency in rats, *Endocrinology* **100**:303–313.
41. Taurog, A., Riesco, G., and Larsen, P. R., 1976, Formation of 3,3′-diiodothyronine and 3′,5′,3-triiodothyronine (reverse T$_3$) in thyroid glands of rats and in enzymatically iodinated thyroglobulin, *Endocrinology* **99**:281–290.
42. Riesco, G., Taurog, A., and Larsen, P. R., 1976, Variations in the response of the thyroid gland of the rat to different low-iodine diets: Correlation with iodine content of diet, *Endocrinology* **99**:270–280.
43. Fragu, P., and Nataf, B. M., 1976, Thyroid peroxidase activity in iodine deficient rats, *Acta Endocrinol.* **82**:535–543.
44. Vagenakis, A. G., and Braverman, L. E., 1975, Adverse effects of iodides on thyroid function, *Med. Clin. North Am.* **59**:1075–1088.
45. Croxson, M. S., Gluckman, P. D., and Ibbertson, H. K., 1976, The acute thyroidal response to iodized oil in severe endemic goiter, *J. Clin. Endocrinol. Metab.* **42**:926–930.
46. Ikeda, H., and Nagataki, S., 1976, Augmentation of thyrotropin responses to thyrotropin-releasing hormone following inorganic iodide, *Endocrinol. Jpn.* **23**:431–433.
47. Lamas, L., and Taurog, A., 1977, The importance of thyroglobulin structure in thyroid peroxidase-catalyzed conversion of diiodotyrosine to thyroxine, *Endocrinology* **100**:1129–1136.
48. Kawada, J., Shindo, T., and Yoshimura, Y., 1976, Further study of the mechanism of thyroid hormone secretion in an *in vitro* model system: Direct evidence for fusion of lysosomes with thyroglobulin liposomes, *Endocrinology* **98**:1425–1429.
49. Pelletier, G., Puviani, R., and Dussault, J. H., 1976, Electron microscope immunohistochemical localization of thyroglobulin in the rat thyroid gland, *Endocrinology* **98**:1253–1259.

50. Taurog, A., 1976, The mechanism of action of the thioureylene antithyroid drugs, *Endocrinology* **98**:1031–1046.

51. Nagasaka, A., and Hidaka, H., 1976, Effect of antithyroid agents 6-propyl-2-thiouracil and 1-methyl-2-mercaptoimidazole on human thyroid iodide peroxidase, *J. Clin. Endocrinol. Metab.* **43**:152–158.

52. Williams, J. A., 1976, *In vitro* studies on the nature of vinblastine inhibition of thyroid secretion, *Endocrinology* **98**:1351–1358.

53. Green, W. L., 1976, Induction of a coupling defect in rats during inhibition of tyrosine dehalogenase, *Endocrinology* **98**:10–19.

54. Pommier, J., Tourniaire, J., Rahmoun, B., Dème, D., Pallo, D., Bornet, H., and Nunez, J., 1976, Thyroid iodine organification defects: A case with lack of thyroglobulin iodination and a case without any peroxidase activity. *J. Clin. Endocrinol. Metab.* **42**:319–329.

55. Cuestas, R. A., Lindall, A., and Engel, R. R., 1976, Low thyroid hormones and respiratory-distress syndrome of the newborn, *N. Engl. J. Med.* **295**:297–302.

56. Burger, A., Nicod, P., Suter, P., Vallotton, M. B., Vagenakis, A., and Braverman, L., 1976, Reduced active thyroid hormone levels in acute illness, *Lancet* **1**:653–655.

57. Naeiji, R., Clumeck, N., Somers, G., Vanhaelst, L., and Golstein, J., 1976, Thyroid hormones in serious non-thyroidal illness, *Lancet* **1**:1070–1971.

58. Brandt, M. R., Kehlet, H., Skovsted, L., and Hansen, J. M., 1976, Rapid decrease in plasma-triiodothyronine during surgery and epidural analgesia independent of afferent neurogenic stimuli and of cortisol, *Lancet* **2**:1333–1335.

59. Burger, A., Dinichert, D., Nicod, P., Jenny, M., Lemarchand-Béraud, T., and Vallotton, M. B., 1976, Effect of aminodarone on serum triiodothyronine, reverse triiodothyronine, thyroxin and thyrotropin: A drug influencing peripheral metabolism of thyroid hormones, *J. Clin. Invest.* **58**:255–259.

60. Bürgi, H., Wimpfheimer, C., Burger, A., Zaunbauer, W., Rösler, H., and Lemarchand-Béraud, T., 1976, Changes of circulating thyroxine, triiodothyronine and reverse triiodothyronine after radiographic contrast agents, *J. Clin. Endocrinol. Metab.* **43**:1203–1210.

61. Verhoeven, R. P., Visser, T. J., Docter, R., Hennemann, G., and Schalekamp, M. A. D. H., 1977, Plasma thyroxine, 3,3′,5-triiodothyronine and 3,3′,5′-triiodothyronine during β-adrenergic blockade in hyperthyroidism, *J. Clin. Endocrinol. Metab.* **44**:1002–1005.

62. Danforth, E., Jr., Tyzbir, E. D., Horton, E. S., Sims, E. A. H., Burger, A. G., Braverman, L. E., Vagenakis, A. G., and Ingbar, S. H., 1976, Reciprocal changes in serum triiodothyronine (T_3) and reverse (r T_3) induced by altering the carbohydrate content of the diet, *Clin. Res.* **24**:271A.

63. Spaulding, S. W., Chopra, I. J., Sherwin, R. S., and Lyall, S. S., 1976, Effect of caloric restriction and dietary composition on serum T_3 and reverse T_3 in man, *J. Clin. Endocrinol. Metab.* **42**:197–200.

64. Balsam, A., Sexton, F. C., and Ingbar, S. H., 1976, *In vitro* generation of T3 from T4 by rat liver: Reversible inhibition by starvation and diabetes mellitus, *Program Am. Thyroid Assoc.*, P. T-16.

65. Harris, A., Fang, S., Ingbar, S., Braverman, L., and Vagenakis, A., 1977, Effect of carbohydrate, protein, and fat infusion on the hepatic T3 generation in the fasted rat, *Clin. Res.* **25**:463A.

66. Bray, G. A., Fisher, D. A., and Chopra, I. J., 1976, Relation of thyroid hormones to body weight, *Lancet* **1**:1206–1208.

67. Hervas, F., Morreale de Escobar, G., and Escobar del Rey, F., 1976, Conversion of L-thyroxine to triiodo-L-thyronine and biological activity of L-thyroxine as measured by changes in growth hormone, *Endocrinology* **98:**77–83.

68. Larsen, P. R., and Frumess, R. D., 1977, Comparison of the biological effects of thyroxine and triiodothyronine in the rat, *Endocrinology* **100:**980–988.

69. Croxson, M. S., and Ibbertson, H. K., 1977, Low serum triiodothyronine (T₃) and hypothyroidism in anorexia nervosa, *J. Clin. Endocrinol. Metab.* **44:**167–174.

70. Boyar, R. M., Hellman, L. D., Roffwarg, H., Katz, J., Zumoff, B., O'Connor, J., Bradlow, H. L., and Fukushima, D. K., 1977, Cortisol secretion and metabolism in anorexia nervosa, *N. Engl. J. Med.* **296:**190–193.

71. Bradlow, H. L., Boyar, R. M., O'Connor, J., Zumoff, B., and Hellman, L., 1976, Hypothyroid-like alterations in testosterone metabolism in anorexia nervosa, *J. Clin. Endocrinol. Metab.* **43:**571–574.

72. Chopra, I. J., 1976, An assessment of daily production and significance of thyroidal secretion of 3,3',5'-triiodothyronine (reverse T₃) in man, *J. Clin. Invest.* **58:**32–40.

73. Burman, K. D., Dimond, R. C., Wright, F. D., Earll, J. M., Bruton, J., and Wartofsky, L., 1977, A radioimmunoassay for 3,3',5'-L-triiodothyronine (reverse T₃): Assessment of thyroid gland content and serum measurements in conditions of normal and altered thyroidal economy and following administration of thyrotropin releasing hormone (TRH) and thyrotropin (TSH), *J. Clin. Endocrinol. Metab.* **44:**660–672.

74. Westgren, U., Melander, A., Ingemansson, S., Burger, A., Tibblin, S., and Wahlin, E., 1977, Secretion of thyroxine, 3,5,3'-triiodothyronine and 3,3',5'-triiodothyronine in euthyroid man, *Acta Endocrinol.* **84:**281–289.

75. Ingbar, S. H., and Braverman, L. E., 1975, Active form of the thyroid hormone, *Annu. Rev. Med.* **26:**443–449.

76. Einsenstein, A., Hagg, S., Vagenakis, A., Fang, S., Ransil, B., Braverman, L., and Ingbar, S., 1977, Observations on the peripheral metabolism of 3,3',5'-triiodothyronine (reverse T3, rT3) in fed and fasted patients, *Clin. Res.* **25:**294A.

77. Suda, A., Chambers, J., Jr., Thurston, C., and Pittman, C., 1977, Thyroid hormone kinetics in the fasting and diabetic subjects, *Clin. Res.* **25:**516A.

78. Gavin, L., Castle, J., McMahon, F., Martin, P., Hammond, M., and Cavalieri, R. R., 1977, Extrathyroidal conversion of thyroxine to 3,3',5'-triiodothyronine (reverse-T₃) and to 3,5,3'-triiodothyronine (T₃) in humans, *J. Clin. Endocrinol. Metab.* **44:**733–742.

79. Smallridge, R. C., Wartofsky, L., Desjardins, R. E., and Burman, K. D., 1977, Reverse T3 (rT3) production rates in thyrotoxic, euthyroid, and hypothyroid subjects, *Clin. Res.* **25:**302A.

80. Nicod, P., Burger, A., Staeheli, V., and Vallotton, M. B., 1976, A radioimmunoassay for 3,3',5'-triiodo-L.thyronine in unextracted serum: Method and clinical results, *J. Clin. Endocrinol. Metab.* **42:**823–829.

81. Ratcliffe, W. A., Marshall, J., and Ratcliffe, J. G., 1976, The radioimmunoassay of 3,3',5'-triiodothyronine (reverse T3) in unextracted human serum, *Clin. Endocrinol.* **5:**631–641.

82. Griffiths, R. S., Black, E. G., and Hoffenberg, R., 1976, Measurement of serum 3,3',5'-(reverse) T3, with comments on its derivation, *Clin. Endocrinol.* **5:**679–685.

83. Gordon, A., and Gross, J., 1976, An inter-laboratory comparison of total serum triiodothyronine determination, *Acta Endocrinol.* **83:**539–548.

84. Smals, A. G. H., Ross, H. A., and Kloppenborg, P. W. C., 1977, Seasonal variations in serum T3 and T4 levels in man, *J. Clin. Endocrinol. Metab.* **44:**998–1001.
85. Papavasiliou, S. S., Martial, J. A., Leetham, K. R., and Baxter, J. D., 1976, Thyroid hormone-like actions of reverse T3 and 3,3′-diiodothyronine (3,3′-T2), *Program Am. Thyroid Assoc.* P. T-18.
86. Chopra, I. J., 1976, Extrathyroid conversion of T4 to T3 *in vitro:* Evidence that reverse T3 is a potent inhibitor of T3 production, *Clin. Res.* **24:**426A.
87. Chopra, I. J., Carlson, H. E., and Solomon, D. H., 1976, Comparison of TSH-suppressive effects of various thyroid hormones *in vitro, Clin. Res.* **24:**270A.
88. Fishman, N., Huang, Y. P., Tergis, D. C., and Rivlin, R. S., 1977, Relation of triiodothyronine and reverse triiodothyronine administration in rats to hepatic L-triiodothyronine aminotransferase activity, *Endocrinology* **100:**1055–1059.
89. Lindstedt, G., Lundberg, P.-A., Olsson, A., and Karlsson, K., 1976, Reverse triiodothyronine in screening for congenital hypothyroidism, *Lancet* **2:**1142.
90. Rudolph, M., Sakurada, T., Vagenakis, A., Fang, S., Braverman, L., and Ingbar, S., 1976, Demonstration of sequential monodeiodination as the major pathway of iodothyronine metabolism, *Clin. Res.* **24:**429A.
91. Wu, S.-Y., Chopra, I. J., Nakamura, Y., Solomon, D. H., and Bennett, L. R., 1976, A radioimmunoassay for measurement of 3,3′-L-diiodothyronine (T$_2$), *J. Clin. Endocrinol. Metab.* **43:**682–685.
92. Burman, K. D., Read, J., Dimond, R. C., Strum, D., Wright, F. D., Patow, W., Earll, J. M., and Wartofsky, L., 1976, Measurements of 3,3′,5′-triiodothyronine (reverse T3), 3,3′-L-diiodothyronine, T3, and T4 in human amniotic fluid and in cord and maternal serum, *J. Clin. Endocrinol. Metab.* **43:**1351–1359.
93. Gavin, L. A., Hammond, M., Castle, J. N., and Cavalieri, R. R., 1977, 3,3′-diiodothyronine production, a major pathway of peripheral iodothyronine metabolism in man, *Clin. Res.* **25:**294A.
94. VanHerle, A. J., Chopra, I. J., Hershman, J. M., and Hornabrook, R. W., 1976, Serum thyroglobulin in inhabitants of an endemic goiter region in New Guinea, *J. Clin. Endocrinol. Metab.* **43:**512–516.
95. Schneider, A. B., Favus, M. J., Stachura, M. E., Arnold, J. E., Ryo, U., Pinsky, S., Colman, M., Arnold, M. J., and Frohman, L. A., 1977, Plasma thyroglobulin in detecting thyroid carcinoma after childhood head and neck irradiation, *Ann. Intern. Med.* **86:**29–34.
96. Takeda, Y., and Kriss, J. P., 1977, Radiometric measurement of thyroglobulin–antithyroglobulin immune complex in human serum, *J. Clin. Endocrinol. Metab.* **44:**46–55.
97. Gershengorn, M. C., Larsen, P. R., and Robbins, J., 1976, Radioimmunoassay for serum thyroxine-binding globulin: Results in normal subjects and in patients with hepatocellular carcinoma, *J. Clin. Endocrinol. Metab.* **42:**907–911.
98. Glinoer, D., McGuire, R. A., Gershengorn, M. C., Robbins, J., and Berman, M., 1977, Effects of estrogen on thyroxine-binding globulin metabolism in rhesus monkeys, *Endocrinology* **100:**9–17.
99. Glinoer, D., Gershengorn, M. C., Dubois, A., and Robbins, J., 1977, Stimulation of thyroxine-binding globulin synthesis by isolated rhesus monkey hepatocytes after *in vivo* β-estradiol administration, *Endocrinology* **100:**807–813.

100. Refetoff, S., Fang, V. S., Marshall, J. S., and Robin, N. E., 1976, Metabolism of thyroxine-binding globulin in man: Abnormal rate of synthesis in inherited thyroxine-binding globulin deficiency and excess, *J. Clin. Invest.* **57**:485–495.

101. Woeber, K. A., 1976, A granule-associated L-thyroxine deiodinating system in the human leukocyte, *Endocrinology* **98**:802–806.

102. Woeber, K. A., 1976, Influence of superoxide dismutase and catalase on the stimulation by phagocytosis of L-thyroxine and L-triiodothyronine deiodination in the human leukocyte, *Endocrinology* **99**:887–890.

103. Woeber, K. A., 1977, Observations concerning the binding of L-triiodothyronine in the human polymorphonuclear leukocyte, *J. Clin. Endocrinol. Metab.* **44**:62–68.

104. Zaninovich, A. A., 1976, Reciprocal effects of thyroxine and triiodothyronine on their deiodination by rat tissues *in vitro*, *Acta Endocrinol.* **82**:510–516.

105. Japundzic, M., M., Bastomsky, C. H., and Japundzic, I. P., 1976, Enchanced biliary thyroxine excretion in rats treated with pregnenolone-16α-carbonitrile, *Acta Endocrinol.* **81**:110–119.

106. Leffert, H. L., and Alexander, N. M., 1976, Thyroid hormone metabolism during liver regeneration in rats, *Endocrinology* **98**:1241–1247.

107. Langer, P., Kokesova, H., and Gschwendtova, K., 1976, Acute redistribution of thyroxine after the administration of univalent anions, salicylate, theophylline and barbiturates in rats, *Acta Endocrinol.* **81**:516–524.

108. Balsam, A., and Sexton, F. C., 1976, Thyroid hormone regulation of extrathyroidal iodoproteins, *Endocrinology* **98**:476–481.

109. Goslings, B., Schwartz, H. L., Dillmann, W., Surks, M. I., and Oppenheimer, J. H., 1976, Comparison of the metabolism and distribution of L-triiodothyronine and triiodothyroacetic acid in the rat: A possible explanation of differential hormonal potency, *Endocrinology* **98**:666–675.

110. Karlsson, F. A., Wibell, L., and Wide, L., 1977, Hypothyroidism due to thyroid-hormone-binding antibodies, *N. Engl. J. Med.* **296**:1146–1148.

111. Wu, S.-Y., and Green, W. L., 1976, Triiodothyronine (T_3)-binding immunoglobulins in a euthyroid woman: Effects on measurement of T_3 (RIA) and on T_3 turnover, *J. Clin. Endocrinol. Metab.* **42**:642–652.

112. Samuels, H. H., and Shapiro, L. E., 1976, Thyroid hormone stimulates *de novo* growth hormone synthesis in cultured GH_1 cells: Evidence for the accumulation of a rate limiting RNA species in the induction process, *Proc. Natl. Acad. Sci., U.S.A.* **73**:3369–3373.

113. Samuels, H. H., Stanley, F., and Shapiro, L. E., 1976, Dose-dependent depletion of nuclear receptors by L-triiodothyronine: Evidence for a role in induction of growth hormone synthesis in cultured GH_1 cells, *Proc. Natl. Acad. Sci. U.S.A.* **73**:3877–3881.

114. Sterling, K., Lazarus, J. H., Milch, P. O., and Rose, H. G., 1976, Nature and significance of the mitochondrial T3 receptor, *Program Am. Thyroid Assoc.*, p. T-7.

115. Asano, Y., Lieberman, U. A., and Edelman, I. S., 1976, Thyroid thermogenesis: Relationships between Na^+-dependent respiration and $Na^+ + K^+$-adenosine triphosphatase activity in rat skeletal muscle, *J. Clin. Invest.* **57**:368–379.

116. Hamada, S., and Fukase, M., 1976, Demonstration and some properties of cytosal-binding proteins for thyroxine and triiodothyronine in human liver, *J. Clin. Endocrinol. Metab.* **42**:302–308.

117. Solomon, D. H., and Kleeman, K. E., 1976, Concepts of pathogenesis of Graves' disease, *Adv. Intern. Med.* **22:**273–299.
118. Volpé, R., 1976, The pathogenesis of Graves disease, *Compr. Ther.* **2:**43–52.
119. Irvine, W. J., and Toft, A. D., 1976, The diagnosis and treatment of thyrotoxicosis, *Clin. Endocrinol.* **5:**687–707.
120. Orgiazzi, J., Williams, D. E., Chopra, I. J., and Solomon, D. H., 1976, Human thyroid adenyl cyclase-stimulating activity in immunoglobulin G of patients with Graves' disease, *J. Clin. Endocrinol. Metab.* **42:**341–354.
121. McKenzie, J. M., and Zakarija, M., 1976, A reconsideration of a thyroid-stimulating immunoglobulin as the cause of hyperthyroidism in Graves' disease, *J. Clin. Endocrinol. Metab.* **42:**778–781.
122. Bryson, J. M., Joasoo, A., and Turtle, J. R., 1976, The thyrotrophin receptor in human thyroid plasma membranes: Effect of serum immunoglobulins, *Acta Endocrinol.* **83:**528–538.
123. Ong, M., Malkin, D. G., Tay, S. K., and Malkin, A., 1976, Activation of thyroid adenyl cyclase by antisera to thyroid plasma membrane preparations, *Endocrinology* **98:**880–885.
124. Clague, R., Mukhtar, E. D., Pyle, G. A., Nutt, J., Clark, F., Scott, M., Evered, D., Rees Smith, B., and Hall, R., 1976, Thyroid-stimulating immunoglobulins and the control of thyroid function, *J. Clin. Endocrinol. Metab.* **43:**550–556.
125. Solomon, D. H., Chopra, I. J., Chopra, U., and Smith, F. J., 1977, Identification of subgroups of euthyroid Graves's ophthalmopathy, *N. Engl. J. Med.* **296:**181–186.
126. Christy, J. H., and Morse, R. S., 1977, Hypothyroid Graves' disease, *Am. J. Med.* **62:**291–296.
127. Mullin, B. R., Levinson, R. E., Friedman, A., Henson, D. E., Winand, R. J., and Kohn, L. D., 1977, Delated hypersensitivity in Graves' disease and exophthalmos: Identification of thyroglobulin in normal human orbital muscle, *Endocrinology* **100:**351–366.
128. Knox, A. J. S., von Westarp, C., Row, V. V., and Volpé, R., 1976, Thyroid antigen stimulates lymphocytes from patients with Graves' disease to produce thyroid-stimulating immunoglobulin (TSI), *J. Clin. Endocrinol. Metab.* **43:**330–337.
129. Knox, A. J. S., von Westarp, C., Row, V. V., and Volpé, R., 1976, Demonstration of the production of human thyroid-stimulating immunoglobulins (HTSI) by Graves' lymphocytes cultured *in vitro* with pyytohaemagglutinin (PHA), *Metabolism* **25:**1217–1223.
130. Amino, N., Miyai, K., Yamamoto, T., Kuro, R., Tanaka, F., Tanizawa, O., and Kumahara, Y., 1977, Transient recurrence of hyperthyroidism after delivery in Graves' disease, *J. Clin. Endocrinol. Metab.* **44:**130–136.
131. Greer, M. A., Kammer, H., and Bouma, D. J., 1976, A simplified short-term technique for treating Graves' disease with antithyroid drugs, *Program Am. Thyroid Assoc.*, p. T-2.
132. Lumholtz, T. B., Loldrup-Poulsen, D., Siersboek-Nielsen, K., Friis, T., Rogowski, P., Kirkegaard, C., and Mølholm Hansen, J. 1977, Outcome of long-term antithyroid treatment of Graves' disease in relation to iodine intake, *Acta Endocrinol.* **84:**538–541.
133. Martino, E., Pinchera, A., Capiferri, R., Machia, E., Sardano, G., Bartalena, L., Mazzanti, F., and Baschieri, L., 1976, Dissociation of responsiveness to thyrotropin-releasing hormone and thyroid suppressibility following anti-

thyroid drug therapy of hyperthyroidism, *J. Clin. Endocrinol. Metab.* **43:**543–549.

134. Buerklin, E. M., Schimmel, M., and Utiger, R. D., 1976, Pituitary–thyroid regulation in euthyroid patients with Graves' disease previously treated with antithyroid drugs, *J. Clin. Endocrinol. Metab.* **43:**419–427.

135. Lebacq, E. G., Therasse, G., Schmitz, A., Delannoy, A., and Destailleurs, C., 1976, Subacute thyroiditis, *Acta Endocrinol.* **81:**707–715.

136. Woolf, P. D., and Daly, R., 1976, Thyrotoxicosis with painless thyroiditis, *Am. J. Med.* **60:**73–79.

137. Dorfman, S. G., Cooperman, M. T., Nelson, R. L., Depuy, H., Peake, R. L., and Young, R. L., 1977, Painless thyroiditis and transient hyperthyroidism without goiter, *Ann. Intern. Med.* **86:**24–28.

138. Toft, A. D., Irvine, W. J., and Hunter, W. M., 1976, A comparison of plasma TSH levels in patients with diffuse and nodular non-toxic goiter, *J. Clin. Endocrinol. Metab.* **42:**973–976.

139. Gemsenjäger, E., Staub, J. J., Girard, J., and Heitz, P. H., 1976, Preclinical hyperthyroidism in multinodular goiter, *J. Clin. Endocrinol. Metab.* **43:**810–816.

140. Miyai, K., Tanizawa, O., Yamamoto, T., Azukizawa, M., Kawai, Y., Noguchi, M., Ishibashi, K., and Kumahara, Y., 1976, Pituitary–thyroid function in trophoblastic disease, *J. Clin. Endocrinol. Metab.* **42:**254–259.

141. Morley, J. E., Jacobson, R. J., Melamed, J., and Hershman, J. M., 1976, Choriocarcinoma as a cause of thyrotoxicosis, *Am. J. Med.* **60:**1036–1040.

142. Nagataki, S., Mizuno, M., Sakamoto, S., Irie, M., Shizume, K., Nakao, K., Galton, V. A., Arky, R. A., and Ingbar, S. H., 1977, Thyroid function in molar pregnancy, *J. Clin. Endocrinol. Metab.* **44:**254–263.

143. Baylis, P. H., 1976, Case of hyperthyroidism due to a chromophobe adenoma, *Clin. Endocrinol.* **5:**145–150.

144. Reschini, E., Giustina, G., Cantalamessa, L., and Peracchi, M., 1976, Hyperthyroidism with elevated plasma TSH levels and pituitary tumor: Study with somatostatin, *J. Clin. Endocrinol. Metab.* **43:**924–927.

145. Horn, K., Erhardt, F., Fahlbusch, R., Pickardt, C. R., von Werder, K., and Scriba, P. C., 1976, Recurrent goiter, hyperthyroidism, galactorrhea, and amenorrhea due to a thyrotropin and prolactin-producing pituitary tumor, *J. Clin. Endocrinol. Metab.* **43:**137–143.

146. Sandler, R., 1976, Recurrent hyperthyroidism in an acromegalic patient previously treated with proton beam irradiation: Graves' disease as probable etiology based on follow-up observations, *J. Clin. Endocrinol. Metab.* **42:**163–168.

147. Gerstner, J. B., and Caplan, R. H., 1976, Hyperthyroidism with normal concentrations of total serum thyroxine and triiodothyronine, *J. Clin. Endocrinol. Metab.* **42:**64–69.

148. Horwitz, D. L., and Refetoff, S., 1977, Graves' disease associated with familial deficiency of thyroxine-binding globulin, *J. Clin. Endocrinol. Metab.* **44:**242–247.

149. Kusakabe, T., Yoshida, M., and Nishikawa, M., 1976, Thyrotoxic periodic paralysis: A peculiar case with unusual dystonic behavior and variable relations of paralysis to serum potassium levels, *J. Clin. Endocrinol. Metab.* **43:**730–740.

150. Takeda, R., Morimoto, S., Uchida, K., and Miyamori, I., 1976. Changes in plasma renin activity and plasma aldosterone in the induced paralytic attack of thyrotoxic periodic paralysis, *Acta Endocrinol.* **82:**715–727.

151. Peterson, D. M., Bounds, J. V., Jr., and Karnes, W. E., 1976, Clinical observations on thyrotoxicosis coexisting with myotonic dystrophy, *Mayo Clin. Proc.* **51**:176–179.
152. Swaminathan, R., Segall, N. H., Chapman, C., and Morgan, D. B., 1976, Red-blood-cell composition in thyroid disease, *Lancet* **2**:1382–1385.
153. Auton, J. A., Barragry, J. M., Carter, N. D., Morris, D. V., and Cohn, R. D., 1976, Rapid diagnosis of thyroid disease using carbonic-anhydrase immunoassay, *Lancet* **2**:1385–1387.
154. Imura, H., Seino, Y., Ikeda, M., Taminato, T., Miyamoto, Y., and Goto, Y., 1976, Impaired plasma insulin response to arginine in hyperthyroidism, *Diabetes* **25**:961–968.
155. Shima, K., Sawazaki, N., Tanaka, R., Morishita, S., Tarui, S., and Nishikawa, M., 1976, The pancreatic alpha and beta cells responses to *l*-arginine and insulin-induced hypoglycaemia in hyperthyroidism, *Acta Endocrinol.* **83**:114–122.
156. Kannan, C., Akbar, M., Begum, F., Dwarakanathan, A., and Burke, G., 1976, Dissociation between TSH and prolactin dynamics in treated thyrotoxicosis, *Clin. Endocrinol.* **5**:331–340.
157. Onishi, T., Itoh, K. F., Miyai, K., Izumi, K., Shima, K., and Kumahara, Y., 1976, Prolactin response to arginine in normal subjects and in patients with hyperthyroidism, *J. Clin. Endocrinol. Metab.* **42**:148–151.
158. Seino, Y., Matsukara, S., Miyamoto, Y., Goto, Y., Taminato, T., and Imura, H., 1976, Hypergastrinemia in hyperthyroidism, *J. Clin. Endocrinol. Metab.* **43**:852–855.
159. Coulombe, P., Dussault, J. H., and Walker, P., 1976, Plasma catecholamine concentrations in hyperthyroidism and hypothyroidism, *Metabolism* **25**:973–979.
160. Coulombe, P., Dussault, J. H., Latarte, J., and Simard, S. J., 1976, Catecholamines metabolism in thyroid diseases. I. Epinephrine secretion rate in hyperthyroidism and hypothyrodism, *J. Clin. Endocrinol. Metab.* **42**:125–131.
161. Carter, D. J., and Heath, D. A., 1977, The effect of treatment of hyper- and hypothyroidism on urinary excretion of cyclic adenosine 3′,5′-monophosphate, *Acta Endocrinol.* **84**:542–547.
162. Mundy, G. R., Shapiro, J. L., Bandelin, J. G., Canalis, E. M., and Raisz, L., 1976, Direct stimulation of bone resorption by thyroid hormones, *J. Clin. Invest.* **58**:529–534.
163. Tougaard, L., 1976, The degree of bone mineralization in hyperthyroidism estimated from the phosphorus to hydroxyproline ratio in bone, *Acta Endocrinol.* **81**:482–486.
164. Burman, K. D., Monchik, J. M., Earll, J. M., and Wartofsky, L., 1976, Ionized and total serum calcium and parathyroid hormone in hyperthyroidism, *Ann. Intern. Med.* **84**:668–671.
165. May, P., and Levy, R. P., 1976, Thyrotoxicosis associated with renal tubular acidosis and acute pancreatitis: A case report, *Ann. Intern. Med.* **84**:569–570.
166. Velentzas, C., Oreopoulos, D. G., From, G., Porret, B., and Rapoport, A., 1977, Vitamin-D levels in thyrotoxicosis, *Lancet* **1**:370–371.
167. Kasai, K., Suzuki, H., Kikuchi, T., Ieiri, T., Takemura, Y., and Shimada, S.-I., 1976, Clinical study on early changes in thyroid function of hyperthyroidism treated with propylthiouracil and a relatively small dose of iodide, *Endocrinol. Jpn.* **23**:347–354.

168. Turner, J. G., Brownlie, B. E. W., Sadler, W. A., and Jensen, C. H., 1976, An evaluation of lithium as an adjunct to carbimazole treatment in acute thyrotoxicosis, *Acta Endocrinol.* **83:**86–92.

169. Boehm, T. M., Burman, K. D., and Wartofsky, L., 1976, Synergystic effects of lithium (Li) and iodine (I) in the treatment of hyperthyroidism (HT), *Program Endocrine Soc.*, p. 366.

170. Spaulding, S. W., Burrow, G. N., Ramey, J. N., and Donabedian, R. K., 1977, Effect of increased iodide intake on thyroid function in subjects on chronic lithium therapy, *Acta Endocrinol.* **84:**290–296.

171. Burman, K. D., Dimond, R. C., Earll, J. M., Wright, F. D., and Wartofsky, L., 1976, Sensitivity to lithium in treated Graves' disease: Effects on serum T_4, T_3, and reverse T_3, *J. Clin. Endocrinol. Metab.* **43:**606–613.

172. Toft, A. D., Irvine, W. J., McIntosh, D., MacLeod, D. A. D., Seth, J., Cameron, E. H. D., and Lidgard, G. P., 1976, Propranolol in the treatment of thyrotoxicosis by subtotal thyroidectomy, *J. Clin. Endocrinol. Metab.* **43:**1312–1316.

173. Toft, A. D., Irvine, W. J., and Campbell, R. W. F., 1976, Assessment by continuous cardiac monitoring of minimum duration of preoperative propranolol treatment in thyrotoxic patients, *Clin. Endocrinol.* **5:**195–198.

174. Ortigosa, J. L., Mendoza, F. A., Argote, R., Garcia, G., Cervantes, C., and Parra, A., 1976, Propranolol effect on plasma glucose, free fatty acid, insulin, and growth hormone in Graves' disease, *Metabolism* **25:**1201–1207.

175. Eriksson, M., Rubenfeld, S., Garber, A. J., and Kohler, P. O., 1977, Propranolol does not prevent thyroid storm, *N. Engl. J. Med.* **296:**263–264.

176. Bremner, W. F., Spencer, C. A., Ratcliffe, W. A., Greig, W. R., and Ratcliffe, J. G., 1976, The assessment of ^{125}I treatment of thyrotoxicosis, *Clin. Endocrinol.* **5:**225–234.

177. McDougall, I. R., and Greig, W. R., 1976, ^{125}I therapy in Graves' disease: Long-term results in 355 patients, *Ann. Intern. Med.* **85:**720–723.

178. Malone, J. F., and Cullen, M. J., 1976, Two mechanisms for hypothyroidism after ^{131}I therapy, *Lancet* **2:**73–75.

179. Creutzig, H., Kallfelz, I., Haindl, J., Thiede, G., and Hundeshagen, H., 1976, Thyroid storm and iodine-131 treatment, *Lancet* **2:**145.

180. Stoffer, S. S., and Hamburger, J. I., 1976, Inadvertent ^{131}I therapy for hyperthyroidism in the first trimester of pregnancy, *J. Nucl. Med.* **17:**146–149.

181. Toft, A. D., McIntosh, D., Cameron, E. H. D., Irvine, W. J., Seth, J., and Lidgard, G. P., 1976, Temporary hypothyroidism after surgical treatment of thyrotoxicosis, *Lancet* **2:**817–821.

182. Wilkin, T. J., Isles, T. E., Paterson, C. R., Crooks, J., and Beck, J. S., 1977, Post-thyroidectomy hypocalcaemia: A feature of the operation or the thyroid disorder?, *Lancet* **1:**621–623.

183. Crowley, W. F., Jr., Ridgway, E. C., Bough, E. W., Francis, G. S., Daniels, G. H., Kourides, I. A., Myers, G. S., and Maloof, F., 1977, Noninvasive evaluation of cardiac function in hypothyroidism, *N. Engl. J. Med.* **296:**1–6.

184. Yamada, T., Tsukui, T., Ikejiri, K., Yukimura, Y., and Kotani, M., 1976, Volume of sella turcica in normal subjects and in patients with primary hypothyroidism and hyperthyroidism, *J. Clin. Endocrinol. Metab.* **42:**817–822.

185. Vagenakis, A. G., Dole, K., and Braverman, L. E., 1976, Pituitary enlargement, pituitary failure, and primary hypothyroidism, *Ann. Int. Med.* **85:**195–198.

186. Favus, M. J., Schneider, A. B., Stachura, M. E., Arnold, J. E., Ryo, U. Y., Pinsky, S. M., Colman, M., Arnold, M. J., and Frohman, L. A., 1976, Thyroid cancer occurring as a late consequence of head-and-neck irradiation, *N. Engl. J. Med.* **294:**1019–1025.
187. Schneider, A. B., Favus, M. J., Stachura, M. E., Arnold, M. J., and Frohman, L. A., 1977, Salivary gland neoplasms as a late consequence of head and neck irradiation, *Ann. Int. Med.* **87:**160–164.
188. McConahey, W. M., and Hayles, A. B., 1976, Radiation and thyroid neoplasia, *Ann. Intern. Med.* **84:**749–750.
189. Busnardo, B., Vangelista, R., Girelli, M. E., Bui, F., and Lazzi, C., 1976, TSH levels and TSH response to TRH as a guide to the replacement treatment of patients with thyroid carcinoma, *J. Clin. Endocrinol. Metab.* **42:**901–906.
190. McCowen, K. D., Adler, R. A., Ghaed, N., Verdon, T., and Hofeldt, F. D., 1976, Low dose radioiodide thyroid ablation in postsurgical patients with thyroid cancer, *Am. J. Med.* **61:**52–58.
191. Mazzaferri, E. L., Young, R. L., Oertel, J. E., Kemmerer, W. T., and Page, C. P., 1977, Papillary thyroid carcinoma: The impact of therapy in 576 patients, *Medicine* **56:**171–196.
192. Holt, P. J. A., Lazarus, J., and Marks, R., 1976, The epidermis in thyroid disease, *Br. J. Dermatol.* **95:**513–518.
193. Shenkman, L., and Bottone, E. J., 1976, Antibodies to *Yersinia enterocolitica* in thyroid disease, *Ann. Intern. Med.* **85:**735–739.
194. Bech, K., Nerup, J., and Larsen, J. H., 1977, *Yersinia enterocolitica* infection and thyroid diseases, *Acta Endocrinol.* **84:**87–92.
195. Konno, N., 1976, Serum thyrotropin response to thyrotropin-releasing hormone and free thyroid hormone indices in patients with familial thyroxine-binding globulin deficiency, *Endocrinol. Jpn.* **23:**313–317.
196. Abreau, C. M., Vagenakis, A. G., Roti, E., and Braverman, L. E., 1977, Clinical evaluation of a hemagglutination method for microsomal and thyroglobulin antibodies in autoimmune thyroid disease, *Ann. Clin. Lab. Sci.* **7:**73–78.
197. Ichikawa, Y., Saito, E., Abe, Y., Homma, M., Muraki, T., and Ito, K., 1976, Presence of TSH receptor in thyroid neoplasms, *J. Clin. Endocrinol. Metab.* **42:**395–398.
198. Ramirez, G., O'Neill, W., Jr., Jubiz, W., and Bloomer, H. A., 1976, Thyroid dysfunction in uremia: Evidence for thyroid and hypophyseal abnormalities, *Ann. Intern. Med.* **84:**672–676.

Parathyroid Hormone
and Calcitonin

Karen Kleeman and Charles R. Kleeman

4.1. Parathyroid Hormone

4.1.1. Introduction

To paraphrase the contemplative White Knight,[1] the *name* of our subject is "parathyroid hormone and calcitonin," but the *subject* is really calcium homeostasis—the control of a major controller of cellular and multicellular life.

Life is impossible without calcium, which seems to couple almost every stimulus and response in the body: nerve to nerve, nerve to muscle, hormone to receptor cell. To be effective, calcium must be released into the cell only in the proper quantity and at the proper time; too much free intracellular calcium can kill cells by disrupting basic metabolic machinery. Cells carefully control their cytoplasmic free calcium ion concentration at a level some 100 times lower than that in the extracellular fluid. Calcium that enters the cell down its concentration gradient is removed, temporarily by mitochondria and other storage organelles, permanently by outward active transport in the cell membrane.

KAREN KLEEMAN • Department of Medicine, Beth Israel Hospital, Boston, Massachusetts. CHARLES R. KLEEMAN • Department of Medicine, UCLA School of Medicine and Center for the Health Sciences, Los Angeles, California.

We are only beginning to learn how cells handle calcium. But most cells probably cannot adapt to large changes in the amount of calcium entering them, either steadily, along its concentration gradient, or in pulses, in response to a stimulus. If extracellular calcium is too low, some stimuli which act via calcium entry will not induce their full cellular responses; if extracellular calcium is excessive, some cells could gradually become overloaded, and their normal function would be aborted.

The purpose of parathyroid hormone (PTH) is to keep indispensable calcium available at the proper concentration, drawing as necessary on the skeleton (where quantities of calcium are stored that far exceed the body stores of any other element). Every one of the hormone's actions is directed toward that end.

4.1.2. Hormone Synthesis, Secretion, and Turnover

This year, a fine comprehensive review of the difficult subject of PTH synthesis and secretion was published by Dr. Joel Habener[2] of the endocrinology group at the Massachusetts General Hospital, whose recent investigations have made the major contribution to our current understanding of that subject. Most details omitted from our discussion can be found in this review.

Intact secreted PTH is an 84-amino-acid polypeptide chain. No smaller forms are secreted. It has been known for some years that full activity resides in the 1–34 peptide sequence and in no smaller peptide, and that carboxy terminal peptides are inactive. A PTH precursor with six additional N-terminal amino acids, proPTH, has been identified in parathyroids of man and animals, and in a cell-free system, it has been shown that the PTH mRNA originally directs the synthesis of an even longer peptide, pre-proPTH,[3] the 25 amino terminal amino acids of which are removed within seconds of its complete synthesis.[4] ProPTH is then converted into PTH after a 20-min delay.[5] This time is probably required for transport of the proPTH from rough endoplasmic reticulum to the Golgi apparatus, because drugs that disrupt microtubular function inhibit the conversion of proPTH to PTH.[6]

Of the small amount of PTH that is normally stored within the cell, only 7% is stored as proPTH. ProPTH tested in an *in vitro* renal adenylate cyclase bioassay had only 2–3% of the activity of PTH, and even this amount was probably due to its conversion.[2] Little if any .proPTH is normally released into the circulation, and there is no evidence that any functionally hypoparathyroid state is due to the release of PTH precursor instead of PTH.

Only a limited amount is known about the actual secretion of PTH. The hormone is packaged into secretory granules that presumably traverse the cell, perhaps via microtubules, to somehow unite with the plasma membrane and release their contents into the circulation. About 30 min is required from packaging to secretion. It has not been conclusively proved that these "secretory granules" are the source of secreted PTH, and it is possible that most hormone may be secreted without prior packaging.[7]

The rate of synthesis and release of PTH is primarily controlled by plasma calcium. This regulation is discussed in Section 4.1.5.1.

Although the intact 1–84 peptide hormone is fully active at all its receptor sites without prior conversion elsewhere to its N- and C-terminal fragments, it was recently shown that the liver will take up and split intact hormone but not C-terminal fragments.[8,9] The significance of this activity is unknown. At its effector cells, the hormone is split into its 1–34 and 35–84 fragments, but is is not certain at what point this occurs or whether it necessarily precedes the response to the hormone. McIntosh and Hesch[10] labeled antibodies to the N- and C-terminal fragments, which they incubated with PTH prebound to renal cortical membranes. Their finding that both types of antibodies would bind to the PTH indicates that at least intact hormone need not be split before it binds to its receptor.

The splitting of the hormone during its career means that circulating "PTH" detected by radioimmunoassay (RIA) may include intact hormone and both terminal fragments. This heterogeneity was observed by Berson and Yalow[11] in their original RIA. Assays specific for both N- and C-terminal fragments have been available for some time, but their sensitivity has been poor. It appears that the N-terminal fragment is present at a very low concentration not only in normal persons, but also in patients with hyperparathyroidism, such that the N-terminal assay is always at the lower limit of its sensitivity and is unable to discriminate between patients with hyperparathyroidism and normals. Even the C-terminal assay has in the past been unable to detect minimal hyperparathyroidism, although the C-terminal fragment is present in the circulation for much longer and at much higher levels than the N-terminal (eventually being excreted by the kidney), and the difference in levels between normal subjects and hyperparathyroid patients is greater. Currently, however, C-terminal assays are available that offer very good discrimination between normal and hyperparathyroid levels,[12] and Christensen[13] has now developed an extremely sensitive assay for intact circulating hormone, using an extraction with microfine precipitated silica that concentrates the hormone 3.2-fold. The reported detection limit with this assay was as low as 10 pg/ml, and the assay was able to detect intact hormone in 95% of normal subjects (mean level 67 pg/ml). PTH by this assay was undetectable in all 18 patients with nonmalignant, nonparathyroid hypercalcemia and in 23 of 25 patients with hypercalcemia of malignancy. Of patients with primary hyperparathyroidism, 96% had hormone values above normal (mean 433 pg/ml). In patients with secondary hyperparathyroidism of renal failure, values ranged from normal to 9000 pg/ml, and 7 of 8 patients with values greater than 3000 had clear radiological evidence of osteitis fibrosa cystica. The normal levels detected by Christensen approached the physiological level calculated by Parsons from the effects of chronic PTH infusion in dogs (see Section 4.1.3.5a).

The rat has been a popular subject for investigations of PTH, but reliable assay of circulating PTH in this animal has been difficult. Fujita *et al.*[14] found that rat PTH was detected by an antibody to bovine *N*-terminal PTH, but not by one to intact PTH, suggesting that the dominant circulating form of PTH in the rat may be unlike that in larger mammals.

4.1.3. Physiological Role of Parathyroid Hormone

PTH exists to maintain a normal concentration of ionized calcium in body fluids. All its effects are coordinated to achieve that end. Five effects dominate at the organ level:

1. PTH increases the remodeling rate, or turnover, of bone, thereby supporting a metabolically active, "youthful" skeleton with more readily accessible mineral stores.
2. It increases the release of calcium from bone by one mechanism that does not break down bone matrix, and by others that do.
3. It increases the renal reabsorption of calcium.
4. It decreases the renal reabsorption of phosphate.
5. By increasing the generation of 1,25-dihydroxycholecalciferol (active vitamin D), it increases the absorption of calcium in the upper small intestine.

Hypoparathyroid patients remodel bone very slowly, but their bones are strong and do not fracture more readily than do normal bones. The bones may be somewhat undermineralized, or conversely somewhat sclerotic, but they are fairly normal bones; they are *not* capable, however, of contributing to the support of plasma calcium at its normal level. For that function, they must be prepared by PTH.

As bone physiology has become better understood, we have learned both that the effects of PTH on bone and bone cells depend on the dose that is used and that the effects of physiologic and pharmacologic doses are very different. Almost all older studies involved the use of massive pharmacologic doses, given in unphysiologic boluses that may have raised blood hormone levels to from 100 to 1000 times normal. Unfortunately, many studies are still being performed in this way. Any such study that purports to explain some action of PTH must be interpreted cautiously.

4.1.3.1. Calcium Homeostasis

Those of us who have not thought critically about calcium homeostasis have probably maintained a rather simple mental picture of it, something like this: when calcium is at a high plasma level, it moves into bones, and when it is at a low level, it moves out of bones via PTH-mediated bone breakdown, with decreased renal loss and increased intestinal absorption making some contribution. Hyperparathyroid hypercalcemia is casually assumed to result from excessive bone breakdown and release of calcium into the system.

This simple and seemingly obvious conception includes no consideration of the complex physiology of bone. Furthermore, the explanation of hyperparathyroid hypercalcemia becomes completely untenable if we heed Parfitt's calculation of the bone mineral that would have to leave the skeleton to maintain, unaided, a 1 mg/dl increase in the serum calcium level. The calculated loss of over 500 mg/day would consume the entire skeleton in about 7 years.[16]

For the sake of our clearer thinking, it is fortunate that in the past year, Dr. Michael Parfitt has published an insightful and encyclopedic four-part review[15-18] of bone physiology and its control for good and ill by PTH. His discussion has redefined our thoughts of PTH and calcium homeostasis. From a wide base of evidence, he convincingly argues two theses: (1) PTH affects bone in two ways: it induces removal of calcium to support the plasma calcium level, and it supports a normal rate of normal skeletal remodeling. These processes are related, but they are also distinct and independent of each other. (2) The steady-state level of plasma calcium is set by the rate of PTH secretion. PTH sets the "calciostat" through the integration of its skeletal and renal effects, both of which are absolutely required. Acute adjustments of the calcium level around the preset point are also accomplished by PTH, through induction of mineral removal.

Because effects of PTH on bone cannot be appreciated without knowledge of the basics of bone physiology, we herewith present them, as derived from Parfitt,[17] whose discussion is much more thorough and complex.

4.1.3.2. Physiology of Bone

Parfitt identifies four bone cell types: (1) The *osteoblast* produces bone matrix or osteoid and rapidly imbues it with 70–75% of its final mineral content. (2) The *osteoclast* simultaneously removes matrix and its mineral. Osteoclasts are not able to initiate removal of osteoid that has never been mineralized; this limitation may contribute to the "resistance" of bone to PTH in chronic vitamin D deficiency, wherein unmineralized osteoid accumulates at free bone surfaces. (3) *Surface osteocytes* line all bone surfaces where neither formation nor resorption is taking place. They may be the progenitors of osteoblasts and osteoclasts, and are probably responsible for pumping calcium out of the bone extracellular fluid (see below). (4) *Deep osteocytes* are osteoblasts that have incorporated themselves into lacunae in the bone they built. These cells communicate with each other and with surface cells via protoplasmic extensions lying in canaliculi. Microcanaliculi radiating from the canaliculi between collagen fiber bundles provide a huge surface area of 35,000 mm^2/mm^3 for exchange between crystal and bone fluid.[19] Outside the lacunar wall of the deep osteocyte is a 1 to 2-μm thick layer of so-called "perilacunar bone," which has fewer collagen fibers and less dense, more soluble mineral than bone elsewhere. Healthy osteocytes maintain this labile mineral by continuously remodeling the perilacunar bone.

Cortical bone can be visualized in three dimensions as a mass of closely packed cylindrical columns (Haversian systems or osteons) running parallel to the long axis of the bone. Each osteon is formed of concentric lamellae of bone around a central canal containing a blood vessel, lymphatics, and nerves. Remodeling of this bone is constant and is carried out by the *coordinated* resorption of a new cylindrical space and its refilling in the form of a new osteon. The coupled resorption and filling is carried out by what Parfitt has called a *cortical remodeling unit* (CRU), which includes an advancing edge of newly formed osteoclasts followed by undifferentiated spindle cells, blood vessels, and, bringing up the rear at some distance, osteoblasts refilling the hole. New osteoclasts and osteoblasts are continuously formed as the CRU travels through the bone; the initiation of CRU activity at each new horizontal level along its course may be called a *cortical remodeling cycle* (CRC).

The delay between resorption and formation varies, and the nature of the coupling is not known. In some cases, the progression of the CRU is somehow aborted, and a permanent space is left in the bone. The bone area over which resorption and formation have been temporarily or permanently "uncoupled" increases with age, so that the process of Haversian remodeling is associated, over the years of adult life, with a slow net loss of bone mass.

Parfitt has demonstrated by careful calculation that variation in the rate of bone remodeling or turnover is almost entirely due to *change in the rate of initiation of new remodeling cycles, accomplished by the formation of new osteoclasts.* Formation is stimulated by PTH (see Section 4.1.3.3c).

4.1.3.2a. Blood–Bone Equilibrium and the Maintenance of Serum Calcium. The extracellular fluid (ECF) bathing bone crystal in canaliculi and lacunae and between surface osteocytes and bone has a different ionic composition from "systemic" ECF. The differences are probably maintained by energy-requiring pumps in surface and deep osteocytes. Bone ECF has a low calcium level because osteocytes actively pump calcium from bone ECF to systemic ECF. This work develops and maintains a concentration gradient for calcium from blood to bone ECF: calcium continuously flows down this gradient and is in turn removed by the osteocytes. The total flux, which is large enough to replace the entire ECF calcium at least once per day, depends on the concentration gradient developed by the osteocytes; acute hypercalcemia will raise inward flux, and acute hypocalcemia decrease it, until the preset concentration gradient is reestablished.

If a piece of bone is removed from an animal and placed in culture, the osteocytes will establish a steady-state level of calcium in the medium. The ultimate steady-state level will be the same *no matter what the original calcium concentration in the medium:* it is the metabolic state of the bone *in vivo* which determines the concentration gradient which will be set by the osteocyte pumps and thus the equilibrium calcium level which the bone will set *in vitro.*

This pumping system will maintain a low but constant serum calcium *in vivo* in the total absence of PTH. In the parathyroidectomized animal baseline serum calcium is about 6 mg/dl; if a hypocalcemia of 4 mg/dl is induced acutely with EDTA, the animal returns its serum calcium to 6 as rapidly as does an intact animal. As a result of the hypocalcemia, the calcium level at the crystal–fluid interface falls; mineral is then released without breakdown of matrix until the previous equilibrium serum calcium level is reached. The speed of this restoration appears to be limited primarily by the bone blood flow, which determines the rate at which released calcium can be carried from the bones to the rest of the body. At a serum calcium level of 6, renal reabsorption of calcium is virtually complete even in the absence of PTH, so that a minimal net drain of calcium occurs by this route, and renal loss does not impede reequilibration.

4.1.3.3. Parathyroid Hormone and the Skeleton[16]

4.1.3.3a. Blood–Bone Equilibrium and Bone Blood Flow. We said above that the equilibrium calcium level that a piece of bone will set in incubation medium is determined by its *in vivo* metabolic state. It appears that this state is determined by PTH. Bone taken from an animal pretreated with PTH will set a higher equilibrium calcium level in culture, and bone from a parathyroidectomized animal will set a low level.

Two mechanisms have been suggested for this effect. One invokes PTH-stimulated organic acid production. Production and release of organic acid into the bone by the osteocyte is known to increase the solubility of the mineral involved in blood–bone transfer, making more mineral more readily available. PTH does increase the production of citrate in osteocytes, though this increase may be a nonspecific reflection of stimulated cellular metabolism. The other theory is that PTH increases outward calcium pumping by the osteocyte, and that the resultant increased calcium concentration gradient in turn increases inward flux. Ramp[20] showed that PTH does increase the activity of the pump. These theories are not mutually exclusive, and both may well apply.

PTH keeps bones "youthful" by supporting a healthy rate of continuous Haversian remodeling and revascularization. Young, recently synthesized bone has a higher water content, and its mineral is more soluble and more available for blood–bone exchange. Without PTH, mean skeletal age increases; bone becomes increasingly dense and gives up mineral less readily. Thus, by stimulating remodeling, PTH maintains a skeleton capable of supporting an equilibrium body fluid calcium in the normal range.

PTH is an arterial vasodilator when given in very large intravenous doses. Boelkins *et al.*[21] recently showed that blood flow in the hindlimb of the hen first decreased, then increased in concert with the hypocalcemic and hypercalcemic phases of the response to PTH. Since the blood–bone equilibration system needs normal bone blood flow to reestablish base-line serum calcium after a disturbance, it seems logical that increased bone blood flow might be an important effector of the hypercalcemic response to PTH. However, Boelkins and co-workers used massive doses of PTH that probably created blood levels 1000 times the physiological; we cannot conclude from their experiments that the observed effect is a physiological one.

4.1.3.3b. Deep Osteocytes. In response to low levels of PTH, the osteocyte removes only mineral from the perilacunar bone; at higher PTH levels, the osteocyte resorbs both matrix and mineral. Chronic stimulation with hypercalcemic doses of PTH leads to an increase in size of the sphere of perilacunar bone, and the rate of periosteocytic remodeling probably increases. At very high, totally nonphysiological PTH concentration, progressive lacunar enlargement may occur, with eventual confluence of lacunae and death of the osteocytes.

4.1.3.3c. Osteoclasts; Bone Resorption and Remodeling. The nature of the acute effect of PTH on osteoclasts depends on its concentration. At a fairly low concentration, it activates "resting" osteoclasts that are not actively resorbing; it stimulates their production and release of organic acid, lysosomes, and collagenase, all of which may be involved in the poorly understood biochemical process of whole bone resorption. When larger amounts of PTH are administered, generation of new osteoclasts can be observed over many hours. When PTH is being given *acutely*, a much higher dose is needed to generate the new osteoclasts of a cortical remodeling cycle (see Section 4.1.3.2) than is needed to stimulate either osteocytes or resting osteoclasts to resorb bone; Parfitt believes, however, that the base-line Haversian remodeling rate responds not to acute changes in PTH secretion, but to the integrated secretion rate over a long period. Thus, he suggests, PTH is able to control serum calcium and bone remodeling simultaneously and independently. Note that these processes *are independent,* whether or not we accept Parfitt's explanation of their control: plasma calcium may be normally maintained in the face of very low bone turnover, as in hypothyroidism, or very high bone turnover, as in Paget's disease; these two conditions may span a 100-fold difference in turnover rate.

4.1.3.4. Parathyroid Hormone and the Kidney

4.1.3.4a. Calcium Clearance. Hyperparathyroidism is the only hypercalcemic disorder in which, given normal kidneys, hypercalciuria in proportion to the serum calcium elevation does not appear. A marked PTH-induced decrease in calcium clearance can be seen in the reported results of Albright's early experiments,[22] but he did not notice the effect. It was first reported by Talmage and Kraintz[23] in rats and by Kleeman *et al.*[24] in humans receiving either human or bovine parathyroid extract. Every species since studied has responded in the same way.

PTH depresses reabsorption of both sodium and calcium (and phosphate and bicarbonate) in the proximal nephron, but it dissociates transport of these ions in the distal nephron, such that acute administration of the hormone increases sodium loss but decreases the loss of calcium. Indirect experiments by the senior author in 1968 suggested the distal nephron as the reabsorptive site.[25] This year, Sutton *et al.,*[26] using nephron micropuncture in the dog, directly showed enhanced tubular reabsorption of calcium both at or beyond the distal convoluted tubule and at a preceding site, perhaps in the thick ascending limb. In a complementary study, Chabardès *et al.,*[27] using physiologic levels of 1–34 bovine PTH, found PTH-sensitive adenylate cyclase activity in five cortical segments of the rabbit nephron: proximal convoluted tubule and pars recta, thick ascending limb, distal convoluted tubule, and branched collecting duct. No medullary nephron segments responded to the hormone. Distal convoluted tubule and branched collecting duct will probably prove to be the dominant sites of PTH-mediated reabsorption.

The widely used thiazide diuretics increase tubular reabsorption of calcium relative to sodium; no other kind of diuretic can produce sustained hypocalciuria in the absence of overt salt depletion with reduced GFR. This unique property of thiazides has led to their successful use in the treatment of recurrent nephrolithiasis.

We have no exact explanation for thiazide hypocalciuria. Previous work[28,29] suggested that the effect requires or is enhanced by PTH; Quamme et al.,[30] however, using micropuncture in thyroparathyroidectomized dogs, recently found that the hypocalciuric effect of chlorothiazide was not increased by concomitant administration of PTH. There were important methodological differences between these two groups of experiments, and we cannot yet reconcile the results. Quamme and co-workers located the effect of chlorothiazide in the distal convoluted tubule, where sodium reabsorption was inhibited but calcium reabsorption was not; PTH could easily have an additive effect in this segment.

4.1.3.4b. Phosphate Clearance. The phosphaturic action of PTH might superficially appear unrelated to its ability to keep up the calcium level in body fluids. It has become clear, however, that any increase in the amount of inorganic phosphate bathing the metabolically active skeleton will cause a net movement of calcium phosphate into the bone, frequently with a fall in the extracellular calcium concentration. The phosphaturic effect of PTH disposes of the phosphate liberated with calcium from the bone, and so prevents an increase in serum phosphate that would tend to thwart the attempt to raise serum calcium.

The mechanism of the increased renal clearance of phosphate is not fully understood. PTH probably inhibits phosphate reabsorption in both the proximal and the distal nephron.[31-33] However, it is the degree of inhibition of distal reabsorption that seems to regulate the net change in phosphate clearance seen at any PTH concentration.

Boudry et al.[34] recently described *secretion* of phosphate in the rat nephron after phosphate loading. Phosphate secretion has often been hypothesized, since net tubular reabsorption of phosphate in animals on high phosphate diets may fall essentially to zero, and total inhibition of phosphate reabsorption is physiologically extremely improbable. It is likely that phosphate secretion is continuous, but is masked by excretion of a much larger amount of filtered phosphate. We cannot exclude the possibility that PTH may actually increase tubular secretion rather than decrease reabsorption, as has been suggested by Tröhler et al.[35]

Renal tubular phosphate reabsorption somehow adapts itself to the level of dietary phosphate.[36,37] Adaptation does not require PTH and can be observed at any steady-state level of hormone. One of us (C.R.K.) has seen many patients with surgically confirmed hyperparathyroidism and normal renal function clear their urine of phosphate almost completely after only 1 week of rigid phosphate restriction (200 mg dietary P + 4 oz. aluminum hydroxide gel/day).

Tröhler et al.[35] recently studied this adaptation in intact and thyro-parathyroidectomized rats fed very small, normal, or large quantities of phosphate for periods of up to 10 days. They found striking adaptation of the phosphate clearance, exceeding that which might be produced merely by change in the filtered phosphate load. The response appeared within 3 days of dietary alteration. It was not delayed or abolished by prior parathyroidectomy, but on a high-phosphate diet the parathyroidectom-ized animals were not able to increase phosphate excretion to the same degree as intact animals. On a low-phosphate diet, both groups of animals could produce urine that was almost free of phosphate. It is known that phosphate-depleted animals producing a phosphate-free urine may be completely unresponsive to the phosphaturic effect of exogenous PTH, even if serum phosphate (and thus filtered load) is normal. Steele[38] showed that the tubules in such animals respond to PTH with normal generation of cAMP (see Section 4.1.4), yet phosphaturia does not occur. Administered dibutyryl cAMP is also without effect.

The mechanism for this remarkable degree of tubular adaptation is unknown. Possibly it is related to a low level of free inorganic phosphate in the renal tubular cell. Further work with the drug disodium etidronate (EHDP) may provide an answer. This drug, a stable form of pyrophos-phate used in the treatment of Paget's disease, produces hyperphospha-temia in man. Walton et al.[39] have now shown that EHDP increases the maximal tubular reabsorption of phosphate for any level of GFR (TmP:GFR[40]) without changing the circulating PTH level.

It is interesting that in the sheep, a ruminant, phosphate excretion seems to be controlled in the saliva, with automatic renal conservation.[41] Clark et al.[42] showed that PTH given to adult sheep produces renal calcium reabsorption and hypophosphatemia but no phosphaturia, while a marked rise in salivary phosphate secretion occurs. This effect repre-sents the first demonstration to our knowledge of hormone influence on phosphate secretion into the GI tract.

4.1.3.4c. Bicarbonate Clearance. PTH produces an alkaline urine[43] by inhibition of hydrogen ion secretion, with consequent bicarbonate wast-ing and sometimes even metabolic acidosis.[44,45] A teleological explana-tion for this effect has not been obvious in the past, but some good possibilities have arisen recently. Froeling and Bijvoet[46] noted that PTH-mediated resorption of bone mineral releases bicarbonate as well as calcium and phosphate, so that increased bicarbonate excretion might protect against alkalosis. Beck and Webster[47] showed that acute meta-bolic acidosis in the rat directly raises the serum calcium and also augments the hypercalcemic effect of PTH, suggesting that PTH might improve its own efficiency by producing bicarbonaturia and a mild drop in systemic pH. The most arresting hypothesis is that the bicarbonaturia itself is the one and only cause of the phosphaturia; the proposed mechanism and evidence in its support are discussed in Section 4.1.4.

The bicarbonaturic effect of PTH is responsible for the fact that 30–35% of patients with hyperparathyroidism will have a mild hyperchloremic acidosis, in contrast to patients with hypercalcemia of any other cause. This fact has applied to the differential diagnosis of hypercalcemia.[48]

The site in the nephron in which bicarbonate reabsorption is inhibited was recently confirmed through micropuncture studies as the proximal tubule,[49] where reabsorption of sodium, calcium, phosphate, chloride, and water is also inhibited.

4.1.3.5. An Integrated Model of Calcium Homeostasis

From myriad wide-ranging studies, Parfitt[16] has developed a model of calcium homeostasis in which mineral flux from the skeleton and renal calcium reabsorption jointly support body fluid calcium, and in which different bone cells are activated in progression to respond to progressively severe degrees of hypocalcemia. We will present this model briefly, as we believe it best accounts for all that is now known about PTH, bone physiology, and bone disease.

Acting on healthy bone, well mineralized with the help of vitamin D and continuously remodeling under the long-term control of PTH, PTH sets the level of calcium flux between the bone and blood. Simultaneously, it fixes the fractional renal calcium reabsorption. The blood–bone equilibration level and calcium reabsorption have similar PTH dose–response curves, so they are always regulated in parallel, and the serum calcium is maintained with almost no calcium loss from the skeleton.

If the serum ionized calcium falls slightly from its normal level, the small parathyroid response induces deep osteocytes to remove mineral without matrix from the perilacunar bone. Resting osteoclasts may also be transiently stimulated. Renal reabsorption of calcium increases concurrently. If the drain on the body fluid calcium is transient and dietary calcium is available, the perilacunar bone will be remineralized; however, if the drain continues or if the acute demand is great, more PTH is released, and this activates osteocytic and osteoclastic resorption of whole bone. Measured urinary hydroxyproline will rise as matrix is broken down, and calcium excretion will fall further. A normal serum calcium concentration will generally be reestablished long before PTH reaches a concentration high enough to stimulate osteoclast proliferation. If the condition tending to lower the serum calcium is a chronic one, however, such as a high-phosphate diet,[50] the increased PTH secretion rate integrated over time will lead to an increased skeletal remodeling rate.

In this model, a chronic calcium drain could lead to osteoporosis by two routes. First, Parfitt postulates that in contrast to osteoclast generation, "resting" osteoclast activation would not be coupled to the formation of new osteoblasts, so that the activated osteoclasts might leave permanent holes in the bone. Second, since the ratio of resorption to formation in the cortical remodeling unit increases with age, any stimulus that increases the bone turnover rate will slowly decrease the total bone mass. Although this is a very neat formula, and although either calcium deficiency or phosphate excess can produce osteoporosis in laboratory animals, we must remember that human senile osteoporosis is a complex disease that has never been definitely linked to any dietary imbalance—not for lack of trying, as Parfitt[18] points out. There does seem to be a subclass of normocalcemic osteoporotics with high circulating PTH; we suspect that most of these patients have secondary hyperparathyroidism due to $1,25-OH_2D_3$ deficiency stemming from either inadequate diet or mild renal disease (see Section 4.1.6.5). Most recently, a small group of such patients was described by Teitelbaum et al.[51]; their bone biopsies revealed both an increased number of osteoclasts and an increase in osteoid, compatible with mild D deficiency with secondary hyperparathyroidism. Accepting Parfitt's convincing arguments for independent control of calcium homeostasis and skeletal remodeling, we can easily imagine that a chronic increase in PTH secretion intended to combat D-deficiency hypocalcemia could lead to increased bone turnover and eventually to osteoporosis. A similar, but more marked, dissociation of serum calcium maintenance and bone remodeling may result in the combination of hypocalcemia and osteitis fibrosa seen in some pseudohypoparathyroid patients (see Section 4.1.7).

Returning to the model, we stress two of its aspects: (1) that PTH has many effects on bone and is not a simple agent of destruction, and (2) that maintenance of body fluid calcium is always a joint effort by kidney and bone (barring primary disease of either).

4.1.3.5a. Hyperparathyroid Hypercalcemia and Bone Disease. Although hyperparathyroidism appears in all degrees of severity, patients tend to fall into two groups.[52] One group has severe disease of short duration, with markedly high serum calcium, prominent osteitis fibrosa cystica, often renal stones, and a comparatively large mass of abnormal parathyroid tissue. The other group has mild disease, often of many years' standing, with recurrent kidney stones the most common complaint, few or no signs of any bone disease, and a smaller, presumably slower-growing abnormal parathyroid mass.

Using the model we have described, Parfitt derived convincing pathophysiologic explanations for what we might call the stable and rapidly progressive forms of hyperparathyroidism.[16,17] The stable form is presumed to begin with a slight, sustained increase in PTH secretion, which resets both the blood–bone equilibrium and renal calcium reabsorption to maintain a higher body fluid calcium. Only a few hundred milligrams of calcium leaving the bone for the ECF and saved by the kidney from excretion would establish a new, mildly hypercalcemic steady state. Once established, the steady state would be maintained without need of further bone breakdown or mineral loss. An increase in the rate of normal skeletal remodeling would occur concurrently, and would lead over months to years to some net bone loss, even symptomatic osteoporosis in a few patients.

Parsons' hyperparathyroid dog[53] is a canine vindicator of Parfitt's human model. The dog is given a chronic, continuous infusion of just enough PTH to sustain mild hypercalcemia. Plasma hydroxyproline does not rise; bone biopsy shows no increased destruction; intestinal calcium absorption rises, calcium clearance falls, and the animal actually goes into *positive* calcium balance. A very small amount of PTH, far less than has been used in the past to produce laboratory hyperparathyroidism, suffices to produce these effects.

Rapidly progressive disease with osteitis fibrosa cystica (of which the well-known phalangeal subperiosteal resorption is a common form) is the postulated result of severe hyperparathyroidism with very high circulating PTH levels. Bone breakdown is rapid; so much calcium is poured into the ECF that renal reabsorption is saturated, and only renal excretion of the excess prevents serum calcium from reaching lethal levels. Renal insufficiency is a great danger to one of these patients; very severe hypercalcemia may develop if dehydration, hypotension, nephrocalcinosis, or any other insult lowers the GFR.

Parfitt suggests that osteitis fibrosa reflects complete uncoupling of bone resorption and formation (see Section 4.1.3.2) under the influence of superpathologic quantities of PTH. Rapidly formed osteoclasts resorb bone, not in neat longitudinal cylinders, but in amorphous chunks extending in all directions. Abnormally stimulated osteoblasts fill the space, not with healthy lamellar bone, but with weak, fragile woven bone. In extremely severe cases, almost the entire skeleton may be resorbed and replaced with woven bone.[17]

4.1.3.6. Parathyroid Hormone and Vitamin D

There can be no doubt that PTH and vitamin D are interdependent. Neither hormone behaves normally when the other is deficient. In all forms of hypoparathyroidism, cholecalciferol (the precursor of active vitamin D) is effective only in huge doses. Conversely, secondary hyperparathyroidism always accompanies vitamin D deficiency, and the hypophosphatemia characteristic of vitamin D deficiency is due to the high renal phosphate clearance produced by PTH. Patients with chronic vitamin D deficiency secondary to malabsorption may even develop frank parathyroid adenomas, called tertiary or "masked" hyperparathyroidism because overt hypercalcemia does not appear until vitamin D deficiency is corrected.[54] Vitamin-D-deficient patients need these high PTH levels to support their serum calcium; D-deficient dogs and rats cannot maintain a normal serum calcium despite prodigious secretion of PTH.

Skeletal resistance to PTH in vitamin D deficiency has been amply demonstrated in a variety of systems,[55] but we do not know exactly how vitamin D "permits" PTH to act on the bone. Although the unmineralized osteoid of classic osteomalacia is known to be resistant to osteoclastic resorption, hypocalcemia occurs in the vitamin-D-deficient dog or rat in the absence of obvious histologic osteomalacia.[55] Recent studies[56,57] indicate that vitamin D deficiency does not interfere with activation of adenyl cyclase in response to PTH (see Section 4.1.4).

The interrelationship of PTH and vitamin D is complex, controversial, and currently confusing. Active vitamin D (1,25-dihydroxycholecalciferol; $1,25\text{-OH}_2D_3$) seems able to mimic some of the effects of PTH on bone, such as "priming" the bone to maintain blood–bone equilibrium at a normal calcium level, and it has recently proved an effective treatment for the hypocalcemia of hypoparathyroidism.[58,60] However, it probably does not affect the renal clearance of either calcium or phosphate.[59-61] Vitamin-D-deficient patients commonly have an almost calcium-free urine with a very high renal clearance of phosphate; conversely, hypoparathyroid patients maintained on vitamin D and calcium therapy are always hypercalciuric.

Recent attempts to clarify the vitamin D–PTH alliance have produced successful studies of vitamin D metabolism[62] and controversial studies of PTH secretion.[63,64] Over the past decade, we have learned that hypocalcemia or calcium deficiency increases production of $1,25\text{-OH}_2D_3$ from the intermediate form 25-OHD_3. PTH, released in response to the hypocalcemia, mediates the active D production by stimulating the mitochondrial enzyme 1α-hydroxylase present in the tubular cells of the renal cortex. Using a new radioreceptor binding assay for 1,25-OH_2D_3, Hughes *et al.*[62] showed that parathyroidectomized hypocalcemic or calcium-depleted rats are unable to generate 1,25-OH_2D_3 and have very low plasma levels of this hormone, even though plenty of cholecalciferol is available in their diet.

Phosphate has a direct effect, independent of PTH, on the 1α-hydroxylase enzyme: phosphate deficiency stimulates 1α-hydroxylase, and phosphate excess inhibits it. Thus, the hypophosphatemia of primary hyperparathyroidism might be a secondary effector, through 1,25-OH_2D_3, of the increased serum calcium. There is recent exciting but still disputable evidence that the 1,25-OH_2D_3 molecule binds to the parathyroid cell and inhibits further secretion.[63,64] Such inhibition would supply another negative-feedback loop to the calcium regulating system. We might more profitably regard it, however, as a way for the body to deal with excess phosphate: phosphate excess that stimulates PTH production and simultaneously inhibits that of 1,25-OH_2D_3 could permit maximum PTH secretion and maximum phosphaturia.

Unfortunately, the inhibitory effect of active D has not proved itself in early *in vivo* tests by Coburn *et al.*[65] Administration of 1,25-OH_2D_3 to humans with secondary hyperparathyroidism of renal failure and to vitamin-D-deficient dogs did not decrease circulating immunoreactive PTH in their studies.

The important physiological action of PTH in increasing the intestinal absorption of calcium is probably mediated through increased production of 1,25-OH_2D_3. Adaptation to low-calcium intake with increased absorption probably occurs by this route,[66] but the requirement for PTH is not yet certain or fully accepted.[67,68]

For those attempting to make teleological sense of all this, we think it is helpful to recall that PTH does not appear in animals lower than the amphibia; in fish, in the watery environment of which calcium is plentiful but phosphate is at a premium,[69] vitamin D probably regulates these divalent ions. We can imagine that PTH appeared only with the move to land, when it became necessary for animals to salvage calcium and dispose of large quantities of phosphate, and that its effects were superimposed on the system controlled by vitamin D. Thus, PTH and vitamin D subtly interact or even duplicate each other's work in bone, while PTH regulates intestinal calcium absorption and functions alone in the kidney.

4.1.3.7. Nature of Active Parathyroid Hormone

Ever since Berson and Yalow originally observed the heterogeneity of circulating PTH, investigators have questioned whether different fragments might be responsible for different effects. Several naturally occurring and substituted fragments have been synthesized and tested in a variety of assays (see Parsons[70]). Although some of the fragments have been variably active from assay to assay, no active fragment has shown an effect qualitatively different from that of intact native PTH. Moreover, Di Bella et al.[71] showed that the effect of a PTH preparation at a receptor site in vitro may be heavily dependent on the species from which the receptor tissue is taken, possibly due to differences in the rate of degradation of the hormone at the receptor site. Thus, we are unlikely to obtain useful information by comparing the effects of a hormone preparation on, for example, rat renal cortex and chick bone, as some have done in the past.

A related question is whether the active 1–34 amino terminal fragment of PTH and the intact hormone behave identically at every receptor site. We now have available for research purposes both synthetic 1–34 PTH and highly purified native hormone extracts. The active fragment has never, in any assay, shown an effect that the purified hormone did not; neither one has any effect that cannot also be produced by the very crude original hydrochloric acid extract of Collip and Clark (Lilly Parathormone®), which is no longer marketed. Most recently, Goltzman et al.[72] studied adenylate cyclase stimulation in response to intact and 1–34 PTH in an in vitro renal cortical membrane assay. The kinetics of the adenylate cyclase responses to the two forms were identical; analysis of membrane-bound hormone following the incubation with intact PTH showed that no proteolysis had occurred, although adenylate cyclase had been stimulated.

Despite all this good in vitro support for the power of intact PTH, there are some interesting bits of evidence suggesting that PTH in vivo must act at or be acted on by some peripheral organ before it can act at its known receptors. Years ago, one of the authors (C.R.K.) made numerous unsuccessful attempts (unpublished!) to decrease calcium clearance in normal and thyroparathyroidectomized dogs by infusing PTH directly into the renal artery, rather than the peripheral circulation. Parsons and Robinson[73] and Mueller et al.[74] similarly found no increase in calcium release from cat tibia and hen femur, respectively, when the bones were perfused directly with PTH; the PTH was effective only after passing through the systemic circulation. Finally, we know that the liver takes up and splits intact PTH,[8,9] presumably with purpose.

The paucity of data in this line invites further research and prevents us from reaching a conclusion this year.

4.1.3.8. A Wider Role for Parathyroid Hormone

PTH may affect a much larger number of tissues than we usually consider its domain. The hormone may enhance calcium entry into skin,[75] cornea,[76] and blood vessels,[77] and it has been shown experimentally that lymphoblast proliferation,[78] hepatic regeneration,[79] and erythropoiesis[80] may be defective in hypocalcemic, hypoparathyroid animals. Studies in 1974 and 1975 by Arieff and Massry[81] and Guisado et al.[82] on acutely uremic dogs with secondary hyperparathyroidism clearly showed that rising brain calcium with associated EEG changes was not related to either serum divalent ion levels or uremia *per se,* but specifically required excess PTH. We can speculate, pleasurably if we are parathyroid enthusiasts, that the hormone may be a more generally important physiological regulator than we have previously supposed.

4.1.4. Cellular Response to Parathyroid Hormone

It seems that in all its major sites of action, PTH binds to a specific receptor in the plasma membrane of effector cells,[55,83] and that receptor binding has two effects: stimulation of adenylate cyclase with an increase in cAMP production, and an increase in membrane permeability to calcium such that more calcium enters the cell along its concentration gradient.[55] This calcium entry may explain the hypocalcemia that appears within the first minutes after PTH administration.

The relationship between cAMP generation and the increase in intracellular calcium is unclear. Both are probably essential mediators of the response to PTH. In what seems to be a very important study (reported in abstract form), Herrmann-Erlee et al.[84] used the calcium antagonist isoptin (Verapamil), which inhibits calcium entry into many cell types including bone, to study the effect of dissociating the calcium entry and cAMP generation produced by PTH. With calcium entry inhibited, PTH-stimulated release of calcium, phosphate, and citrate from cultured fetal mouse calvaria was significantly reduced, while cAMP generation and PTH-dependent lactate release were stimulated. These results suggest that two groups of cellular responses to PTH may exist and support the hypothesis that cAMP might not mediate the response of all effector cells to PTH. This hypothesis is unlikely, but it is not untenable. In 1975, two groups reported apparent dissociation of cAMP production and response to PTH, one group studying the phosphaturic response in humans,[85] the other studying the hypercalcemic response in rats.[86] It is possible, but we cannot assume, that the results might have been due to insensitivity of the cAMP measurement. The rat study is also interesting in that the dissociation was found only at low levels of PTH and not at pharmacologic levels. This result underlines the necessity of using PTH in physiologic doses to define physiologic effects.

Little is known about the intracellular events that follow calcium entry and cAMP generation and that result in the many biochemical, morphological, and functional changes observed in various cells after PTH stimulation.[18,19] The increased outward calcium pumping observed by Ramp[20] in the osteocyte is probably induced by the calcium entry.

In secretory cells, an increase in intracellular calcium is required for secretion to occur; the calcium may be needed for microtubular structures to be built in the cytoplasm. Colchicine is a potent inhibitor of microtubule formation. Heath et al.[87] showed in 1972 that hypocalcemia resistant to correction by PTH developed in nephrectomized rats given colchicine. Recently, Dousa et al.[88] observed that colchicine disruption of cytoplasmic microtubules in renal cortical cells interfered with phosphate transport and its regulation by PTH. It is possible that one effect of the increased intracellular calcium induced by PTH may be the formation of specific microtubular structures.

The phosphaturic response to PTH was first reported in 1911, but we have not understood it. We know that the phosphaturia, which follows an increase in cAMP generation, is accompanied by inhibition of hydrogen ion secretion and increase in the excretion of $NaHCO_3$. Puschett and Goldberg[89] and Beck and Goldberg[90] suggested that inhibition of proximal tubular reabsorption of bicarbonate increases luminal pH and so increases the ratio of urinary HPO_4^{2-} to $H_2PO_4^-$; since the more highly charged HPO_4^{2-} molecule diffuses less easily across the tubular membrane, the increased luminal pH would reduce phosphate reabsorption. Uchikawa et al.[91] studied the flux of $H^{32}PO_4^{2-}$ and $H_2^{32}PO_4^-$ across kidney cells and slices and the effect of PTH on their H^+ production. $H_2PO_4^-$ entered kidney cells 12 times more readily than did HPO_4^{2-}. H^+ production fell by 35% during incubation with PTH; the fall was probably due to cAMP generation, since it was duplicated by aminophylline and dibutyryl cAMP. Uchikawa calculated that a proximal tubular luminal pH change of only 0.4 units, from 6.8 to 7.2, well within the probable capacity of PTH, would alter the $HPO_4^{2-}/H_2PO_4^-$ ratio enough to decrease tubular reabsorption of phosphate from 87 to 60%. They concluded that the phosphaturic effect of PTH is entirely due to its bicarbonaturic effect. Beck et al.[92] have since shown that carbonic anhydrase activity in renal cortical homogenates is inhibited by both PTH and cAMP; bicarbonaturia and subsequent phosphaturia might be produced in this way.

4.1.5. Regulation of Hormone Synthesis and Secretion

To succeed in their appointed function, normal parathyroid cells must be able to continuously secrete enough hormone to set and sustain the steady-state serum calcium; they must increase secretion rapidly in response to acute hypocalcemic stress; and they must divide and hypertrophy to master chronic hypocalcemic stress. We do not know how any of these is accomplished—only that they are all controlled by free calcium ion.

Calcium ion—or its absence—could theoretically regulate any step from hormone synthesis to secretion. Only a few points in the sequence have been studied. Cleavage of hormone precursors is probably not regulated[2]; intracellular degradation of hormone appears to be.[93] High extracellular calcium stimulates, and low extracellular calcium inhibits, hormone degradation. Habener *et al.*[93] suggested that this "salvaged" hormone may be that which acutely combats acute hypocalcemia, since changes in the rate of hormone synthesis become manifest only after some hours.[2]

Almost nothing is known about the adaptive response to chronic hypocalcemia, other than that it occurs. Parathyroid cells cultured in a low-calcium medium will increase their contingent of many subcellular organelles.[94] The links between low calcium and organelle synthesis are undiscovered.

There is some evidence that all parathyroid activators may work through cAMP.[95-97] We cannot yet go farther within the cell.

Magnesium ion can evoke parathyroid secretory responses *in vitro* that parallel the responses to calcium ion, but only at 2–3 times the molar concentration required of calcium.[98] In these artificial systems, magnesium may be "accidentally" getting caught in a regulatory mechanism intended for use only by calcium. There is no evidence that magnesium is a physiologic regulator of PTH secretion, or conversely that PTH controls magnesium balance.

It has been thought in the past that PTH secretion was a linear function of the serum calcium, i.e., that the parathyroid cell would always respond identically to a given absolute change in the calcium ion concentration, regardless of the prevailing serum calcium around which the change took place. This concept is incorrect. As we can see in Fig. 1,[2,99] secretion rate is a sigmoid function of the calcium level; this is much more suitable than a linear function for keeping the serum calcium within normal range. Between 9 and 11 mg/dl, PTH secretion changes only slightly with a change in serum calcium, indicating that the system maintains a rather casual attitude toward fluctuations within the normal range. Secretion increases very sharply, however, as soon as the calcium level falls below normal. Hormone secretion reaches a maximum and levels off at a serum calcium level between 6 and 7 mg/dl; note that this is the level that a normal subject can maintain without PTH, purely on the basis of blood–bone equilibration.

Observe further in Fig. 1 that PTH secretion also levels off at a plasma calcium above 11 mg/dl, and it never reaches zero. Normal para-

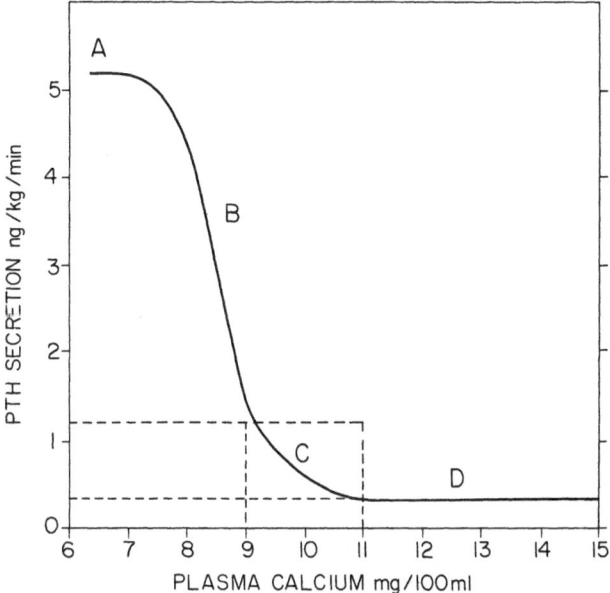

Fig. 1. PTH secretion as a function of total blood calcium concentration. (Reproduced from Habener.[2])

thyroid glands *in vivo* maintain a certain degree of continuous secretion that will not be suppressed by calcium, even at very high concentrations.[100] Habener[2] suggested that this nonsuppressible component may be responsible for hyperparathyroid hypercalcemia: hypercalcemia would simply result from a much-increased number of cells, each one suppressed, but continuing to secrete the nonsuppressible quantity of hormone. Although this theory seems to us inadequate, since a quite small mass of abnormal tissue can produce hypercalcemia, it certainly remains to be disproved.

The nonsuppressible component of secretion is very likely maintained by physiologic β-adrenergic stimulation,[101] probably from circulating catecholamines. A number of recent *in vivo* and *in vitro* studies using both β-adrenergic agonists and antagonists clearly indicate that β activity not only stimulates secretion, but is also necessary for the full secretory response to acute hypocalcemia.[102–105]

4.1.5.1. Why Do Parathyroid Cells React to Calcium?

Parathyroid cells are a most unusual sort. They sense and respond to changes in the extracellular calcium level that other cells don't even notice; and they seem to be "turned on" to secrete by a decrease, rather than an increase, in their intracellular free calcium.

Most types of secretory cells require an increase in intracellular free calcium for secretion to occur. We can imagine that a similar requirement for parathyroid cells might interfere with their ability to respond to a drop in the extracellular calcium. It is interesting that most PTH may be secreted directly from the cell without prior packaging into secretory granules[7]; perhaps for this reason, secretion is not dependent on microtubules, as Chertow et al.[94] showed. Going out on a limb, we suggest that parathyroid cells, in contrast to other secretory cells, may not need calcium ions for secretion because they do not need calcium-dependent microtubule formations.

As we mentioned in the introduction, most cells carefully maintain their intracellular free calcium at a level orders of magnitude lower than the extracellular concentration. Excess calcium that enters the cell down its concentration gradient is rapidly removed from the cytoplasm by intracellular organelles (mitochondria, sarcoplasmic reticulum) and outward calcium pumps in the plasma membrane. We find it intriguing that parathyroid chief cells—the cells that secrete hormone—have a very small number of mitochondria. Might these cells be sensitive to the extracellular free calcium concentration because, when it is high, they haven't the capacity to rapidly sequester the increased calcium that enters the cell, and when the extracellular calcium is low, they haven't enough stored intramitochondrial calcium to release to the cytoplasm? Thus, in parathyroid cells, the intracellular free calcium might change instantaneously in parallel with the extracellular free calcium, whereas other cells, with more mitochondria, could hold their intracellular calcium steady.

Besides active chief cells, parathyroid glands contain a quiet, nonsecretory cell type, the oxyphil cell. Oxyphil cells have many mitochondria. Boquist[106] showed that chief cells appear to transform into oxyphil cells when gland tissue is incubated in a high-calcium medium. This suggests to us that exposure to a high-calcium concentration may induce multiplication of the mitochondria in the chief cell. As the number of mitochondria increased, the cell would develop the same ability to control its intracellular free calcium that nonparathyroid cells have, and it would no longer be responsive to changes in the extracellular calcium; eventually it would become a nonsecreting oxyphil cell.

4.1.5.2. Is Hyperparathyroidism a Primary Mitochondrial Disease?

We propose the following theory in the spirit of intellectual sport: If mitochondria do in fact control the response of the parathyroid cell to calcium, we can imagine that an abnormality of these complex organelles might interfere with the normal reactions of the cell. Suppose that the parathyroid cell contained either too many mitochondria, or mitochondria abnormally avid for calcium: these organelles could lower the intracellular/extracellular calcium ratio below that existing in a normal parathyroid cell at the same extracellular calcium level. Thus, whatever cell structure it is that (we postulate) senses and responds to intracellular free calcium would "see" hypocalcemia, where none, in fact, existed, and would increase hormone production. When hypercalcemia had, in turn, been produced and more calcium was entering the cell, the intracellular free calcium could reach the usual "normal" level, and hormone overproduction would cease, but the serum calcium would then be regulated around a higher level, as is seen in stable hyperparathyroidism.

Nothing is known about the multiplication of parathyroid cells, except that it can be induced by low extracellular calcium. If the signal for division were actually low *intracellular* calcium, our theoretical cells with the numerous or hungry mitochondria would not only secrete too much hormone, but also multiply.

This theory is armchair speculation, pure and pleasant, without support other than the observation of Thliveris and Dube[107] that hyperplastic parathyroid chief cells have an abnormally large number of mitochondria. Still, we think that further electron-microscopic studies of normal and abnormal glands and studies of calcium flux in parathyroid cells might yield some interesting results.

4.1.6. Hyperparathyroidism

4.1.6.1. Pathology of Classic Hyperparathyroidism

Hyperparathyroidism may result from a single tumor or from hyperplasia of all four glands; a small intermediate group of patients has mild generalized parathyroid hyperplasia with more than one adenoma. In a recent large series spanning 43 years, the incidence of tumor vs. hyperplasia remained constant at about 85/15, the tumors comprising 81% adenomas and 4% carcinomas.[108]

It is interesting and definite that patients with hyperparathyroidism have an abnormally high incidence of thyroid pathology, including malignancies of all kinds. LiVolsi and Feind[109] reported an 11.4% incidence of non-medullary thyroid carcinoma in 272 consecutive cases of parathyroid adenoma. Petro and Hardy[110] reported a 9% incidence in 56 hyperparathyroid patients, and they stressed the importance of biopsying thyroid nodules discovered during parathyroidectomy. Unfortunately, multinodular goiter is also very common in these patients, so that adequate biopsy may be very difficult.

We have recently recognized the development of thyroid and other head and neck tumors as an unfortunate sequela of neck irradiation in childhood. Distressingly, it now seems that hyperparathyroidism may be similarly induced.[111,112] In a recent series of 69 consecutive patients with surgically proved hyperparathyroidism, 20 had a history of radiation to the head and neck at some age.[112]

4.1.6.2. Clinical Presentation and Diagnosis

4.1.6.2a. Presentation. All the signs and symptoms of hyperparathyroidism result from either bone disease or hypercalcemia. Unfortunately, the patient is almost never aware of hyperparathyroid bone disease, except for drastically severe osteitis fibrosa, unless a pathologic fracture or large bone cyst intrudes. And although serum calcium presumably rises slowly over years in most cases,[52] most patients feel fine until the serum calcium rises above 12. Even then, despite careful questioning, many patients will steadfastly deny all the classic vague GI, urinary, neuromuscular, and mental symptoms of hypercalcemia; only after surgery do they suddenly become aware that they were always thirsty, or tired, or forgetful, or never felt hungry, before.

A recent study compared 68 hyperparathyroid patients detected by routine biochemical screening with 68 normocalcemic controls; only renal calculi, constipation, and mental blunting (i.e., forgetfulness, slowing of thought) were more common in the patients. Gastritis or ulcer, hypertension, polyuria, and weakness were not more common.[113]

The existence of the entity called *normocalcemic hyperparathyroidism* is disputed. Can a primary excess of PTH, while exerting the usual effects on all the hormone receptors, fail to raise the serum calcium? No: such "normocalcemic" patients have an elevated serum calcium, but it simply remains within the "normal range." These patients maintain an average serum calcium, on repeated testing, at the upper limit of normal; normal subjects do not do this. Muldowney *et al.*[114] also found that every one of a series of these patients had abnormally high PTH and ionized calcium levels, although their total calcium values were within normal limits. In the author's experience (C.R.K.), if such patients come to surgery their serum calcium always falls postoperatively, and once they have reequilibrated, they maintain serum calcium at significantly lower than preoperative values.

There may be, however, a group of truly normocalcemic hyperparathyroid patients hidden under the label of *idiopathic hypercalciuria with recurrent nephrolithiasis.*[115] These patients seem to absorb dietary calcium avidly and lose most of it in the urine. We speculate that some of them may have kidneys that do not respond to the calcium-retaining effect of PTH. These patients would maintain normocalcemia in the face of a large urinary calcium drain by increasing PTH secretion, thereby increasing their absorption of dietary calcium. It is not surprising that parathyroidectomy may fail to cure many of these patients of their nephrolithiasis.[115]

Hyperparathyroidism in pregnancy or in infancy is dangerous, but it is rare and therefore often not diagnosed immediately. Pedersen and Permin[116] reviewed the literature on hyperparathyroidism in pregnancy; they conclude that pregnancy may exacerbate hyperparathyroidism and that the disease is associated with a much-increased incidence of spontaneous abortion, perinatal and neonatal death, and premature birth. Hyperparathyroidism should be considered in a pregnant patient with a history of unsuccessful pregnancies, renal calculi, or hyperemesis gravidarum, and it should be surgically corrected as early in the pregnancy as is safe.

Neonatal hyperparathyroidism is rare and extremely serious. There are two forms, one secondary to maternal hypoparathyroidism, the other familial with autosomal dominant inheritance. In both forms, the babies look the same at birth, with poor suck and feeding, hypotonia, severe bone demineralization on X ray, and even multiple fractures, and both forms require prompt diagnosis and surgery; at least 50% of the reported cases died before surgery could be performed. All have chief cell hyperplasia, and three and one-half glands should be removed.

In a fascinating family reported by Spiegel et al.,[117] 15 of 31 family members, including 5 children under 6, had definite hypercalcemia, and 5 others had serum calcium at the upper limit of normal. Serum phosphate levels in the 15 hypercalcemic subjects were low normal or low. Extensive evaluation of this family failed to turn up evidence of multiple endocrine neoplasia, although 3 members had Hashimoto's thyroiditis.

4.1.6.2b. Diagnosis. The quality of diagnostic PTH assays is steadily improving. The C-terminal assay, which detects intact hormone and C-terminal fragments, has the greatest discrimination of the commonly used assays; it is the current choice for diagnosis, though we can foresee its replacement by Christensen's intact hormone assay (see Section 4.1.2). Most clinical laboratories now supply not only an isolated absolute PTH value, but also a graph of PTH values against serum calcium for their own assay; the graph identifies patients whose PTH values may be inappropriately high, though still within the "normal" range.

The myriad older, indirect tests of parathyroid activity are out of favor today, but almost all of them, if carefully performed, can provide support for the diagnosis in a questionable case. Drezner et al.[118] developed a simple test that discriminated with 100% accuracy between normal, hyperparathyroid, nonparathyroid hypercalcemic, and hypoparathyroid subjects in their series. These authors took the well-known, but not overly sensitive, total urinary cAMP value and subtracted the amount calculated to represent cAMP filtered from the plasma; the resulting "renal cAMP" value was a completely accurate reflection of PTH activity. If the discrimination of this measurement holds true in further studies, it could be used interchangeably with the PTH assay.

4.1.6.3. Surgery

Before the advent of mass screening, almost every hyperparathyroid patient was operated on when the diagnosis was made, even if the disease seemed mild. We now detect so many more "asymptomatic" patients that the question of when surgery is indicated has arisen. All who have seen and followed many hyperparathyroid patients know of cases in which an untreated patient has lived for years without evidence of skeletal or soft tissue disease and without recognized symptoms. Nevertheless, the author (C.R.K.) still feels that almost all patients should have surgery at the time of diagnosis: because the patients are often unaware of subtle symptoms before surgery but recognize marked improvement afterward; because untreated patients may gradually develop subtle renal impairment or hypertension and risk renal stones or pancreatitis[119]; and because over 90% can be completely cured by a single operation.

Once the decision for surgery is made, it is absolutely necessary that a surgeon specifically experienced in parathyroid surgery be consulted. A general, head and neck, or even thyroid surgeon without specific knowledge of parathyroid surgery is not adequate. Size, shape, color, number, location, and circulation of normal and abnormal parathyroid glands vary enormously[120] (Fig. 2). Three, five, or six glands may be present, rather than four. Most upper glands are in the cricothyroid junction, but they may be found behind the thyroid, behind the esophagus, or within the

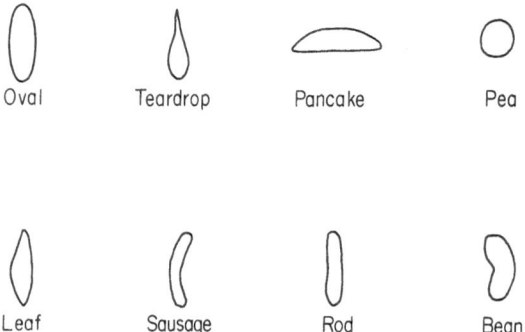

Fig. 2. A child's garden of parathyroid glands: normal variations in gland shape. (Reproduced from Wang.[120])

thyroid.[121] Lower glands wander farther, about half developing adjacent to the thyroid, but *40%* in Wang's series[120] being found within the thymus. The occasional development of a parathyroid gland low in the anterior mediastinum is a well-known cause of the failure of "first-look" surgery for hyperparathyroidism, and Rothmund et al.[122] advocate an inch-by-inch sternotomy and mediastinal exploration during the original operation if neither proved hyperplasia nor tumor has been found after meticulous neck exploration.

Currently accepted surgical practice calls for removal of either the adenoma, or three and one-half hyperplastic glands, without resection of any normal gland tissue. Unfortunately, the differentiation at surgery between normal, hyperplastic, and adenomatous glands may be difficult or impossible, even by frozen section. Roth and Gallagher[123] have made an important contribution to the success of future parathyroid surgery by developing a staining technique that renders their interpretation of frozen-section biopsy virtually infallible. When parathyroid tissue is stained with Sudan, suppressed normal tissue shows prominent intracellular fat droplets, while hyperplastic cells have no intracellular fat.* Using this method for tissue diagnosis, an adequate exploration for an adenoma could comprise simply finding the adenoma itself plus one biopsy-proved normal gland.

Adequate surgery for parathyroid hyperplasia, or multiple adenomas on a background of mild hyperplasia, requires greater skill, meticulous technique, and difficult decisions if both surgical failure and complications are to be avoided. We quote Mason et al.[124]:

> No parathyroid tissue should be removed until an estimated 50 mg of the gland that appears most normal, well-vascularized and accessible has been selected, marked and established as the patient's probable lifetime solitary source of parathyroid hormone. To remove three or even two normal parathyroid glands from the neck during exploration and before all glands have been located is a frequent temptation, particularly during a prolonged, frustrating search. This temptation must be resisted if the development of hypoparathyroidism is to be prevented in some of those patients who present the more difficult diagnostic and therapeutic problems.

Autotransplantation of some hyperplastic parathyroid tissue to an intramuscular site at the time of surgery has been much discussed recently[125-128] and even recommended as a routine procedure.[126] Although transplanted parathyroid tissue clearly functions and may be able to support normal calcium homeostasis,[127, 128] we can see no advantage to the procedure. Once a definite diagnosis of hyperplasia is made

---

*The striking appearance of the stained sections is demonstrated in Roth and Gallagher's original paper.[123]

and three and one-half glands resected, a clip can be placed to mark the location of the remaining half-gland in case more tissue must later be removed; however, a second operation is rarely needed.

4.1.6.4. Preoperative Localization of Pathological Glands

When parathyroid surgery is meticulously performed by an experienced surgeon, the cure rate for first-look cervical exploration should be well over 90%.[129] Numerous papers continue to appear on the use of techniques to locate pathological glands prior to surgery; the methods include ultrasound, radioisotope scans,[130,131] thermography,[132] angiography,[133-135] and sampling from veins draining the parathyroids with RIA for PTH.[134,136] Unfortunately, these techniques reliably detect only those glands that are large enough to be easily found by the surgeon without prior knowledge of their whereabouts. The more sensitive techniques— venous sampling and arteriography—are also difficult, invasive, and costly. At present, therefore, use of these techniques is indicated only when a painstaking and thorough first operation has failed. Under these circumstances, selective arteriography followed by venous sampling will probably give the best results.[134]

Doppman *et al.*[137] recently reported the attempted embolic infarction of ectopic glands located by arteriography in three patients after unsuccessful surgery. Two mediastinal adenomas were infarcted, one with apparent cure of the patient. This technique, if further developed, could cure selected patients without a difficult second-look operation.

4.1.6.5. Renal Osteodystrophy

In the course of chronic renal failure, secondary hyperparathyroidism develops very early—when GFR has fallen by only 20-30%. The biochemical pattern in these mildly diseased patients closely resembles that of vitamin D deficiency: barely normal to low serum calcium, mild hypophosphatemia, reduced renal clearance of calcium and increased clearance of phosphate, and a blunted bone response to PTH; impaired intestinal absorption of calcium is common.

Hypophosphatemia in these patients casts doubt on the theory that primary phosphate retention leading to hypocalcemia is the stimulus to parathyroid overactivity. Casting yet more, Massry *et al.*[138] have now shown that patients with early renal failure given phosphate infusions actually reach a *lower,* not a higher, serum phosphate level than do control subjects; i.e., they dispose of serum phosphate more, not less, efficiently than normal.

There is very good evidence that the early hyperparathyroidism of renal failure is secondary to active vitamin D deficiency.[139] The 1α-hydroxylase enzyme in the renal tubular cells is a very sensitive one, its activity readily disrupted,[139] so that loss of 1α-hydroxylating ability does not parallel, but far outstrips, the loss of functioning kidney mass; thus, the patient with early renal failure may be deficient in 1,25-OH$_2$D$_3$ despite an adequate intake of inactive D precursors. Although Slatopolsky and DeLuca[140] measured "normal" levels of 1,25-OH$_2$D$_3$ in these patients, "normal" levels are inappropriate in subjects who are hypocalcemic, hypophosphatemic, and hyperparathyroid; such a biochemical milieu should induce *high* levels of 1,25-OH$_2$D$_3$ if vitamin D metabolism is normal.

4.1.7. Hypoparathyroidism

New insight into the workings of PTH has produced a better pathophysiological classification of the hypoparathyroid states and a better treatment.

Table I, modified from the recent review of Nusynowitz *et al.*,[141] contains a classification of the myriad hypoparathyroid states that have been observed clinically. If we consider all the known steps in PTH synthesis, secretion, receptor binding, and target cell activation, we can postulate all sorts of specific defects that could lead to hypoparathyroidism and that will undoubtedly be described in the future, as we learn how to find them.

4.1.7.1. Postsurgical Hypoparathyroidism

This disorder may be very subtle. Some patients can produce enough hormone to maintain an unstressed steady state, but not to meet an acute, marked demand for calcium. When pressed, as by an EDTA infusion or a low-calcium, high-phosphate diet, they will respond with an abnormally severe hypocalcemia, which they will need a long time to reverse when the stress is removed.[142] These patients may turn up months after surgery complaining of fatigue, vague GI symptoms, perhaps mild extremity cramps, with serum calcium near the low, and phosphate near the high, borderline of normal. In the past, we have not been able to diagnose postsurgical hypoparathyroidism by the serum PTH level, because PTH assays have been so insensitive as to detect no hormone even in many normal subjects. However, the new intact hormone assay of Christensen[13] (see Section 4.1.2) is sensitive enough to separate normal and hypoparathyroid subjects, so that in the near future we should be able to dispense

Table I. A Classification of the Hypoparathyroid States[a]

I. Hormone-deficiency hypoparathyroidism
   A. Iatrogenic
      1. Postoperative: thyroid, parathyroid, or radical neck surgery
      2. Postirradiation: [131]I
   B. Absence, damage, or insufficiency of glands
      1. Idiopathic hypoparathyroidism
         a. Familial
            1. Sex-linked
            2. Heredofamilial, ?transmission
         b. Sporadic (?autoimmune): isolated or associated with Addison's disease, pernicious anemia, or moniliasis
      2. Branchial dysembryogenesis—DiGeorge syndrome
      3. Replacement: hemochromatosis, invasive metastatic cancer, or amyloid
      4. Inadequate hormone synthesis: neonatal hypoparathyroidism
   C. Suppression of secretion
      1. Neonatal, from maternal hypercalcemia
      2. Physiological, from nonparathyroid hypercalcemia
      3. Post-resection of parathyroid adenoma
      4. Magnesium deficiency (severe)
II. Hormone-resistance hypoparathyroidism
   A. Hereditary
      1. Pseudohypoparathyroidism, type 1: defect in cAMP generation in response to PTH
         a. Complete osteocytic, osteoclastic, and renal tubular resistance, with Albright's Hereditary osteodystrophy (AHO)
         b. Subnormal osteocytic, osteoclastic, and renal tubular responsiveness, with AHO
         c. Osteocytic and renal resistance; osteoclastic responsiveness:
            1. with AHO ("pseudohypohyperparathyroidism," "pseudohypoparathyroidism with osteitis fibrosa")
            2. without AHO ("hypohyperparathyroidism," "pseudohypoparathyroidism with osteitis fibrosa")
         d. Osteocytic and osteoclastic resistance; renal responsiveness:
            1. with AHO
            2. without AHO
      2. Pseudohypoparathyroidism, type II: defect in intracellular response to cAMP
   B. Acquired
      1. 1,25-Dihydroxycholecalciferol (active vitamin D) deficiency
         a. Deficient vitamin D ingestion
         b. Deficient vitamin D absorption
         c. Renal osteodystrophy
         d. Liver disease (25-hydroxylase deficiency)
         e. Chronic anticonvulsant therapy (hydantoins or barbiturates; disrupt 25-hydroxylase activity)
      2. Magnesium deficiency
      3. Osteosclerosis and osteopetrosis
      4. Pseudoidiopathic hypoparathyroidism
      5. PTH antagonists
         a. Phosphates, diphosophonates, and analogues
         b. Corticosteroids
      6. Hypothyroidism

[a]Modified from Nusynowitz *et al.*[141]

with the cumbersome indirect stress tests through which diagnosis has previously been attempted.

4.1.7.2. Hormone-Resistant Hypoparathyroidism

In all the hormone-resistant states, both congenital and acquired, hypocalcemia occurs and the parathyroid glands pour out hormone in an ineffective response. In the classic pseudohypoparathyroidism described by Albright (II, A, 1, a in Table I), all the PTH receptor cells are unresponsive to the hormone, so that despite high hormone levels, no bone mineral removal, no osteoclastic skeletal remodeling, no phosphate excretion, and no calcium reabsorption is stimulated. In most of the hormone-resistant states, however, only some types of target cells are resistant; the responsive cells then have to contend with very high hormone levels, and the result is a "paradoxical" picture of hypoparathyroidism and hyperparathyroidism combined. Naming these states for their mixed clinical appearance has resulted in such apparent absurdities as "pseudohypohyperparathyroidism" (II, A, 1, c in Table I). A common combination is resistant osteocytes and responsive osteoclasts; this dissociation occurs in renal osteodystrophy and some of the congenital states. Normal serum calcium cannot be maintained, but the heavy overstimulation of osteoclasts can eventually lead to osteitis fibrosa.

Classic pseudohypoparathyroidism comprises both hormone resistance and the conjunction of short stature, round face, and foreshortened metacarpals (often accompanied by mental retardation) that has been termed *Albright's hereditary osteodystrophy* (AHO).[143] We now know that AHO and hormone resistance may be inherited independently; "pseudopseudohypoparathyroidism" is not hypoparathyroidism at all, but simply AHO inherited alone.

4.1.7.2a. Magnesium Deficiency. PTH does not seem to control, or even affect, magnesium homeostasis. Hyper- and hypoparathyroidism have no effect on magnesium balance, unless either marked hypercalciuria or hypercalcemic renal injury intervenes and prevents normal magnesium reabsorption. Nevertheless, it is well known that acute magnesium deficiency, like acute calcium deficiency, stimulates PTH secretion in all species. In the rat, chronic magnesium deficiency continues to stimulate PTH secretion and its target cell response,[144] and the rat develops hypercalcemia, increased calcium absorption, and widespread metastatic calcifications, all preventable or reversible by parathyroidectomy.

Humans (and dogs and chickens), however, do not respond this way. In man, chronic magnesium deficiency produces a combined state of

PTH deficiency and PTH resistance. Both these derangements have now been amply documented; past arguments in the literature, debating the existence of one or the other, can be ascribed to faults in interpretation and experimental method.*

Magnesium deficiency inhibits the response of the parathyroid glands to hypocalcemia, and the calcium-suppressible component of secretion can be suppressed by quite a low concentration of calcium.[145,146] Acute release of hormone always follows magnesium infusion.

All target cells become resistant to PTH in experimental magnesium deficiency. The renal responses may be interfered with in variable degree. Bone seems to become resistant, not only to PTH, but also to doses of vitamin D sufficient to treat hormone-deficiency hypoparathyroidism.[147] Magnesium deficiency may alter the structure of the bone mineral, making it less soluble and resistant to breakdown and turnover. Experimental magnesium deficiency actually produces osteopetrosis in the chick.[148]

4.1.7.3. Treatment

The recent successful treatment of hypoparathyroidism[58-60] and one case of pseudohypoparathyroidism[58] with $1,25\text{-}OH_2D_3$ or its analogue $1\alpha\text{-}OHD_3$ has shown us that the supposed "resistance" of the hypoparathyroid to vitamin D is due to impaired 1α-hydroxylase activity. In hypoparathyroidism, this enzyme not only remains unstimulated by PTH, but is also suppressed by high serum phosphate. Hypoparathyroid patients will respond to physiologic doses of active D, the same doses as are needed to prevent rickets.

Once we seek to distinguish them, we will probably find, along the spectrum of pseudohypoparathyroid states, some patients with and some without a 1α-hydroxylase system responsive to PTH.

4.1.7.4. Pancreatitis

In a recent study, 7 of 8 patients with acute pancreatitis with hypocalcemia had only normal serum PTH levels, rather than the high levels that would have been predicted.[149] Since neither calcitonin nor glucagon

---

*Some of those who measured "normal" PTH levels in these patients failed to recognize that a "normal" hormone level, in the face of hypocalcemia and hyperphosphatemia, is not, in fact, normal: it indicates both deficient secretion—since PTH should be high if calcium is low—and deficient responsiveness—since a normal amount of PTH should produce normal serum calcium and phosphate levels. In addition, some of the experiments purporting to demonstrate "normal" responsiveness to exogenous PTH used massive bolus doses of hormone, large enough to overcome nearly any degree of hormone resistance less than total.

seemed to be responsible for the hypocalcemia, and since there is no evidence that normal glands cannot sustain high rates of secretion when the demand is great, it appears that something in the blood in acute pancreatitis interferes with PTH synthesis or secretion. We have no idea what the interfering element could be. Nor do we know whether PTH target cells are fully responsive in pancreatitis; although the investigators cited observed rising ionized calcium and urinary cAMP in response to administered hormone, they used massive doses to obtain these effects.

4.1.8. Interaction of Parathyroid Hormone with Other Hormones

4.1.8.1. Thyroid Hormone

Thyroid hormone in excess greatly speeds the rate and quantity of normal skeletal remodeling. Osteoporosis (usually asymptomatic) develops in hyperthyroidism because the small net bone loss that normally occurs in the adult with each remodeling cycle—a slightly greater amount of bone resorbed than reformed—is multiplied by a much larger than normal number of cycles.[17] The hyperactive bone remodeling removes a large amount of calcium from the skeleton to the ECF. As a result, all hyperthyroid patients have a heavy urinary calcium load, and many— 47% in a recent series[150]—have mild to marked hypercalcemia. The hypercalcemia is always accompanied by high-normal or minimally elevated serum phosphate, which is not due to hypercalcemic renal injury. It is clear now that hyperthyroid hypercalcemia is not produced by PTH, but suppresses PTH secretion, so that circulating levels of PTH are low or undetectable.[13,150,151]

In contrast, hypothyroidism is characterized by sluggish skeletal remodeling and metabolically torpid bone that neither gives up nor accepts calcium readily. As a rule, serum calcium is barely normal, and ionized calcium is low; PTH levels, in response, are high, but cannot induce normal mineral removal from bone. These quantities of PTH do, however, enhance dietary calcium absorption, and since the hypothyroid skeleton cannot buffer a calcium load as normal bones will, a high-calcium meal can produce frank hypercalcemia in these patients.

Castro et al.[152] demonstrated that the skeletal and renal responses (measured as change in serum calcium and phosphate) to large doses of PTH are enhanced in hyperthyroidism and depressed in hypothyroidism. We can perhaps explain the differences in skeletal response by comparing the metabolic activity of the hyperthyroid and hypothyroid bones. Since rapidly remodeling hyperthyroid bone will be "young," with a high water content, more labile mineral, and greater vascularity, one might expect that the bone cells, in response to a given dose of PTH, would readily be able to dissolve a large amount of bone mineral, whereas in hypothyroidism, the cells, even if activated to the same degree, might be unable to dissolve much mineral from the dense, "locked-in" crystals of the hypothyroid bone. This difference in the availability of bone mineral probably explains why hyperthyroid patients, despite low steady-state PTH levels, recover rapidly from EDTA-induced hypocalcemia, while hypothyroid patients recover slowly despite high PTH levels.

4.1.8.2. Growth Hormone and Somatostatin

The effects of growth hormone (GH) on the kidney are the opposite of those of PTH, and GH will antagonize the efforts of administered or endogenous PTH at the renal level. The effects of GH on the bone, however, mimic those of PTH, with increased bone turnover and a resultant tendency to hypercalcemia. In the past, it has not been clear whether GH stimulated parathyroid cells or produced its bony effects directly. Lancer et al.[153] have now followed circulating PTH in rats receiving GH for several weeks: PTH levels rose progressively, and hypercalcemia developed. The parathyroid glands of these animals were slightly heavier than those of controls.

Extrapolated to acromegaly, these findings suggest that a kind of hyperparathyroidism produces hypercalcemia in this disease. The antagonistic effect of GH on the kidney would blunt the biochemical manifestations of hyperparathyroidism—the hypercalcemia and hypophosphatemia—but might paradoxically aggravate bone disease: acromegalic patients would never reach the steady state characteristic of "stable" hyperparathyroidism, but would drain off bone mineral continuously.

Lancer's findings may not be applicable to humans. Aloia et al.[154] found PTH increased in only 1 of 6 acromegalic patients. Their findings have not, to our knowledge, been confirmed.

Somatostatin, which suppresses the secretion of many other hormones, failed in a recent study to suppress PTH secretion.[155]

4.1.8.3. Glucocorticoids

Glucocorticoid deficiency may produce hypercalcemia, associated with an enhanced hypercalcemic response to PTH. Conversely, glucocorticoids in acute or chronic excess tend to lower serum calcium and oppose the hypercalcemic effect of PTH. Glucocorticoids lower serum calcium by a direct effect on bone, which somehow makes PTH less effective. Two recent publications[156,157] described serum calcium and PTH measurements in patients on long-term prednisone therapy (15–80 mg/day) and in normal men given 200 mg cortisol in a 4-hr infusion. Serum calcium was normal and PTH significantly elevated in all subjects, indicating that glucocorticoid excess causes a state of secondary hyperparathyroidism. Although we cannot describe the hypocalcemic effect of glucocorticoids at the tissue level, we would suspect that only mineral removal, and not osteoclastic remodeling, is depressed; thus, the bone loss induced in humans by excess glucocorticoids could be due to PTH-stimulated remodeling.

Au[158] showed that cortisol stimulates hormone secretion by rat parathyroid glands in tissue culture, so the hyperparathyroidism of glucocorticoid excess may be primary as well as secondary.

4.1.9. Hypercalcemia of Malignancy

The incidence of ectopic "hyperparathyroidism" as a cause of hypercalcemia in cancer is very much open to question. The frequency with which elevated levels of circulating "PTH" are found in hypercalcemic cancer patients varies enormously from laboratory to laboratory,[159] and some even measure high levels in many normocalcemic cancer patients. The latter finding suggests that many tumors may produce a peptide immunologically similar to normal PTH, but with enough differences that most antisera do not detect it. Although there is no way to prove, without isolating it, that such a peptide is active or even that it really exists, we feel that the weight of evidence speaks against the secretion of an active ectopic PTH by more than a very small number of tumors.[13,160] These few, however, indubitably exist.[161,162]

4.2. Calcitonin

4.2.1. Introduction

The existence of the hypocalcemic substance later shown to be calcitonin was first disclosed when Copp[163] produced acute, marked hypocalcemia in dogs by perfusing the thyroid *in vivo* with hypercalcemic blood; thyroparathyroidectomy produced a much more gentle fall in the serum calcium. Almost simultaneously, Hirsch *et al.*[164] serendipitously produced the same acute hypocalcemia by damaging the thyroid gland in the course of parathyroidectomy by cautery. These experiments showed that a hypocalcemic substance existed and that it came from the thyroid, not the parathyroid glands. Within seven years, calcitonin had been isolated from

parafollicular cells and from the ultimobranchial body in lower vertebrates and had been completely characterized and synthesized in the
laboratory.[165]

Calcitonin is a hormone that may be of great physiological import in
fish—which have to contend with a very high-calcium environment—but
it has yet to prove itself in most mammals. Although it is active, there is no
evidence that it is necessary. Of all mammals studied, only the rat seems to
need calcitonin to control its serum calcium: after removal of the parafollicular cells, the rat cannot keep serum calcium down to normal, either
immediately postoperation or when faced with a calcium load.[166,167] In
man, neither thyroidectomy, with removal of the parafollicular cells, nor
medullary carcinoma, with soaring calcitonin levels, has any effect on
calcium homeostasis or the state of the bones. In man as in all mammals,
fish calcitonins are much more potent than are their own endogenous
mammalian hormones. We believe that there is almost enough evidence to
permit labeling human calcitonin a vestigial hormone.

4.2.2. Hormone Synthesis and Secretion

In last year's volume of this series, Avioli[168] discussed the assay,
structure, and synthesis of calcitonin in detail; we have nothing new to add
this year, so our discussion will be confined largely to secretion.

The RIA of calcitonin in human serum seems to be as complicated as
that of PTH, what with marked differences in hormone structure from
species to species, heterogeneity of circulating calcitonin, variable affinity
of different antisera for different parts of the hormone, and nonspecific
interference by plasma proteins in the final assay.[168] Hence, there is no
agreement on the normal range or even the normal detectability of
calcitonin in human serum. Because calcitonin cannot be reliably detected
in normal subjects, most studies of hormone secretion in man are performed in patients with calcitonin-secreting medullary carcinoma of the
thyroid.

In contrast to parathyroid cells, which never store much hormone but
contain the most when demand is high, mammalian parafollicular cells
store large quantities of hormone and grow larger when the hormone is
not needed, i.e., during sustained hypocalcemia.[169] In response to hypercalcemia or to GI hormones—gastrin, pentagastrin, glucagon, secretin,
and cholecystokinin[170]—calcitonin is secreted in bursts.[168] Rapid infusions
of calcium and pentagastrin are therefore used to diagnose latent medullary carcinoma of the thyroid.[171] The purpose of calcitonin release by GI
hormones seems to be the prevention of postprandial hypercalcemia,[69]
and in the rats, feeding *per se* will induce calcitonin release; i.e., hypercalcemia need not occur to stimulate the parafollicular cells.[172] Continuous

calcitonin secretion is probably regulated by an interplay of the plasma calcium and circulating GI hormones.[168] Conversely, calcitonin, with an as yet undefined purpose, feeds back to inhibit either the release, or the "hypercalcitoninemic" effect, of the GI hormones.[173]

In animals, both calcium and magnesium will stimulate calcitonin release, but Anast et al.[174] surprisingly found that magnesium infusion consistently decreased plasma calcitonin in patients with medullary carcinoma. Calcium and magnesium may compete for entry into parafollicular cells, and they are probably interchangeable stimulants in normal cells; Anast's work suggests that medullary carcinoma cells are not normal, in that they will not respond to magnesium. Without studies of the effect of magnesium in normal humans, however, we cannot draw such a conclusion.

4.2.3. Physiological Role of Calcitonin in Mammals

We quote Kalu and Foster[69]: "The only two generally accepted roles for calcitonin in mammals are to confer protection against postprandial hypercalcemia and to preserve the integrity of the skeleton during pregnancy and lactation." No new findings dispute this statement, though in the rat—an anomalous mammal, as far as concerns the need for calcitonin—the hormone seems to help with normal mineralization and modeling of fetal and growing bones.[175,176]

The possible role of calcitonin in the physiology of digestion and absorption is not well defined. The interplay of calcitonin and the GI hormones has already been referred to (see Section 4.2.2). In addition to preventing postprandial hypercalcemia, calcitonin induces intestinal secretion of water and electrolytes when it is present at the supernormal levels that may occur in patients with medullary carcinoma. The unexplained diarrhea present in 30% of such patients might be so explained.[173]

Toverud et al.[177] recently showed that calcitonin decreases postprandial hypercalcemia much more effectively in lactating than in nonlactating rats, suggesting a specific physiological effort to salvage all dietary divalent ions during a time of heavy drain on the maternal stores.

We repeat that there is no evidence for a physiologic role of calcitonin in the normal human adult. The human neonatal thyroid, however, has a very high calcitonin content,[178] and plasma calcitonin levels, normal to high at birth, increase to a maximum at about 24 hr of age.[179] Premature infants with hypocalcemia may have particularly high calcitonin levels and may respond to stress with an outpouring of calcitonin.[180] These findings suggest the possibility that calcitonin may promote growth and mineralization in human, as in rat, fetal bone, or may otherwise participate in controlling body fluid calcium in the fetus.

4.2.4. Mechanism of Hormone Action

In pharmacologic doses, calcitonin produces hypocalcemia and hypophosphatemia; it opposes the effect of PTH on bone and enhances its effect on the kidney.

Milhaud *et al.*[181] first pointed to inhibition of mineral release from the skeleton as the *modus operandi* of calcitonin. The hormone has since been shown to suppress osteocyte activity and osteoclast number and activity. In the kidney, calcitonin enhances the excretion of calcium, phosphorus, sodium, chloride, and potassium, as recently reviewed by Katz and Lindheimer.[182] There is no evidence that this effect plays a physiologic role in any mammalian species, though it is possible that hypercalciuria may be thus produced in an occasional patient with medullary carcinoma of the thyroid.[171]

Calcitonin appears to exert all its effects by binding to specific membrane receptors and stimulating a membrane-bound adenylate cyclase.[168,182] Chabardès *et al.*[183] recently located the calcitonin-sensitive adenylate cyclase in the distal convoluted tubule and thick ascending limb of the rabbit nephron. It is interesting that calcitonin, unlike PTH, does not produce a rise in urinary cAMP, even though this nucleotide apparently mediates its effect.[182]

Borle[184] made the fascinating observation that calcitonin greatly stimulates mitochondrial calcium uptake, decreasing intracellular free calcium ion. Our knowledge of cell physiology is insufficient to carry us on into speculation, but we remark again that PTH has the opposite effect on intracellular free calcium ion (see Section 4.1.4).

Kalu and Foster[69] suggested that the original purpose of calcitonin may have been to salvage scarce phosphate for marine animals, and Talmage *et al.*[185] proposed that the hypophosphatemic effect of administered hormone might be due to removal of phosphate from plasma. Meyer and Meyer[186] recently showed that thyrocalcitonin injection increased liver inorganic phosphate in rats. This effect could be advantageous to marine animals and physiological in the rat, but would probably be vestigial in any other mammal in which it was demonstrated.

4.2.5. Multiple Endocrine Neoplasia

We have little new to add to the discussion by Lewis Landsberg[171] in last year's volume. One question that has come up for some discussion of late is the proper handling of the parathyroid glands at the time of thyroidectomy for medullary carcinoma.[187,188] Ideally, one would like to avoid both the removal of normal glands and a difficult later neck exploration for previously latent hyperparathyroidism. Grossly enlarged glands should be removed at surgery[187]; however, we do not yet know enough to predict which normocalcemic patients with grossly normal or hyperplastic glands will later become hyperparathyroid. Heath *et al.,*[188] measuring serum PTH levels after calcium infusion, correctly diagnosed parathyroid hyperplasia before thyroid surgery in 6 of 6 patients with multiple endocrine neoplasia (MEN), type 2A. Their follow-up of such patients should begin to show us the natural history of the parathyroid disease of MEN.

4.2.6. Calcitonin and Renal Failure

Hypocalcemia is a virtually constant concomitant of all renal failure. Since hypocalcemia suppresses calcitonin secretion, it is surprising that elevated calcitonin levels have recently been measured in both acute[189] and chronic[190] renal failure. We have no ready explanation for this finding; Ardaillou *et al.*[189] suggested that a combination of decreased renal clearance of calcitonin, decreased renal clearance of the stimulatory hormones gastrin and glucagon, and the enhanced calcitonin release that these agents will evoke in the presence of hypocalcemia[191] may be responsible.

The patients with end-stage chronic renal failure described by Heynen *et al.*[190] fell into two groups: one with calcitonin levels 6–7 times greater than normal control levels, and one with only minimally elevated values. The group with near-normal calcitonin had very high alkaline phosphatase and PTH levels; in contrast, the group with high calcitonin had near-normal alkaline phosphatase and only slightly elevated PTH levels. We cannot explain why some patients did not raise their calcitonin levels, but Heynen and co-workers suggest that failure to do so may contribute to renal bone disease. Their hypothesis implies a purposeful role for calcitonin in humans, i.e., that of protection against excessive osteoclast stimulation by PTH—though we might expect this "protection" to result in lower serum calcium, as well as less bone disease. The hypothesis of Ardaillou and co-workers, in which high calcitonin is naught but a by-product of renal failure, may well prove to be the true one; however, if calcitonin secretion could be shown to be a protective response to renal failure, that would be the first demonstration of a purpose for human calcitonin.

Whether calcitonin secretion proves to be responsive, or merely incidental, other investigators must try to verify its proposed protective effect in renal bone disease. In the future, we will need to consider whether calcitonin therapy for renal osteodystrophy may be indicated in those patients who fail to raise their own calcitonin levels.

4.2.7. Paget's Disease

Calcitonin can be an effective treatment for the bone pain, neurological abnormalities,[192] or high-output cardiac failure[193] of severe Paget's disease of bone; its use has been endorsed by *The Medical Letter*.[194] The indications for treatment of this usually asymptomatic disease were outlined by Wallach[195]:

1. Disabling pain not relieved by analgesics or antiinflammatory agents.
2. Progression of the skeletal disease: increasing deformity, increasing skull or appendicular bone size, frequent fractures, vertebral compression, acetabular protrusion.
3. Neurologic complications.
4. High-output congestive heart failure.
5. Serum alkaline phosphatase or urinary hydroxyproline excretion increased to 4 or more times above normal in symptomatic patients.

Avramides *et al.*[196] made the interesting observation that for up to 1 year after stopping therapy, 10 of 13 of their formerly calcitonin-treated patients remained asymptomatic and without biochemical evidence of high bone turnover. How long-since metabolized calcitonin might be exerting a long-term effect, we have no idea. The discovery will interest students of bone and calcitonin, but it should not be taken to imply that these patients may not need chronic calcitonin therapy.

A goodly minority of patients will respond poorly or not at all to calcitonin. Diphosphonates may be of great value in relieving symptoms, but their use has not been accepted, because in therapeutic doses they produce a picture of bone demineralization resembling osteomalacia. Now, Hosking *et al.*[197] have found that low-dose synthetic human calcitonin seems to prevent diphosphonate-induced demineralization, and that the combination is effective therapy for Paget's disease. Calcitonin and diphosphonate may have complementary suppressive effects on bone resorption, and may prove together to be a better treatment than calcitonin alone.

4.2.8. Calcitonin as a Tumor Marker

Several peptide hormones are produced by a variety of tumors. Calcitonin is produced by a very large number,[173] of which the most striking seems to be breast cancer. Coombes *et al.*[198] found high plasma calcitonin levels in 23 of 28 patients with metastatic breast cancer and 1 of 13 with localized disease. Calcitonin production by these cancers persisted in monolayer cell cultures maintained for up to 10 weeks. Calcitonin levels may prove useful for staging and following patients with breast cancer.

ACKNOWLEDGMENT

Research for this chapter was supported by the James and Barbara Fleming Fund.

References

1. Carroll, L. (C. L. Dodgson), 1872, *Through the Looking Glass and What Alice Found There,* 1976 Ed., Grossett & Dunlap, New York.
2. Habener, J. F., 1976, New concepts in the formation, regulation of release, and metabolism of parathyroid hormone, in: *Polypeptide Hormones: Molecular and Cellular Aspects,* pp. 197–224, Elsevier/Excerpta Medica, Amsterdam and New York.
3. Habener, J. F., Kemper, B., Potts, J. T., Jr., and Rich, A., 1975, Parathyroid mRNA directs the synthesis of pre-proparathyroid hormone and proparathyroid hormone in the Krebs ascites cell-free system, *Biochem. Biophys. Res. Commun.* **67:**1114–1121.
4. Habener, J. F., Potts, J. T., Jr., and Rich, A., 1976, Pre-proparathyroid hormone, *J. Biol. Chem.* **251:**3893–3899.
5. MacGregor, R. R., Chu, L. L. H., and Cohn, D. V., 1976, Conversion of proparathyroid hormone to parathyroid hormone by a particulate enzyme of the parathyroid gland, *J. Biol. Chem.* **251:**6711–6716.
6. Kemper, B., Habener, J. F., Rich, A., and Potts, J. T., Jr., 1975, Microtubules and the intracellular conversion of proparathyroid hormone to parathyroid hormone, *Endocrinology* **96:**903–912.
7. MacGregor, R. R., Hamilton, J. W., and Cohn, D. V., 1975, The by-pass of tissue hormone stores during the secretion of newly snythesized parathyroid hormone, *Endocrinology* **97:**178–188.
8. Catherwood, B. D., Friedler, R. M., and Singer, F. R., 1976, Sites of clearance of endogenous parathyroid hormone in the vitamin D-deficient dog, *Endocrinology* **98:**228–232.
9. Martin, K., Hruska, K., Greenwalt, A., Klahr, S., and Slatopolsky, E., 1976, Selective uptake of intact parathyroid hormone by the liver. Differences between hepatic and renal uptake, *J. Clin. Invest.* **58:**781–788.
10. McIntosh, C. H. S., and Hesch, R.-D., 1975, Labelled antibody membrane assay for parathyroid hormone. A new approach to the measurement of receptor bound hormone, *Biochem. Biophys. Res. Commun.* **64:**376–383.
11. Berson, S. A., and Yalow, R. S., 1968, Immunochemical heterogeneity of parathyroid hormone in plasma, *J. Clin. Endocrinol. Metab.* **28:**1037–1047.
12. Fischer, J. A., Binswanger, U., and Dietrich, F. M., 1974, Human parathyroid hormone. Immunological characterization of antibodies against a glandular extract and the synthetic amino-terminal fragments 1–12 and 1–34 and their use in the determination of immunoreactive hormone in human sera, *J. Clin. Invest.* **54:**1382–1394.

13. Christensen, M. S., 1976, A sensitive radioimmunoassay of parathyroid hormone in human serum using a specific extraction procedure, *Scand. J. Clin. Lab. Invest.* **36:**313–322.
14. Fujita, T., Okano, K., Ohata, M., and Yoshikawa, M., 1975, A radioimmunoassay for rat serum parathyroid hormone using N-terminal of PTH, *Endocrinol. Jpn.* **22:**159–162.
15. Parfitt, A. M., 1976, The actions of parathyroid hormone on bone: Relation to bone remodeling and turnover, calcium homeostasis, and metabolic bone disease. I. Mechanisms of calcium transfer between blood and bone and their cellular basis: Morphological and kinetic approaches to bone turnover, *Metabolism* **25:**809–844.
16. Parfitt, A. M., 1976, The actions of parathyroid hormone on bone: Relation to bone remodeling and turnover, calcium homeostasis, and metabolic bone disease. II. PTH and bone cells: Bone turnover and plasma calcium regulation, *Metabolism* **25:**909–955.
17. Parfitt, A. M., 1976, The actions of parathyroid hormone on bone: Relation to bone remodeling and turnover, calcium homeostasis, and metabolic bone disease. III. PTH and osteoblasts, the relationship between bone turnover and bone loss, and the state of the bones in primary hyperparathyroidism, *Metabolism* **25:**1033–1069.
18. Parfitt, A. M., 1976, The actions of parathyroid hormone on bone: Relation to bone remodeling and turnover, calcium homeostasis, and metabolic bone disease. IV. The state of the bones in uremic hyperparathyroidism—the mechanisms of skeletal resistance to PTH in renal failure and pseudohypoparathyroidism and the role of PTH in osteoporosis, osteopetrosis, and osteofluorosis, *Metabolism* **25:**1157–1188.
19. Vose, G. P., and Baylink, D. J., 1970, Effect of fibrillar structure of pericanalicular and intercanalicular bone on x-ray absorption, *Anat. Rec.* **166:**239–245.
20. Ramp, W. K., 1975, Cellular control of calcium movements in bone, *Clin. Orthop.* **106:**311–322.
21. Boelkins, J. N., Mazurkiewicz, M., Mazur, P. E., and Mueller, W. J., 1976, Changes in blood flow to bones during hypocalcemic and hypercalcemic phases of the response to parathyroid hormone, *Endocrinology* **98:**403–412.
22. Albright, F., Bauer, W., Cockrill, J. R., and Ellsworth, R., 1931, Studies on the physiology of the parathyroid glands. II. The relation of the serum calcium to the serum phosphorus at different levels of parathyroid activity, *J. Clin. Invest.* **9:**659–677.
23. Talmage, R. V., and Kraintz, F. W., 1954, Progressive changes in renal phosphate and calcium excretion in rats following parathyroidectomy or parathyroid administration, *Proc. Soc. Exp. Biol. Med.* **87:**263–267.
24. Kleeman, C. R., Bernstein, D., Rockney, R., Dowling, J. T., and Maxwell, M. H., 1961, Studies on the renal clearance of diffusible calcium and the role of the parathyroid glands in its regulation, in: *The Parathyroids* (R. O. Greep and R. V. Talmage, eds.), pp. 353–382, Charles C. Thomas, Springfield, Illinois.
25. Massry, S. G., Coburn, J. W., Chapman, L. W., and Kleeman, C. R., 1968, Role of serum Ca, parathyroid hormone and NaCl infusion on renal Ca and Na clearances, *Am. J. Physiol.* **214:**1403–1409.
26. Sutton, R. A. L., Wong, N. L. M., and Dirks, J. H., 1976, Effects of

parathyroid hormone on sodium and calcium transport in the dog nephron, *Clin. Sci. Mol. Med.* **51:**345–351.

27. Chabardès, D., Imbert, M., Clique, A., Montégut, M., and Morel, F., 1975, PTH sensitive adenyl cyclase activity in different segments of the rabbit nephron, *Pfluegers Arch.* **354:**229–239.

28. Brickman, A. S., Massry, S. G., and Coburn, J. W., 1972, Changes in serum and urinary calcium during treatment with hydrochlorothiazide. Studies on mechanisms, *J. Clin. Invest.* **51:**945–954.

29. Parfitt, A. M., 1972, The interactions of thiazide diuretics with parathyroid hormone and vitamin D. Studies in patients with hypoparathryroidism, *J. Clin. Invest.* **51:**1879–1888.

30. Quamme, G. A., Wong, N. L. M., Sutton, R. A. L., and Dirks, J. H., 1975, Interrelationship of chlorothiazide and parathyroid hormone: A micropuncture study, *Am. J. Physiol.* **229:**200–205.

31. Knox, F. G., and Lechene, C., 1975, Distal site of action of parathyroid hormone on phosphate reabsorption, *Am. J. Physiol.* **229:**1556–1560.

32. Beck, L. H., and Goldberg, M., 1974, Mechanism of the blunted phosphaturia in saline-loaded thyroparathyroidectomized dogs, *Kidney Int.* **6:**18–23.

33. Schneider, E. G., Goldsmith, R. S., Arnaud, C. D., and Knox, F. G., 1975, Role of parathyroid hormone in the phosphaturia of extracellular fluid volume expansion, *Kidney Int.* **7:**317–324.

34. Boudry, J.-F., Tröhler, U., Touabi, M., Fleisch, H., and Bonjour, J.-P., 1975, Secretion of inorganic phosphate in the rat nephron, *Clin. Sci. Mol. Med.* **48:**475–489.

35. Tröhler, U., Bonjour, J.-P., and Fleisch, H., 1976, Inorganic phosphate homeostasis. Renal adaptation to the dietary intake in intact and thyroparathyroidectomized rats, *J. Clin. Invest.* **57:**264–273.

36. Bernstein, D., Kleeman, C. R., Rockney, R., Dowling, J. T., and Maxwell, M. H., 1962, Studies on the renal clearance of phosphate and the role of the parathyroid glands in its regulation, *J. Clin. Endocrinol. Metab.* **22:**641–654.

37. Parfitt, A. M., and Frame, B., 1975, Phosphate loading and depletion in vitamin D-treated hypoparathyroidism: Implications for different physiological models of phosphate reabsorption, Paper presented at International Workshop on Phosphate, Paris.

38. Steele, T. H., 1976, Renal resistance to parathyroid hormone during phosphorus deprivation, *J. Clin. Invest.* **58:**1461–1464.

39. Walton, R. J., Smith, R., and Russell, R. G. G., 1976, Effects of diphosphonate (disodium etidronate; EHDP) on phosphate metabolism in Paget's disease of bone, primary hyperparathyroidism and type I hypophosphataemic rickets, *Calcif. Tissue Res.* **21**(Suppl.):339–343.

40. Bijvoet, O. L. M., 1969, Relation of plasma phosphate concentration to renal tubular reabsorption of phosphate, *Clin. Sci.* **37:**23–36.

41. Clark, R. C., Budtz-Olsen, O. E., Cross, R. B., Finnamore, P., and Bauert, P. A., 1973, The importance of the salivary glands in the maintenance of phosphorus homeostasis in the sheep, *Aust. J. Agric. Res.* **24:**913–919.

42. Clark, R. C., French, T. J., Beal, A. M., Cross, R. B., and Budtz-Olsen, O. E., 1975, The acute effects of intravenous infusion of parathyroid hormone on urine plasma and saliva in the sheep, *Q. J. Exp. Physiol.* **60:**95–106.

43. Kleeman, C. R., and Cooke, R. E., 1951, The acute effects of parathyroid hormone on the metabolism of endogenous phosphate, *J. Lab. Clin. Med.* **38:**112–127.

44. Muldowney, F. P., Carroll, D. V., Donohoe, J. F., and Freaney, R., 1971, Correction of renal bicarbonate wastage by parathyroidectomy, *Q. J. Med.* **40**:487–498.

45. Fourman, P., McConkey, B., and Smith, J. W. G., 1960, Defects of water reabsorption and of hydrogen-ion excretion by the renal tubules in hyperparathyroidism, *Lancet* **1**:619–623.

46. Froeling, P. G. A. M., and Bijvoet, O. L. M., 1974, Kidney-mediated effects of parathyroid hormone on extracellular homeostasis of calcium, phosphate and acid-base balance in man, *Neth. J. Med.* **17**:174–183.

47. Beck, N., and Webster, S. K., 1976, Effects of acute metabolic acidosis on parathyroid hormone action and calcium mobilization, *Am. J. Physiol.* **230**:127–131.

48. Reeves, C. D., Palmer, F., Bacchus, H., and Longerbeam, J. K., 1975, Differential diagnosis of hypercalcemia by the chloride/phosphate ratio, *Am. J. Surg.* **130**:166–171.

49. Puschett, J. B., and Zurbach, P., 1976, Acute effects of parathyroid hormone on proximal bicarbonate transport in the dog, *Kidney Int.* **9**:501–510.

50. Jowsey, J., Reiss, E., and Canterbury, J. M., 1974, Long-term effects of high phosphate intake on parathyroid hormone levels and bone metabolism, *Acta Orthop. Scand.* **45**:801–808.

51. Teitelbaum, S. L., Rosenberg, E. M., Richardson, C. A., and Avioli, L. V., 1976, Histological studies of bone from normocalcemic post-menopausal osteoporotic patients with increased circulating parathyroid hormone, *J. Clin. Endocrinol. Metab.* **42**:537–543.

52. Lloyd, H. M., 1968, Primary hyperparathyroidism: An analysis of the role of the parathyroid tumor, *Medicine* **47**:53–71.

53. Parsons, J. A., and Reit, B., 1974, Chronic response of dogs to parathyroid hormone infusion, *Nature (London)* **250**:254–257.

54. Dent, C. E., Jones, P. E., and Mullen, D. P., 1975, Masked primary (or tertiary) hyperparathyroidism, *Lancet* **1**:1161–1169.

55. Rasmussen, H., and Bordier, P., 1974, *The Physiological and Cellular Basis of Metabolic Bone Disease*, Williams & Wilkins Co., Baltimore.

56. Peck, W. A., and Dowling, I., 1976, Failure of 1,25-dihydroxycholecalciferol [1,25-$(OH)_2$-D_3] to modify cyclic AMP levels in parathyroid hormone-treated and untreated bone cells, *Endocr. Res. Commun.* **3**:157–166.

57. Kakuta, S., Suda, T., Sasaki, S., Kimura, N., and Nagata, N., 1975, Effects of parathyroid hormone on the accumulation of cyclic AMP in bone of vitamin D-deficient rats, *Endocrinology* **97**:1288–1293.

58. Kooh, S. W., Fraser, D., DeLuca, H. F., Holick, M. F., Belsey, R. E., Clark, M. B., and Murray, T. M., 1975, Treatment of hypoparathyroidism and pseudohypoparathyroidism with metabolites of vitamin D: Evidence for impaired conversion of 25-hydroxyvitamin D to 1α, 25-dihydroxyvitamin D, *N. Engl. J. Med.* **293**:840–844.

59. Neer, R. M., Holick, M. F., DeLuca, H. F., and Potts, J. T., Jr., 1975, Effects of 1 α-hydroxy-vitamin D_3 and 1,25-dihydroxy-vitamin D_3 on calcium and phosphorus metabolism in hypoparathyroidism, *Metabolism* **24**:1403–1413.

60. Davies, M., Hill, L. F., Taylor, C. M., and Stanbury, S. W., 1977, 1,25-Dihydroxycholecalciferol in hypoparathyroidism, *Lancet* **1**:55–59.

61. Bernstein, D., Kleeman, C. R., and Maxwell, M. H., 1963, The effect of calcium infusions, parathyroid hormone and vitamin D on renal clearance of calcium, *Proc. Soc. Exp. Biol. Med.* **112**:353–355.

62. Hughes, M. R., Baylink, D. J., Jones, P. G., and Haussler, M. R., 1976, Radioligand receptor assay for 25-hydroxyvitamin D_2/D_3 and 1α, 25-dihydroxyvitamin D_2/D_3. Application to hypervitaminosis D, *J. Clin. Invest.* **58:**61–70.

63. Brumbaugh, P. F., Hughes, M. R., and Haussler, M. R., 1975, Cytoplasmic and nuclear binding components for 1α,25-dihydroxyvitamin D_3 in chick parathyroid glands, *Proc. Natl. Acad. Sci. U.S.A.* **72:**4871–4875.

64. Chertow, B. S., Baylink, D. J., Wergedal, J. E., Su, M. H. H., and Norman, A. W., 1975, Decrease in serum immunoreactive parathyroid hormone in rats and in parathyroid hormone secretion *in vitro* by 1,25-dihydroxycholecalciferol, *J. Clin. Invest.* **56:**668–678.

65. Coburn, J. W., Hartenbower, D. H., and Kleeman, C. R., 1977, Divalent ion metabolism, in: *The Year in Metabolism 1977* (N. Freinkel, ed.) Chapter 9, Plenum, New York (in press).

66. Ribovich, M. L., and DeLuca, H. F., 1976, Intestinal calcium transport: Parathyroid hormone and adaptation to dietary calcium, *Arch. Biochem. Biophys.* **175:**256–261.

67. Kemm, J. R., 1976, The effect of parathyroidectomy and large doses of cholecalciferol on the ability of rats to adapt to changes in dietary intake of calcium, *J. Physiol.* **256:**103–115.

68. Bonjour, J.-P., Fleisch, H., and Trechsel, U., 1977, Calcium absorption in diphosphonate-treated rats: Effect of parathyroid function, dietary calcium and phosphorus, *J. Physiol.* **264:**125–139.

69. Kalu, D. N., and Foster, G. V., 1976, Calcitonin: Its physiologic roles, *N. Y. State J. Med.* **76:**230–233.

70. Parsons, J. A., 1976, Parathyroid physiology and the skeleton, in: *Biochemistry and Physiology of Bone*, Vol. IV (G. H. Bourne, ed.), Academic Press, New York.

71. DiBella, F. P., Arnaud, C. D., and Brewer, H. B., Jr., 1976, Relative biologic activities of human and bovine parathyroid hormones and their synthetic NH_2-terminal (1-34) peptides, as evaluated *in vitro* with renal cortical adenylate cyclase obtained from three different species, *Endocrinology* **99:**429–436.

72. Goltzman, D., Peytremann, A., Callahan, E. N., Segre, G. V., and Potts, J. T., Jr., 1976, Metabolism and biological activity of parathyroid hormone in renal cortical membranes, *J. Clin. Invest.* **57:**8–19.

73. Parsons, J. A., and Robinson, C. J., 1968, A rapid indirect hypercalcemic action of parathyroid hormone demonstrated in isolated blood-perfused bone, in: *Parathyroid Hormone and Thyrocalcitonin (Calcitonin)* (R. V. Talmage and L. F. Bélanger, eds.), pp. 329–331, Excerpta Medica, Amsterdam and New York.

74. Mueller, W. J., Brubaker, R. L., Gay, C. V., and Boelkins, J. N., 1973, Mechanisms of bone resorption in laying hens, *Fed. Proc. Fed. Am. Soc. Exp. Biol.* **32:**1951–1954.

75. Massry, S. G., Coburn, J. W., Hartenbower, D. L., Shinaberger, J. H., DePalma, J. R., Chapman, E., and Kleeman, C. R., 1970, Mineral contents of human skin in uremia: Effect of secondary hyperparathyroidism and hemodialysis, *Proc. Eur. Dial. Transplant Assoc.* **7:**146–150.

76. Berkow, J. W., Fine, B. S., and Zimmerman, L. E., 1968, Unusual ocular calcification in hyperparathyroidism, *Am. J. Ophthalmol.* **66:**812–824.

77. Bernstein, D. S., Pletka, P., Hattner, R. S., Hampers, C. L., and Merrill, J. P., 1971, Effect of total parathyroidectomy and uremia on the chemical composition of bone, skin and aorta in the rat, *Isr. J. Med. Sci.* **7:**513–517.

78. Perris, A. D., Weiss, L. A., and Whittfield, J. F., 1968, Parathyroidectomy and the induction of thymic atrophy in normal, adrenalectomized and orchidectomized rats, *J. Cell. Physiol.* **76**:141–150.
79. Rixon, R H., and Whittfield, J. F., 1976, The control of liver regeneration by parathyroid hormone and calcium, *J. Cell. Physiol.* **87**:147–156.
80. Rixon, R. H., 1968, Mitotic activity in the bone marrow of rats and its relation to the level of plasma calcium, *Curr. Mod. Biol.* **2**:68–74.
81. Arieff, A. I., and Massry, S. G., 1974, Calcium metabolism of brain in acute renal failure. Effects of uremia, hemodialysis, and parathyroid hormone, *J. Clin. Invest.* **53**:387–392.
82. Guisado, R., Arieff, A. I., and Massry, S. G., 1975, Changes in the electroencephalogram in acute uremia. Effects of parathyroid hormone and brain electrolytes, *J. Clin. Invest.* **55**:738–745.
83. Malbon, C. C., and Zull, J. E., 1974, Interactions of parathyroid hormone and plasma membranes from rat kidney, *Biochem. Biophys. Res. Commun.* **56**:952–958.
84. Herrmann-Erlee, M. P. M., Hekkelman, J. W., Heersche, J. N. M., and Nijweide, P. J., 1975, The role of Ca^{2+} and cyclic AMP in the action of parathyroid hormone on embryonic bone *in vitro*, *J. Endocrinol.* **64**:69P.
85. Tomlinson, S., Hendy, G. N., Pemberton, D. M., and O'Riordan, J. L. H., 1976, Reversible resistance to the renal action of parathyroid hormone in man, *Clin. Sci. Mol. Med.* **51**:59–69.
86. Nagata, N., Sasaki, M., Kimura, N., and Nakane, K., 1975, The hypercalcemic effect of parathyroid hormone and skeletal cyclic AMP, *Endocrinology* **96**:725–731.
87. Heath, D. A., Palmer, J. S., and Aurbach, G. D., 1972, The hypocalcemic action of colchicine, *Endocrinology* **90**:1589–1593.
88. Dousa, T. P., Duarte, C. G., and Knox, F. G., 1976, Effect of colchicine on urinary phosphate and regulation by parathyroid hormone, *Am. J. Physiol.* **231**:61–65.
89. Puschett, J. B., and Goldberg, M., 1969, The relationship between the renal handling of phosphate and bicarbonate in man, *J. Lab. Clin. Med.* **73**:956–969.
90. Beck, L. H., and Goldberg, M., 1973, Effects of acetazolamide and parathyroidectomy on renal transport of sodium, calcium, and phosphate, *Am. J. Physiol.* **224**:1136–1142.
91. Uchikawa, T., Borle, A. B., and Midgett, R. J., 1976, Parathyroid hormone and phosphaturia, *Calcif. Tissue Res.* **21**(Suppl.):284–287.
92. Beck, N., Kim, K. S., Wolak, M., and Davis, B. B., 1975, Inhibition of carbonic anhydrase by parathyroid hormone and cyclic AMP in rat renal cortex *in vitro*, *J. Clin. Invest.* **55**:149–156.
93. Habener, J. F., Kemper, B., and Potts, J. T., Jr., 1975, Calcium-dependent intracellular degradation of parathyroid hormone: A possible mechanism for the regulation of hormone stores, *Endocrinology* **97**:431–441.
94. Chertow, B. S., Buschmann, R. J., and Henderson, W. J., 1975, Subcellular mechanisms of parathyroid hormone secretion: Ultrastructural changes in response to calcium, vitamin A, vinblastine, and cytochalasin B, *Lab. Invest.* **32**:190–200.
95. Williams, G. A., Hargis, G. K., Bowser, E. N., Henderson, W. J., and Martinez, N.J., 1973, Evidence for a role of adenosine $3^1,5^1$-monophosphate in parathyroid hormone release, *Endocrinology* **92**:687–691.
96. Abe, M., and Sherwood, L. M., 1972, Regulation of parathyroid hormone secretion by adenyl cyclase, *Biochem. Biophys. Res. Commun.* **48**:396–401.

97. Bowser, E. N., Hargis, G. K., Henderson, W. J., and Williams, G. A., 1975, Parathyroid hormone secretion in the rat: Effect of aminophylline, *Proc. Soc. Exp. Biol. Med.* **148**:344–346.

98. Habener, J. F., and Potts, J. T., Jr., 1976, Relative effectiveness of magnesium and calcium on the secretion and biosynthesis of parathyroid hormone *in vitro, Endocrinology* **98**:197–202.

99. Mayer, G. P., 1973, Parathyroid hormone secretion rate in calves, *Endocrinology* **92**(Suppl.):A-160 (abstract 224).

100. Mayer, G. P., Habener, J. F., and Potts, J. T., Jr., 1976, Parathyroid hormone secretion *in vivo.* Demonstration of a calcium-independent nonsuppressible component of secretion, *J. Clin. Invest.* **57**:678–683.

101. Williams, G. A., Kukreja, S. C., Hargis, G. K., Bowser, E. N., Banerjee, P., Vora, N., and Henderson, W. J., 1976, Dual control of suppressibility of parathyroid hormone secretion by calcium and β-adrenergic blockade in man, *Clin. Res.* **24**:585A.

102. Shah, J. H., Motto, G. S., Kukreja, S. C., Hargis, G. K., and Williams, G. A., 1975, Stimulation of the secretion of parathyroid hormone during hypoglycemic stress, *J. Clin. Endocrinol. Metab.* **41**:692–696.

103. Kukreja, S. C., Hargis, G. K., Bowser, E. N., Henderson, W. J., Fisherman, E. W., and Williams, G. A., 1975, Role of adrenergic stimuli in parathyroid hormone secretion in man, *J. Clin. Endrocrinol. Metab.* **40**:478–481.

104. Kukreja, S. C., Johnson, P. A., Ayala, G., Banerjee, P., Bowser, E. N., Hargis, G. K., and Williams, G. A., 1976, Role of calcium and beta-adrenergic system in control of parathyroid hormone secretion, *Proc. Soc. Exp. Biol. Med.* **151**:326–328.

105. Brown, E. M., Hurwitz, S., and Aurbach, G. D., 1976, Preparation of viable isolated bovine parathyroid cells, *Endocrinology* **99**:1582–1588.

106. Boquist, L., 1975, Occurrence of oxyphil cells in suppressed parathyroid glands, *Cell Tissue Res.* **163**:465–470.

107. Thliveris, J. A., and Dube, W. J., 1975, Fine-structural alterations of the chief cells in primary hyperparathyroidism in man, in: *Electron Microscopic Concepts of Secretion* (M. Hess, ed.), John Wiley & Sons, New York.

108. Castleman, B., Schantz, A., and Roth, S. I., 1976, Parathyroid hyperplasia in primary hyperparathyroidism. A review of 85 cases, *Cancer* **38**:1008–1075.

109. LiVolsi, V. A., and Feind, C. R., 1976, Parathyroid adenoma and nonmedullary thyroid carcinoma, *Cancer* **38**:1391–1393.

110. Petro, A. B., and Hardy, J. D., 1975, The association of parathyroid adenoma and non-medullary carcinoma of the thyroid, *Ann. Surg.* **181**:118–119.

111. Rosen, I. B., Strawbridge, H. G., and Bain, J., 1975, A case of hyperparathyroidism associated with radiation to the head and neck area, *Cancer* **36**:1111–1114.

112. Prinz, R., Paloyan, E., Lawrence, A. M., Brooks, M. H., Braithwaite, S., and Pickleman, J. R., 1976, Radiation exposure and hyperparathyroidism, *Clin. Res.* **24**:530A.

113. Christensson, T., Hellström, K., and Wengle, B., 1976, Clinical and laboratory findings in subjects with hypercalcaemia. A study including cases with primary hyperparathyroidism detected in a health screening, *Acta Med. Scand.* **200**:355–360.

114. Muldowney, F. P., Freaney, R., Spillane, E. A., and O'Donohoe, P., 1973, Ionised calcium levels in "normocalcaemic" hyperparathyroidism, *Ir. J. Med. Sci.* **142**:223–229.

115. Grimelius, L., Ejerblad, S., Johansson, H., and Werner, I., 1976, Parathyroid

adenomas and glands in normocalcemic hyperparathyroidism. A light microscopic study, *Am. J. Pathol.* **83:**475–484.

116. Pedersen, N. T., and Permin, H., 1975, Hyperparathyroidism and pregnancy, *Acta Obstet. Gynecol. Scand.* **54:**281–283.

117. Spiegel, A. M., Harrison, H. E., Marx, S. J., Brown, E. M., and Aurbach, G. D., 1977, Neonatal primary hyperparathyroidism with autosomal dominant inheritance, *J. Pediatr.* **90:**269–272.

118. Drezner, M. K., Neelon, F. A., Curtis, H. B., and Lebovitz, H. E., 1976, Renal cyclic adenosine monophosphate: An accurate index of parathyroid function, *Metabolism* **25:**1103–1112.

119. Rosin, R. D., 1976, Pancreatitis and hyperparathyroidism, *Postgrad. Med. J.* **52:**95–101.

120. Wang, C.-A., 1976, The anatomic basis of parathyroid surgery, *Ann. Surg.* **183:**271–275.

121. Spiegel, A. M., Marx, S. J., Doppman, J. L., Beazley, R. M., Ketcham, A. S., Kasten, B., and Aurbach, G. D., 1975, Intrathyroidal parathyroid adenoma or hyperplasia. *J. Am. Med. Assoc.* **234:**1029–1033.

122. Rothmund, M., Diethelm, L., Brünner, H., and Kümmerle, F., 1976, Diagnosis and treatment of mediastinal parathyroid tumors, *Ann. Surg.* **183:**139–145.

123. Roth, S. I., and Gallagher, M. J., 1976, The rapid identification of "normal" parathyroid glands by the presence of intracellular fat, *Am. J. Pathol.* **84:**521–527.

124. Mason, E. E., Hoines, J., and Freeman, J. B., 1975, Hyperparathyroidism: Evaluation of four decades of parathyroid surgery, *Can. J. Surg.* **18:**422–429.

125. Wells, S. A., Jr., Ellis, G. J., Gunnells, J. C. Schneider, A. B., and Sherwood, L. M., 1976, Parathyroid autotransplantation in primary parathyroid hyperplasia, *N. Engl. J. Med.* **295:**57–62.

126. Alveryd, A., El-Zawahry, M. D., Herlitz, P., and Nordenstam, H., 1975, Primary hyperplasia of the parathyroids, *Acta Chir. Scand.* **141:**24–30.

127. Hickey, R. C., and Samaan, N. A., 1975, Human parathyroid autotransplantation. Proved function by radioimmunoassay of plasma parathyroid hormone, *Arch. Surg.* **110:**892–895.

128. Wells, S. A., Jr., Gunnells, J. C., Shelburne, J. D., Schneider, A. B., and Sherwood, L. M., 1975, Transplantation of the parathyroid glands in man: Clinical indications and results, *Surgery* **78:**34–44.

129. Satava, R. M., Jr., Beahrs, O. H., and Scholz, D. A., 1975, Success rate of cervical exploration for hyperparathyroidism, *Arch. Surg.* **110:**625–628.

130. Arkles, L. B., 1975, Experience in parathyroid scanning, *Am. J. Roentgenol.Radium Ther.* **125:**634–639.

131. Burckhardt, P., Bischof-Delaloye, A., Ruedi, B., and Delaloye, B., 1976, Preoperative localization of hyperfunctioning parathyroid tissue by parathyroid scintigraphy, *Acta Endocrinol.* **81:**298–309.

132. Samuels, B. I., 1975, The present status of parathyroid thermography. *J. Am. Med. Assoc.* **233:**907–908.

133. Doppman, J. L., Mallette, L. E., Marx, S. J., Monchik, J. M., Broadus, A., Spiegel, A. M., Beazley, R., and Aurbach, G. D., 1975, The localization of abnormal mediastinal parathyroid glands, *Radiology* **115:**31–36.

134. Doppman, J. L., 1976, Parathyroid localization: Arteriography and venous sampling, *Radiol. Clin. North Am.* **14:**163–188.

135. Tegtmeyer, C. J., Alrich, E. M., and Keats, T. E., 1976, Angiography of

mediastinal parathyroid adenomas, *Am. J. Roentgenol. Radium Ther.* **127**:243–246.

136. Hjern, B., Almqvist, S., Granberg, P.-O., Lindvall, N., and Wästhed, B., 1975, Pre-operative localization of parathyroid tissue by selective neck vein catheterization and radioimmunoassay of parathyroid hormone, *Acta Chir. Scand.* **141**:31–39.

137. Doppman, J. L., Marx, S. J., Spiegel, A. M., Mallette, L. E., Wolfe, D. R., Aurbach, G. D., and Geelhoed, G., 1975, Treatment of hyperparathyroidism by percutaneous embolization of a mediastinal adenoma, *Radiology* **115**:37–42.

138. Massry, S. G., Ritz, E., and Verberckmoes, R., 1977, Role of phosphate in the genesis of secondary hyperparathyroidism of renal failure, *Nephron* **18**:77–81.

139. Massry, S. G., Stein, R., Garty, J., Arieff, A. I., Coburn, J. W., Norman, A. W., and Friedler, R. M., 1976, Skeletal resistance to the calcemic action of parathyroid hormone in uremia: Role of 1,25(OH)$_2$D$_3$, *Kidney Int.* **9**:467–474.

140. Slatopolsky, E., and DeLuca, H. F., Unpublished observations.

141. Nusynowitz, M. L., Frame, B., and Kolb, F. O., 1976, The spectrum of the hypoparathyroid states: A classification based on physiologic principles, *Medicine* **55**:105–119.

142. Parfitt, A. M., 1972, The spectrum of hypoparathyroidism, *J. Clin. Endocrinol. Metab.* **34**:152–158.

143. Frame, B., and Parfitt, A. M., 1973, The syndromes of parathyroid hormone resistance, in: *Clinical Aspects of Metabolic Bone Disease* (B. Frame, A. M. Parfitt, and H. Duncan, eds.), pp. 454–464, Excerpta Medica, Amsterdam.

144. Ashby, J. P., and Heaton, F. W., 1975, Effect of magnesium deficiency and parathyroid hormone on cyclic AMP metabolism in rat renal cortex, *J. Endocrinol.* **67**:105–112.

145. Takatsuki, K., Hanley, D. A., Schneider, A. B., and Sherwood, L. M., 1976, The effects of magnesium depletion on secretion of parathyroid hormone (PTH) *in vitro*, *Clin. Res.* **24**:585A.

146. Anast, C. S., Winnacker, J. L., Forte, L. R., and Burns, T. W., 1976, Impaired release of parathyroid hormone in magnesium deficiency, *J. Clin. Endocrinol. Metab.* **42**:707–717.

147. Medalle, R., Waterhouse, C., and Hahn, T. J., 1976, Vitamin D resistance in magnesium deficiency, *Am. J. Clin. Nutr.* **29**:854–858.

148. Reddy, C. R., Coburn, J. W., Hartenbower, D. L., Friedler, R. M., Brickman, A. S., Massry, S. G., and Jowsey, J., 1973, Studies on mechanisms of hypocalcemia of magnesium depletion, *J. Clin. Invest.* **52**:3000–3010.

149. Robertson, G. M., Jr., Moore, E. W., Switz, D. M., Sizemore, G. W., and Estep, H. L., 1976, Inadequate parathyroid response in acute pancreatitis, *N. Engl. J. Med.* **294**:512–516.

150. Burman, K. D., Monchik, J. M., Earll, J. M., and Wartofsky, L., 1976, Ionized and total serum calcium and parathyroid hormone in hyperthyroidism, *Ann. Intern. Med.* **84**:668–671.

151. Bouillon, R., and De Moor, P., 1974, Parathyroid function in patients with hyper- or hypothyroidism, *J. Clin. Endocrinol. Metab.* **38**:999–1004.

152. Castro, J. H., Genuth, S. M., and Klein, L., 1975, Comparative response to parathyroid hormone in hyperthyroidism and hypothyroidism, *Metabolism* **24**:839–848.

153. Lancer, S. R., Bowser, E. N., Hargis, G. K., and Williams, G. A., 1976, The

effect of growth hormone on parathyroid function in rats, *Endocrinology* **98:**1289–1293.

154. Aloia, J., Powell, D., Mendizibal, E., and Roginsky, M., 1975, Parathyroid function in acromegaly, *Horm. Res.* **6:**145–149.

155. Deftos, L. J., Lorenzi, M., Bohanon, N., Tsalakian, E., Schneider, V., and Gerich, J. E., 1976, Somatostatin does not suppress plasma parathyroid hormone, *J. Clin. Endocrinol. Metab.* **43:**205–207.

156. Fucik, R. F., Kukreja, S. C., Hargis, G. K., Bowser, E. N., Henderson, W. J., and Williams, G. A., 1975, Effect of glucocorticoids on function of the parathyroid glands in man, *J. Clin. Endocrinol. Metab.* **40:**152–155.

157. Lukert, B. P., and Adams, J. S., 1976, Calcium and phosphorus homeostasis in man: Effect of corticosteroids, *Arch. Intern. Med.* **136:**1249–1253.

158. Au, W. Y. W., 1976, Cortisol stimulation of parathyroid hormone secretion by rat parathyroid glands in organ culture, *Science* **193:**1015–1017.

159. Seyberth, H. W., Segre, G. V., Hamet, P., Sweetman, B. J., Potts, J. T., Jr., and Oates, J. A., 1976, Characterization of the group of patients with the hypercalcemia of cancer who respond to treatment with prostaglandin synthesis inhibitors, *Trans. Assoc. Am. Physicians* **89:**92–104.

160. Robertson, R. P., Baylink, D. J., Metz, S. A., and Cummings, K. B., 1976, Plasma prostaglandin E in patients with cancer with and without hypercalcemia, *J. Clin. Endocrinol. Metab.* **43:**1330–1335.

161. Grajower, M., and Barzel, U. S., 1976, Ectopic hyperparathyroidism (pseudohyperparathyroidism) in esophageal malignancy, *Am. J. Med.* **61:**134–135.

162. Deftos, L. J., McMillan, P. J., Sartiano, G. P., Abuid, J., and Robinson, A. G., 1976, Simultaneous ectopic production of parathyroid hormone and calcitonin, *Metabolism* **25:**543–550.

163. Copp, D. H., 1964, Parathyroids, calcitonin and control of plasma calcium, *Recent Prog. Horm. Res.* **20:**59–88.

164. Hirsch, P. F., Gauthier, G. F., and Munson, P. L., 1963, Thyroid hypocalcemic principle and recurrent laryngeal nerve injury as factors affecting the response to parathyroidectomy in rats, *Endocrinology* **73:**244–252.

165. Potts, J. T., Jr. and Deftos, L. J., 1974, Parathyroid hormone, calcitonin, vitamin D, bone and mineral metabolism, in: *Duncan's Diseases of Metabolism,* 7th Ed. (P. K. Bondy and L. E. Rosenberg, eds.), pp. 1225–1413, W. B. Saunders Co., Philadelphia.

166. Kalu, D. N., Hadji-Georgopoulos, A., and Foster, G. V., 1975, Evidence for physiological importance of calcitonin in the regulation of plasma calcium in rats, *J. Clin. Invest.* **55:**722–727.

167. Kalu, D. N., Hadji-Georgopoulos, A., and Foster, G. V., 1976, Further studies on the hypercalcemic effect of acute calcitonin deficiency in rats, *Endocrinology* **98:**534–539.

168. Avioli, L. V., 1976, Calcitonin, in: *The Year in Endocrinology 1975–1976* (S. H. Ingbar, ed.), pp. 233–248, Plenum, New York.

169. Hirsch, P. F., and Munson, P. L., 1969, Thyrocalcitonin, *Physiol. Rev.* **49:**548–622.

170. Barlet, J.-P., and Garel, J.-M., 1976, Effect of an intravenous injection of cholecystokinin-pancreozymin on plasma calcium and calcitonin levels in newborn lambs, *J. Endocrinol.* **70:**151–152.

171. Landsberg, L., 1976, Catecholamines and the sympathoadrenal system, in: *The Year in Endocrinology 1975–1976* (S. H. Ingbar, ed.), pp. 177–231, Plenum, New York.

172. Talmage, R. V., Doppelt, S. H., and Cooper, C. W., 1975, Relationship of blood concentrations of calcium, phosphate, gastrin and calcitonin to the onset of feeding in the rat, *Proc. Soc. Exp. Biol. Med.* **149:**855–859.
173. Gray, T. K., and Ontjes, D. A., 1975, Clinical aspects of thyrocalcitonin, *Clin. Orthop.* **111:**238–256.
174. Anast, C., David, L., Winnacker, J., Glass, R., Baskin, W., Brubaker, L., and Burns, T., 1975, Serum calcitonin-lowering effect of magnesium in patients with medullary carcinoma of the thyroid, *J. Clin. Invest.* **56:**1615–1621.
175. Peshin, J., Ornoy, A., and Menczel, J., 1976, Transplacental effects of thyrocalcitonin on intestinal calcium-binding protein, alkaline phosphatase activity and ossification of long bones in rat fetuses, *Isr. J. Med. Sci.* **12:**248–256.
176. Whalen, J. P., Krook, L., MacIntyre, I., and Nunez, E. A., 1975, Calcitonin, parathyroidectomy and modelling of bones in the growing rat, *J. Endocrinol.* **66:**207–212.
177. Toverud, S. U., Harper, C., and Munson, P. L., 1976, Calcium metabolism during lactation: Enhanced effects of thyrocalcitonin, *Endocrinology* **99:**371–378.
178. Wolfe, H. J., DeLellis, R. A., Voelkel, E. F., and Tashjian, A. H., Jr., 1975, Distribution of calcitonin-containing cells in the normal neonatal human thyroid gland: A correlation of morphology with peptide content, *J. Clin. Endocrinol. Metab.* **41:**1076–1081.
179. Tsang, R. C., Donovan, E. F., and Steichen, J. J., 1976, Calcium physiology and pathology in the neonate, *Pediatr. Clin. North Am.* **23:**611–626.
180. Cannarozzi, D. B., Canale, D. D., and Donabedian, R. K., 1976, Hypercalcitoninemia in infancy, *Clin. Chim. Acta* **66:**387–392.
181. Milhaud, G., Calmettes, C., Julienne, A., Tharaud, D., Bloch-Michel, H., Cavaillon, J. P., Colin, R., and Moukhtar, M. S., 1972, A new chapter in human pathology: Calcitonin disorders and therapeutic use, in: *Calcium Parathyroid Hormone and the Calcitonins* (R. V. Talmage and P. L. Munson, eds.), pp. 56–70, Excerpta Medica, Amsterdam.
182. Katz, A. I., and Lindheimer, M. D., 1977, Actions of hormones on the kidney, *Annu. Rev. Physiol.* **39:**97–134.
183. Chabardès, D., Imbert-Teboul, M., Montégut, M., Clique, A., and Morel, F., 1976, Distribution of calcitonin-sensitive adenylate cyclase activity along the rabbit kidney tubule, *Proc. Natl. Acad. Sci. U.S.A.* **73:**3608–3612.
184. Borle, A. B., 1975, Regulation of cellular calcium metabolism and calcium transport by calcitonin, *J. Membr. Biol.* **21:**125–146.
185. Talmage, R. V., Whitehurst, L. A., and Anderson, J. J. B., 1973, Effect of calcitonin and calcium infusion on plasma phosphate, *Endocrinology* **92:**792–798.
186. Meyer, R. A., Jr., and Meyer, M. H., 1975, Thyrocalcitonin injection to rats increases the liver inorganic phosphate, *Endocrinology* **96:**1048–1050.
187. Block, M. A., Jackson, C. E., and Tashjian, A. H., Jr., 1975, Management of parathyroid glands in surgery for medullary thyroid carcinoma, *Arch. Surg.* **110:**617–624.
188. Heath, H., III, Sizemore, G. W., and Carney, J. A., 1976, Preoperative diagnosis of occult parathyroid hyperplasia by calcium infusion in patients with multiple endocrine neoplasia, type 2a, *J. Clin. Endocrinol. Metab.* **43:**428–435.
189. Ardaillou, R., Beaufils, M., Nivez, M.-P., Isaac, R., Mayaud, C., and Sraer, J.-

D., 1975, Increased plasma calcitonin in early acute renal failure, *Clin. Sci. Mol. Med.* **49:**301–304.

190. Heynen, G., Kanis, J. A., Oliver, D., Ledingham, J. G. G., and Russell, R. G. G., 1976, Evidence that endogenous calcitonin protects against renal bone disease, *Lancet* **2:**1322–1326.

191. Deftos, L. J., Powell, D., Parthemore, J. C., and Potts, J. T., Jr., 1973, Secretion of calcitonin in hypocalcemic states in man, *J. Clin. Invest.* **52:**3109–3114.

192. DeRose, J., Singer, F. R., Avramides, A., Flores, A., Dziadiw, R., Baker, R. K., and Wallach, S., 1974, Response of Paget's disease to porcine and salmon calcitonins: Effects of long-term treatment, *Am. J. Med.* **56:**858–866.

193. Woodhouse, N. J. Y., Crosbie, W. A., and Mohamedally, S. M., 1975, Cardiac output in Paget's disease: Response to long-term salmon calcitonin therapy, *Br. Med. J.* **4:**686.

194. Calcitonin in the treatment of Paget's disease of bone, *Med. Lett.* **17:**97–98.

195. Wallach, S., 1976, When should Paget's disease be treated?, *Current Concepts in Bone Disease 1*, Professional Communications Associates.

196. Avramides, A., Flores, A., DeRose, J., and Wallach, S., 1976, Paget's disease of the bone: Observations after cessation of long-term synthetic salmon calcitonin treatment, *J. Clin. Endocrinol. Metab.* **42:**459–463.

197. Hosking, D. J., van Aken, J., Bijvoet, O. L. M., and Will, E. J., 1976, Paget's bone disease treated with diphosphonate and calcitonin, *Lancet* **1:**615–617.

198. Coombes, R. C., Easty, G. C., Detre, S. I., Hillyard, C. J., Stevens, U., Girgis, S. I., Galante, L. S., Heywood, L., MacIntyre, I., and Neville, A. M., 1975, Secretion of immunoreactive calcitonin by human breast carcinomas, *Br. Med. J.* **4:**197–199.

The Adrenal Cortex

John T. Gwynne and Robert L. Ney

5.1. Introduction

The aim of this chapter is to review advances made within the last year in understanding normal and pathological function of the adrenal cortex. The initial sections deal primarily with events that occur at the molecular and cellular levels, while subsequent sections deal with disorders of adrenal function in the intact organism. An appreciation of the former is essential to clear understanding of the latter. In addition, examination of the action of adrenocorticotropin (ACTH) on specific molecular events within adrenal cells may result in better understanding of polypeptide hormone action in general.

The intent in writing this chapter has been to review selected areas in which several observations by one or more workers have led to the emergence of new concepts. Thus, unitary observations of limited general interest have frequently not been cited. In considering areas of basic investigation, an attempt has been made to relate reported observations to recognition and treatment of adrenal dysfunction. Although major advances have occurred in many areas, little activity has been reported in several areas of clinical importance. Thus, considerable space has been devoted to Cushing's disease, while discussions of Addison's disease, congenital adrenal hyperplasia, and adrenal tumors have not been included in this year's review.

JOHN T. GWYNNE and ROBERT L. NEY • Departments of Medicine and Physiology, University of North Carolina, Chapel Hill, North Carolina.

Since both normal and, in many cases, abnormal adrenal growth and function are dependent on stimulation by ACTH, the structure and function of ACTH and related peptides will first be considered.

5.2. ACTH: Structure and Function

5.2.1. "Big" ACTH and Related Peptides

The predominant circulating adrenocorticotropic peptide, ACTH, is a single chain of 39 residues with a molecular weight of approximately 4500. There are, however, several additional proteins of both larger and smaller molecular weight that have sequence homologies with $ACTH_{1-39}$. Included among this group are "big" ACTH, the melanocyte-stimulating hormones (α- and β-MSH), and β-lipotropin (β-LPH). In many cases, these peptides cross-react with antibodies raised against ACTH. "Big" ACTH is an apparent prohormone to $ACTH_{1-39}$, while the relationship of MSH and β-LPH is less clearly understood.

Elucidation of the structure, function, and relationship of various peptides with ACTH cross-immunoreactivity is currently forthcoming and represents one of the most exciting recent advances in endocrinology. For a complete review of earlier studies in this area, the reader is referred to the papers by Oelofsen[1] and Felber.[2]

The occurrence of "big" ACTH in man was first noted by Yalow and Berson,[3] who observed high-molecular-weight peptides with ACTH cross-immunoreactivity in tissue extracts of normal pituitary, in an ACTH-producing thymoma, and in plasma from patients with Nelson's syndrome, Addison's disease, and Cushing's disease. In addition, they noted that metyrapone stimulation of a normal subject caused the appearance of "big" ACTH in the systemic circulation. Furthermore, trypsin treatment of "big" ACTH caused release of ACTH of normal size, suggesting that the larger form was a precursor peptide.[4]

Subsequent studies of "big" ACTH in many species have relied mainly on gel-filtration chromatography to distinguish large from small forms of radioimmunoreactive ACTH (RIA-ACTH). The conditions employed have not previously permitted precise definition of the peptide species being studied. Eipper and her colleagues, using guanidine hydrochloride or sodium dodecyl sulfate (SDS) to effect complete denaturation, examined the forms of RIA-ACTH produced by cultured mouse pituitary cells.[5-7] Four species of RIA-ACTH were found; these species have molecular weights of 31,000, 23,000, 13,000, and 4500. To determine whether these peptides are metabolically related, cells growing in monolayer cultures were pulsed with tritiated amino acids and the rate of appearance of label in each peptide examined. Labeled amino acids appeared first in the highest-molecular-weight species (mol. wt. 31,000) and subsequently in the smaller forms. Peak labeling of the 23,000-molecular-weight species occurred when activity of the 31,000-molecular-weight species was decreasing, but before peak activity of the 13,000- and 4500-molecular-weight peptides was reached. The latter two peptides became labeled at approximately the same rate. The largest molecular weight peptide therefore appears to be the parent molecule, while the peptide of 23,000 molecular weight is an intermediate in the formation of the two smaller peptides. The relationship of the 13,000- and 4500-molecular-weight species is not yet defined.

The initial gene product for corticotropic activity thus appears to be a high-molecular-weight peptide (mol. wt. 30,000–35,000). This view is supported by the work of Nakanishi et al.,[8] who obtained polyadenylate-containing RNA from bovine anterior pituitary glands and characterized the major peptide with ACTH cross-immunoreactivity produced by translation in a cell-free system. This peptide was shown to have a molecular weight of approximately 35,000 by disk-gel electrophoresis in SDS. In addition to immunological cross-reactivity with ACTH, this large protein was shown to possess a methionine-containing peptide, identified by incorporation of [^{35}S]methionine and derived by chymotryptic digestion, that comigrated with the methionine-containing peptide of $ACTH_{1-39}$.

The physiological function of these large precursor peptides is not yet known. The intracellular mechanisms and regulation of production and release of large and intermediate RIA-ACTH are as yet unexplored. It is of interest, however, that ectopic sources of RIA-ACTH frequently have a much greater percentage of "big" ACTH than of $ACTH_{1-39}$.

The larger forms of RIA-ACTH have generally low ratios of biological to immunological ACTH-like activity.[5] In addition, their reactivity toward ACTH antibodies varies depending on the region of ACTH molecule that is being recognized. Kreiger et al.[9] characterized, for the first time, ACTH produced by cultured corticotrophs removed from a patient with Cushing's disease. Both high- and low-molecular-weight forms were observed by gel filtration on Sephadex G-50. The ratios of biological to immunological activity were less for the high- than for the low-molecular-weight forms, while C-terminal immunoreactivity was fivefold greater than N-terminal immunoreactivity for both. These observations point out the potential difficulty in using many currently available radioimmunoassays to determine biologically effective corticotropic activity.

An additional structural feature of high-molecular-weight ACTH-like peptides is the presence of carbohydrate. This feature was recently reported by Eipper et al.[7] for ACTH from mouse pituitary tumor and has subsequently been demonstrated in man by Orth and Nicholson.[10] The latter workers examined tissue extracts from normal pituitary, an epithelial thymoma, and two islet-cell carcinomas, as well as plasma from a patient with Nelson's syndrome. In both studies, the presence of carbohydrate was demonstrated by adsorption of RIA-ACTH to concanavalin A and subsequent elution with α-methyl-D-mannopyranoside. As with other proteins in serum, the amount and type of carbohydrate may play an important role in cellular release or subsequent hepatic uptake and degradation of "big" ACTH.

Although the relationship of "big" ACTH to $ACTH_{1-39}$ appears to be that of precursor to product, the relationship of ACTH to other peptides with partial sequence homology is less clear. Pelletier et al.[11] recently examined, by immunohistochemical techniques, the distribution of both ACTH and β-LPH within the pituitary of several species, including man. They found that the two peptides are found in secretory granules of the same cell. This observation is of particular interest, since β-LPH is the apparent precursor for the endogenous opiatelike peptides, the endorphins and enkephalins.[12] In addition, β-LPH contains a segment with complete sequence homology to β-MSH, which in turn shares partial sequence homology with $ACTH_{1-39}$.[1] These observations raise several extremely interesting questions of importance to adrenal function. Is pituitary secretion of ACTH coupled to secretion of β-LPH? If not, how are they regulated independently, and if they are, what effects do β-LPH or the endogenous opiates have on the hypothalamic–pituitary–adrenal axis?

5.2.2. $ACTH_{1-39}$: Structure and Function

Although other forms of RIA-ACTH are present, $ACTH_{1-39}$ is responsible for the majority of biological corticotropic activity. To better understand polypeptide hormone action in general and the action of ACTH in particular, the contributions of specific amino acid residues to various ACTH activities have been examined in vitro and in vivo. These studies have generally relied on a comparison of the activity of native $ACTH_{1-39}$ with the activity of synthetic ACTH analogues with specific amino acid substitutions, deletions, or alterations. In addition to providing information about native ACTH function, this approach could also result in identification of therapeutically useful ACTH analogues. A specific synthetic antagonist could, for instance, be useful in treating nonresectable tumors producing ectopic ACTH. Several studies published within the last year have contributed to an understanding of the relationship of the structure of $ACTH_{1-39}$ to its function.

The role of residues 25–39 in ACTH function has not previously been understood. Residues 1–24 are species-invariant and sufficient for maximal biological activity in vivo and in vitro. Baumann and Filber[13] reported studies that suggest that the C-terminal residues (25–39) are important in regulating the duration of ACTH action. Synthetic human $ACTH_{1-24}$ and $ACTH_{1-39}$ were given in supermaximal doses either intravenously or intramuscularly to normal male volunteers, and plasma 11-hydroxycorticosteroids were subsequently measured. The maximal response to each peptide was the same; however, the duration of response to $ACTH_{1-39}$ was significantly longer than to $ACTH_{1-24}$. It is not known whether this extended stimulation results from a decreased clearance rate or changes in other properties of the peptide. It no longer appears, however, that the C-terminal residues are merely a nonfunctional genetic vestige.

Previous studies have indicated that amino acid residues 1–11 are most important for adenylate cyclase activation, while residues 16–24 are most important for membrane binding. For a more complete discussion of previous work, the reader is referred to the recent review by Otsuka and Inouye.[14] The tryptophan residue at position 9 is also important for adrenal cyclase activation. Both chemical modification to produce o-nitrophenyl-sulphenyl-tryptophan at position 9 (NPS-ACTH) and specific amino acid replacements at position 9 result in ACTH analogues that, in broken-cell preparation, have no inherent stimulatory effect and also antagonize the action of $ACTH_{1-24}$. In whole-cell suspensions, however, NPS-ACTH was reported by Moyle[15] to stimulate steroidogenesis. These observations were confirmed and extended by Ramachandran et al.,[16] who examined steroid and adrenal cyclic 3',5'-adenosine monophosphate (cAMP) production in vivo by rats treated with ACTH and NPS-ACTH. In this sytem, as in cell suspensions, NPS-ACTH is about 1.25% as potent as $ACTH_{1-24}$ in stimulating steroid production, but several orders of magnitude less potent in stimulating cAMP production. Similar observations using ACTH analogues with substitutions for tryptophan at position 9 were reported by Finn et al.[17] In particular, synthetic $ACTH_{1-24}$ with glutamine at position 5 and phenylalanine at position 9 $[(Gln^5,Phe^9)ACTH_{1-24}]$ does not itself stimulate adenylate cyclase and also prevents $ACTH_{1-24}$ stimulation in broken-cell preparations. In cell suspensions, however, it produces maximal steroidogenic response and does not antagonize the action of the $ACTH_{1-24}$. Furthermore $(Gln^5,Phe^9)ACTH_{1-24}$ stimulates cAMP production in intact cells, but only at much higher concentrations than are required for stimulation of steroidogenesis.

These apparent discrepancies between observations in broken-cell preparations and in intact cells do not eliminate cAMP as a secondary messenger in the action of ACTH, since full steroidogenic response occurs at much lower levels of stimulation than full cAMP response does (see Section 5.3). They do suggest, however, that in addition to the amount of cAMP produced, other factors such as structural organization or compartmentalization may be important in modulating the steroidogenic response to ACTH. They further suggest caution in extending conclusions derived from studies involving broken-cell preparations to the intact animal.

Finally, the importance of specific residues to membrane binding and adenylate cyclase activation was further examined by Ways and Ontjes,[18] using broken-cell preparations of rat adrenal glands. The ability of a series of $ACTH_{1-24}$ analogues, with either carboxyl- or amino-terminus deletions, to prevent $[^{125}I]ACTH_{1-24}$ binding and unlabeled $ACTH_{1-24}$ stimulation of adenylate cyclase was determined. A good correlation between inhibition of binding and inhibition of cyclase activation was observed. In addition, these studies confirmed both the importance of residues 1–5 in cyclase activation and the role of the charged basic residues in positions 16–18 in promoting binding.

5.2.3. Ectopic ACTH

Numerous ectopic sources of corticotropic activity have previously been identified. In many cases, peptides with ACTH cross-immunoreactivity but without significant biological activity are produced. In others, however, ectopic peptides have both biological and immunological activity, resulting in clinically apparent Cushing's syndrome. Since pituitary corticotrophs and cells responsible for ectopic ACTH production are related embryologically, their peptide products might be expected to be similar. Except for the identification of large and small forms, however, the structure of ectopic ACTH has not previously been examined. Lowry *et al.*[19] obtained sufficient immunoreactive ACTH from a thymic tumor to permit chemical characterization. Determinations of the amino acid composition and of the carboxyl- and amino-terminal residues indicate that the ectopic peptide is identical in structure to residues 2–38 of pituitary $ACTH_{1-39}$. Unfortunately, such subtle differences in structure cannot be exploited at present to differentiate patients with the ectopic ACTH syndrome from those with pituitary-dependent Cushing's disease.

5.3. Cyclic Nucleotides in the Adrenal

The role of cAMP as an intermediate or "second message" in ACTH stimulation of adrenal steroidogenesis is only partially understood. The ability of cAMP to activate adrenal protein kinase is well established; however, the precise mechanism by which this activation leads to enhanced steroidogenesis is not known. Furthermore, maximum steroidogenic response to ACTH is elicited at much lower levels of ACTH than is maximum production of cAMP. Finally, the role of cAMP in mediating the tropic effects of ACTH remains unclear. Questions such as these have led to continued studies of intracellular cAMP metabolism in the adrenal. Within the last year, such studies have centered mainly on the properties of membrane-bound adenylate cyclase and cAMP-sensitive protein kinases.

5.3.1. Adenylate Cyclase

Intracellular cAMP is produced from ATP by membrane-bound adenylate cyclase. In addition to ACTH, guanine nucleotides and various bacterial toxins, such as cholera toxin, also stimulate the enzyme both in broken-cell preparations and in intact cells. It now appears that each of these stimuli enhances the activity of the enzyme by a different mechanism and that each may modulate the response to the others. These observations raise the possibility that *in vivo* many factors in addition to ACTH may be important in modulating adrenocortical cAMP production.

Recently, Wolff and Cook[20] reported that adenosine is also capable of stimulating adenylate cyclase in broken-cell preparations and steroidogenesis in intact cells of the cultured mouse Y1 adrenal tumor. These cells, which have maintained hormonal responsiveness in culture, are frequently used as a model for study of ACTH action, and have been carefully characterized in the past.[21]

In addition to adenosine, a number of phosphorylated adenosine compounds, including ATP, adenyl-5'-yl imidophosphate, ADP, AMP, NAD, and FAD, were also able to stimulate steroidogenesis in the intact cells. It would appear, however, that these phosphorylated derivatives must first be converted to adenosine to be effective. The enzyme adenosine deaminase (ADA) inhibits stimulation of steroidogenesis by adenosine. This enzyme is active only against adenosine, and its inability to hydrolyze 5'-esterified adenosine derivatives was confirmed in this study. One would therefore not expect ATP stimulation of steroidogenesis in Y1 cells to be inhibited by ADA. The opposite, however, was observed, namely, that ADA inhibits the ability of ATP to stimulate steroidogenesis. This finding suggests that ATP must first be converted to adenosine before stimulation can occur.

Stimulation of steroidogenesis in the intact cell by adenosine may result from activation of adenylate cyclase. The ability of adenosine to stimulate adenylate cyclase in broken-cell preparations was shown directly. In addition, dipyridamole, which inhibits membrane transport of adenosine, increased the effectiveness of low concentrations of adenosine in stimulating steroidogenesis. This finding suggests that adenosine produces its effects by acting outside the cell.

These studies are of importance for two reasons. First, they indicate a possible role for adenosine in modulation of cyclase activity. Second, they suggest that the ability of added extracellular cAMP to stimulate end-organ response may result, not from its cellular uptake and activation of protein kinase, but rather by some action on membrane cyclase. If this were so, it would weaken one of the main arguments commonly used to establish cAMP as a second message.

An additional factor that plays an important role in ACTH stimulation of steroidogenesis is the concentration of available divalent cations. Within the last year, two groups have reexamined the role of Ca^{2+} in ACTH activation of adrenal adenylate cyclase. To study the effects of Ca^{2+} or other divalent cations on enzyme function in both broken-cell and intact-cell preparations, investigators have either added chelating agents such as ethyleneglycol bis(β-aminoethylether),N,N'-tetraacetic acid (EGTA) to bind free calcium or have performed their studies in calcium-free media. Either approach may lead to possible artifacts, however, as suggested by the studies cited below. Glossman and Gips,[21] using partially purified adrenal cell membranes, reported that not only Ca^{2+} but also Mn^{2+}, Co^{2+}, Sr^{2+}, and Ni^{2+}, but not Zn^{2+}, Ac^{2+}, Fe^{2+}, or La^{2+}, are able to reverse the inhibitory effect of added EGTA on ACTH stimulation of adenylate cyclase. Complete reversal occurs at a cation concentration just sufficient to completely complex the added EGTA. Further addition of Ca^{2+} results in inhibition of activity. Interestingly, however, further additions of Mn^{2+} are stimulatory. The authors suggest that the inhibitory effects of EGTA may be mediated by binding of this agent to metal ions complexed to the enzyme, not by chelation of free cations in solution. If this were so, examination of the effects of EGTA on enzyme kinetics under various condition might shed additional light on enzyme structure and functions. There seems little doubt, however, that Ca^{2+} plays a role in coupling ACTH binding to cyclase activation. The importance of Ca^{2+}, as well as of other divalent cations, particularly Mn^{2+}, *in vivo* is not yet clear.

Haksar *et al.*[22] used the calcium antagonist lanthanum (La^{3++}) to examine the role of Ca^{2+} in ACTH stimulation of steroidogenesis in rat adrenal cell suspensions. They showed, by electron micrography, that lanthanum is found in high concentration at the cell membrane. They further showed that its inhibitory effects are on cyclase activation, not on subsequent intracellular events. The use of calcium-free medium or extracellular calcium chelators in studies employing whole-cell preparations may result in depletion of intracellular as well as extracellular Ca^{2+}. This problem appears to be avoided with the use of lanthanum. These authors hypothesize that Ca^{2+} may exert its effects by stimulating contractile membrane proteins that bring the ACTH receptor and adenylate cyclase enzyme in contact. No direct data bearing on this hypothesis are yet available.

The studies discussed above serve to emphasize the as yet incomplete understanding of the regulation of membrane adenylate cyclase in the adrenal as well as in other hormonally responsive tissues. They also demonstrate the possibilities for very fine modulation of activity that exist in the intact organism.

5.3.2. cAMP-Dependent Protein Kinase

Adrenal cAMP-dependent protein kinase is composed of two regulatory and two catalytic subunits. Cyclic AMP is believed to produce its effects in the adrenal by binding to the regulatory subunit, with resultant dissociation and activation of the catalytic subunit. Phosphorylation effected by the catalytic subunit is believed to be necessary for ACTH stimulation of steroidogenesis. The critical protein undergoing phosphorylation has not been identified. Indeed, its precise mechanism of action is also unresolved. Alternatively, phosphorylation by cAMP-dependent protein kinase may stimulate steroidogenesis by enhancing synthesis of an essential peptide with a short half-life (see Section 5.4.1) or by activating a previously formed peptide that also has a short half-life.

Moyle et al.[23] questioned the role of protein kinase in ACTH activation of adrenal steroidogenesis by correlating kinase activity, bound cAMP, and corticosterone content in adrenal glands excised from hypophysectomized rats treated with ACTH, NSP-ACTH, or dibutyryl-cyclic 3′,5′-adenosine monophosphate (db-cAMP). These workers observed that following administration of ACTH to rats hypophysectomized 24 hr before treatment, the corticosterone content of excised adrenal glands increased to near maximal levels before any increase in protein kinase or bound cAMP could be detected. In addition, the corticosterone content increased to high levels in glands from rats treated with increasing doses of NPS-ACTH before any increase in bound cAMP or protein kinase activity was noted. With db-cAMP stimulation, however, the kinetic and dose responses of corticosterone content paralleled the increase in kinase activity. These results suggest that ACTH stimulation of steroidogenesis may not be mediated by cAMP activation of protein kinase. No definitive conclusion is possible, however, for several reasons. Histones, which were used as substrate in the kinase activity assay, may not be an appropriate substrate. More than one type of kinase is found in adrenal tissue, and activation of compartmentalized or specific kinases would not be observed by the experimental techniques employed. These studies do point out, however, the complexity of the mechanism by which

ACTH activates steroidogenesis and should stimulate attempts at further purification and characterization of adrenal kinase. It is still likely that protein kinases do play an obligatory role in ACTH stimulation of steroidogenesis.

This conclusion is supported by the observations of Riou et al.,[24] who examined protein kinase activity in human adrenal tumors unresponsive to ACTH in vivo and in vitro. One tumor studied had previously been shown to respond to ACTH stimulation with an increased production of cAMP, indicating that the activities of the membrane ACTH receptor and adenylate cyclase were intact. Total protein kinase activity, however, was found to be decreased. When total kinase activity was separated into several fractions by DEAE chromatography and compared with activity from hormonally responsive tissue, one fraction was absent from the unresponsive tumor. The correlation between loss of ACTH responsiveness and absence of at least one form of protein kinase supports the contention that protein kinase and cAMP play obligatory intermediate roles in ACTH-induced activation of steroidogenesis.

5.4. Adrenal Metabolism

5.4.1. Steroidogenesis

The rate-limiting step in steroid hormone synthesis is formation of pregnenolone from cholesterol. This step requires cleavage of the cholesterol side chain between carbons 20 and 22 and results in release of isocaproic acid. The enzyme that performs this function is located only within mitochondria. It is a mixed-function oxidase containing cytochrome P_{450} and requires reduced NADPH as well as adrenodoxin and adrenodoxin reductase to transfer electrons from NADPH to the cytochrome moiety. The precise mechanism by which ACTH regulates cholesterol side-chain cleavage (SCC) is not known. Current evidence suggests that this regulation occurs through control of available substrate cholesterol, although direct effects on the enzyme or on the availability of a cofactor, such as adrenodoxin, must also be considered. Considerable effort has recently been devoted to elucidating the structure and regulation of the SCC enzyme.

Wang and Kimura[25] reported the results of their purification and characterization of a mitochondrial cytochrome P_{450} containing an enzyme specific for cholesterol SCC activity. The enzyme, which was solubilized from bovine adrenal mitochondria by treatment with cholate and purified by affinity chromatography using an octylamine-substituted Sepharose column, was found to have a molecular weight of 60,000 by polyacylamide disk-gel electrophoresis. The enzyme was more than 90% pure as judged from disk-gel electrophoresis and contained 4.9 mol heme/mg protein. The purified protein possessed no 11-β-hydroxylase activity. The availability of the enzyme in purified form will permit further studies of its functional properties, and these studies should help in understanding the stimulatory effects of ACTH.

It has recently been possible to examine in intact mitochondria the interaction of substrate cholesterol with the cytochrome P_{450} that contains SCC enzyme. Two techniques have been employed. Cytochrome P_{450} absorbs light in the ultraviolet range. The amount of light absorbed and the wavelength of maximum absorption change with cholesterol binding. Also, the electron paramagnetic resonance (EPR) signal generated by the iron in SCC cytochrome P_{450} changes with binding of cholesterol. Thus, these two spectral properties can be measured to determine whether cholesterol is bound to the enzyme. Furthermore, EPR studies can be performed on intact tissue. Paul et al.[26] examined the effects of temperature on cholesterol binding by cytochrome P_{450} in isolated mitochondria obtained from hypophysectomized rats either treated with ACTH or left untreated. Both changes in the high-spin EPR signal of the ferric state of cytochrome P_{450} and Type I spectral changes, changes due to cholesterol binding, were reported. The increase in EPR signal and the Type I spectral change resulting from substrate cholesterol binding showed reversible changes with temperatures. At low temperatures, no binding could be detected for either treated or untreated rats, while at 22°C, spectral changes in mitochondria from ACTH-treated rats were four- to fivefold greater than in mitochondria from untreated rats. Reversibility could be demonstrated over several cycles of temperature change, and ACTH stimulation of enhanced binding could be prevented by cyclohexmide. Thus, the temperatures at which Type I heat-induced spectral changes are examined are important in estimating binding by this technique. In addition, by assuming that total mitochondrial cholesterol is available for cytochrome P_{450} binding, these authors extended their observations at various temperatures to allow calculations of the enthalpy and entropy of cholesterol binding. They conclude that cholesterol binding is largely entropically driven. This observation suggests that the action of ACTH may be to remove cholesterol from the mitochondrial membrane matrix and deliver it to the enzyme. The current data do not allow one to determine whether this movement requires a transport protein, as has been previously suggested.

Additional studies by Williams-Smith et al.[27] examined the EPR signals generated by intact adrenals from ACTH-treated and untreated hypophysectomized rats. The findings indicated that the amounts of adrenodoxin present were equal, and that all adrenodoxin was in the reduced form. Thus, the stimulatory effects of ACTH are probably not mediated by availability of adrenodoxin. Furthermore, in the intact gland, in contrast to isolated mitochondria, cytochrome P_{450} remains in the reduced ferrous state. Thus, in the intact tissue, binding of cholesterol leads to SCC, and measurements of EPR more clearly reflect the activity of the enzyme than in isolated mitochondria.

Together, these and previous studies[28] strongly indicate that it is the availability of substrate cholesterol for SCC that is regulated by ACTH. Many questions regarding this process, however, remain unanswered. Is it delivery to the mitochondria—which was previously shown to be enhanced by ACTH[28]—or is it subsequent intramitochondrial movement that is rate-limiting?

The stimulatory effect of ACTH on steroidogenesis can be rapidly inhibited by cycloheximide, indicating a requirement for new protein synthesis in this action of the hormone. For a more complete discussion, the reader is referred to the recent review by Gill.[29] In addition, ACTH stimulates total adrenal protein synthesis (see Section 5.5.1). The identity and precise function of the peptide with a short half-life that is demonstrable by cycloheximide inhibition and required for ACTH stimulation of steroidogenesis are unknown. Asano and Harding[30] recently showed, in the Y1 line of mouse adrenal tumor cells, that ACTH stimulates the synthesis of adrenodoxin within the cell cytosal. They also observed that ACTH stimulation of mitochondrial protein synthesis is required for incorporation of adrenodoxin into the mitochondria. It seems unlikely from the results of EPR studies cited above that adrenodoxin is the "labile" protein intermediate in the steroidogenic action of ACTH. Further studies will be necessary to resolve this question. Dazord et al.[31] further examined ACTH stimulation of protein synthesis in cultured Y1 mouse adrenal tumor cells by comparing the incorporation of labeled amino acids into specific peptides obtained from ACTH-stimulated and unstimulated cells. They reported that $ACTH_{1-24}$, as well as other stimuli to steroidogenesis such as NPS-ACTH, cAMP, and cholera toxin, enhance synthesis of a specific peptide of molecular weight 3500. Of particular interest was their further observation that only $ACTH_{1-24}$ and not the other stimuli tested caused an increase in total protein synthesis. The others appeared to stimulate only the synthesis of the low-molecular-weight peptide. Further identification of the structure and function of this peptide will be quite interesting.

5.4.2. Cholesterol Metabolism

Increasing interest has focused on adrenal cholesterol metabolism, not only because availability of substrate cholesterol is rate-limiting in ACTH-stimulated steroidogenesis, but also because investigation of cholesterol metabolism in the adrenal may help elucidate several general features of cellular cholesterol metabolism. Substrate cholesterol for mitochondrial SCC can be synthesized intracellularly, taken up from plasma lipoproteins, or mobilized by the action of cholesterol esterase from intracellular "lipid droplets." The mechanism of intracellular movement is not understood, but is of great importance not only in the adrenal, but also in other tissues.

Anderson and Dietschy[32-34] recently showed that in the rat adrenal, sterol synthesis from acetate is normally suppressed by circulating serum lipoproteins. Administration of the agent 4-aminopyrazolopyrimidine (4-APP), which is known to prevent hepatic release of serum lipoproteins, caused an almost 90% reduction in serum cholesterol and a greater than 50-fold enhancement in adrenal sterol synthesis. Reinfusion of either serum high-density (HDL) or low-density lipoprotein (LDL) caused inhibition of previously enhanced sterol synthesis. Balasubramanian et al.[35,36] subsequently showed that suppression of adrenal sterol synthesis by extracellular lipoproteins results from a decrease in the activity of the rate-limiting enzyme 3-hydroxy-3-methylglutaryl CoA (HMG-CoA) reductase, and is associated with changes in intracellular content of esterified, but not free, cholesterol. They observed that rats given 4-APP to lower serum cholesterol levels did not exhibit enhanced sterol synthesis unless ACTH was also available to deplete intracellular adrenal cholesterol content. In addition, these authors reported[36] that not only HMG-CoA reductase but also the enzyme immediately preceding it in the sterol biosynthetic pathway, HMG-CoA synthetase, respond to diurnal variations in the light–dark cycle and to depletion of cell cholesterol. Under these circumstances, the enzymes appear to be regulated coordinately. Thus, in the absence of extracellular cholesterol, the adrenal is capable of synthesizing the steroidogenic substrate, cholesterol.

When available, however, extracellular lipoprotein cholesterol is taken up into the cells. Gwynne et al.[37] showed that ACTH stimulates the uptake of cholesterol from HDL, but not from LDL, by quartered rat adrenal glands. The uptake process exhibited saturation kinetics and was greatly inhibited at low temperatures. Labeled cholesterol taken up from HDL was shown to be converted to pregnenolone by isolated mitochondria. Gwynne and Hess[38] further demonstrated the presence of a specific, reversible HDL membrane receptor site in the adrenal. It appears that ACTH stimulates adrenal HDL-receptor-site activity. Thus, one point at which ACTH may stimulate delivery of substrate cholesterol is by stimulating uptake from extracellular lipoproteins.

Additional sites of regulation also exist. One such site is in the stimulation of cholesterol esterase and mobilization of cholesterol ester stores.[39] Pittman and Steinberg[40] recently examined rat adrenal choles-

terol esterase activity. They reported the presence of two forms of cholesterol esterase, one with high and one with a low K_m for substrate. Both
forms were found in the 100,000 g supernatant of adrenal homogenates,
but could be separated not only kinetically, but also by gel filtration on 6%
agarose. The significance of these two forms of cholesterol esterase activity is not yet known. Both forms were activated by preincubation with
cAMP and Mg^{2+}-ATP in the presence of endogenous protein kinases.
Inhibition of protein kinase activity prevented activation. The two forms
of the enzyme may act on different endogenous substrates.

Stylianopoulou and Clayton[41] examined the effects of ACTH stimulation on cholesterol ester content and composition in males and females
of two strains of mice. Neither male nor female C57B1 mice showed
depletion, while cholesterol esters were acutely and markedly depleted in
both sexes of DBA/2 mice. They also observed, as was previously reported
in the rat,[42,43] that cholesterol arachidonate (C 20:4) appears to be preferentially hydrolyzed. No explanation for this observation is available. It
could reflect the structure of the various esters within lipid droplets, or
perhaps substrate specificity of the cholesterol esterases. It is clear from
the studies cited above that regulation of adrenal cholesterol metabolism is
complex and involves both hormonal and metabolic controls.

Little is yet known about the intracellular movement of cholesterol in
the adrenal. Recent studies by Falke et $al.$[44,45] examined adrenal metabolism of 25-OH-cholesterol. In other tissues, this cholesterol analogue
appears to move more freely than the less soluble parent cholesterol.
Falke and his co-workers observed that addition of 25-OH-cholesterol to
suspensions of rat adrenal cells results in enhanced corticosterone synthesis. Aminoglutethimide, but not cycloheximide, prevents this enhancement. Enhancement of corticosterone production by 25-OH-cholesterol
persists in the presence of submaximal but not maximal ACTH stimulation. These studies are consistent with the following formulation: Access
of cholesterol, but not of its 25-OH derivative, to mitochondria for SCC is
regulated by ACTH. At submaximal ACTH stimulation, the SCC enzyme
is not yet saturated with substrate, and consequently 25-OH-cholesterol
causes enhancement of activity, while at maximal ACTH stimulation,
endogenous cholesterol saturates the enzyme. These studies reinforce
studies of cytochrome P_{450} SCC activity cited earlier that indicate that the
delivery of cholesterol is rate-limiting. They further indicate that the
mechanism of delivery is specific for free cholesterol.

5.4.3. Prostaglandins

Prostaglandins (PGs) were previously shown to enhance steroid production in $vitro$ by bovine, murine, and feline adrenal preparations.[46] In

bovine adrenal slices, PGE_1 also increases intracellular levels of cAMP, suggesting that the stimulatory effects on steroidogenesis may be mediated, as with ACTH, by activation of adenylate cyclase. Honn and Chavin[47] extended these observations to human adrenals. They showed that both PGE_1 and PGE_2 enhance cortisol output and cAMP levels in diced normal human adrenal tissue. In addition, they observed that preincubation of adrenal fragments with indomethacin delayed the onset of subsequent ACTH stimulation of steroidogenesis, suggesting a link between PG function and the action of ACTH. Additional observations that suggest such a link were reported by Laychock and Rubin,[48] using isolated cat adrenal cells. At submaximal levels of ACTH stimulation, low concentrations of indomethacin (10^{-8} M) stimulate and high concentrations of indomethacin (10^{-5} M) inhibit stimulation of steroidogenesis. These authors further note, however, that PGs probably do not play an obligatory role in ACTH action, since at maximal ACTH doses, indomethacin has very little effect.

In addition to responding to PGs with enhanced steroid production, adrenal tissue also synthesizes PGs. Laychock and colleagues[49,50] showed that isolated cat adrenocortical cells synthesize PGs of both the E and the F series, and that ACTH enhances their rate of release. At low ACTH doses (10^{-9} M), indomethacin enhanced ATCH-stimulated PG synthesis, while at 10^{-5} M, significant inhibition occurred. In superfused adrenal glands, both NPS-ACTH and $ACTH_{1-24}$ were shown to enhance $PGF_2\alpha$ and PGE_2 release. Calcium deprivation prevented both enhanced steroidogenesis and PG release. The role of PGs in the steroidogenic actions of ACTH is not yet clear. Prostaglandins are probably not obligatory intermediates, but may play a role in modulating ACTH effects.

5.5. Regulation of Normal Adrenal Growth

5.5.1. ACTH Regulation

The trophic effects of ACTH on the adrenal are well known. In rats, *in vivo* administration of ACTH results in rapid stimulation of protein synthesis, followed at 3 hr by an increase in RNA content and finally at 16 hr by an increased incorporation of [³H]thymidine into DNA.[51] The mechanisms by which ACTH stimulates these processes are only poorly understood. To learn more about ACTH stimulation of RNA and protein synthesis, the effects of ACTH on various adrenal RNA polymerase activities in the guinea pig were recently examined by Fuhrman and Gill.[52-54] As in other tissues, three classes of RNA polymerase are recognized in the adrenal: RNA polymerase I, responsible for synthesis of ribosomal RNA; RNA polymerase II, responsible for synthesis of heterogeneous nuclear and messenger RNA; and RNA polymerase III, responsible for synthesis of pre-4 S-RNA, the precursor of transfer RNA, and 5 S-RNA. ACTH and db-cAMP administered *in vivo* stimulate by at least twofold the activity of nuclear RNA polymerase I when assayed *in vitro* using endogenous nuclear template. This enhancement of activity results from an increase in the rate of RNA chain elongation without a change in the numbers of chains being synthesized. That there was no change was ascertained by comparing both chain length and the number of chains being made *in vitro* by adrenal nuclei obtained from ACTH-treated and untreated guinea pigs.

Endogenous RNA polymerase II activity assayed *in vitro* is not stimulated, although a 50% increase in activity is observed if exogenous rather than endogenous DNA is used as the template. This finding suggests that template availability may be rate-limiting. Furthermore, the amount of extractable nuclear RNA polymerase II is increased by hormonal stimulation, suggesting that ACTH causes an increase in the actual number of RNA polymerase II molecules, even though endogenous activity appears not to be increased.

Finally, *in vivo* ACTH treatment also results in an increase in nuclear RNA polymerase III activity, as shown by the increase in synthesis of pre-4 S-RNA and 5 S-RNA. This enhancement in RNA polymerase III activity, like that of RNA polymerase II, results from an increase in the actual amount of the enzyme present. Interestingly, a second cytosolic pool of RNA polymerase III is unaffected by hormonal stimulation. Fuhrman and Gill[54] point out that ACTH stimulation of adrenal RNA polymerase activity is similar to the stimulation of fibroblast RNA polymerase activity induced in resting fibroblasts by addition of serum, and may represent a general pattern of cellular growth response. The mechanisms responsible for ACTH stimulation of RNA polymerase activity are not completely known, but are of broad interest in understanding not only adrenal growth but also regulation of growth in other tissues.

Saez *et al.*[55] further examined the effects of ACTH and glucocorticoids on adrenal DNA synthesis *in vivo*. As has been previously observed, either single or multiple *in vivo* injections of ACTH result in increased DNA synthesis, as indicated either by an increase in incorporation of [³H]thymidine into DNA or by an increase in DNA polymerase activity. Surprisingly, administration of dexamethasone caused a decrease in DNA synthesis. Consistent with this observation was the observation that aminoglutethimide causes increased [³H]thymidine incorporation, presumably as a result of its ability to decrease endogenous production of glucocorticoids. Finally, both actinomycin D and cycloheximide were effective in preventing ACTH stimulation of DNA synthesis.

The inhibitory effects of dexamethasone were further examined.

Since steroid hormone action requires binding to cytosolic proteins, these investigators sought to determine whether a steroid-binding protein was present in guinea pig adrenals. Only when adrenal homogenates were prepared from rats given aminoglutethimide and were subsequently treated with charcoal to remove as much endogenous glucocorticoid as possible was a binding protein consistently demonstrable. Nonetheless, such a steroid-binding protein appears to be present. The results cited above not only further confirm previous studies of the stimulatory effects of ACTH on DNA synthesis *in vivo,* but also indicate a possible role for glucocorticoids in regulation of adrenal growth.

Thus, *in vivo,* ACTH appears to stimulate both adrenal hypertrophy and hyperplasia. *In vitro,* however, ACTH was reported to cause cellular hypertrophy, but to inhibit DNA synthesis and cell division.[56,57] Weidman and Gill[58,59] examined the effects of ACTH and an analogue of cAMP, 8-Br-cAMP, on cell growth and division in the Y1 line of functional mouse adrenal cells in monolayer cultures. Either serum deprivation or addition of ACTH to complete media results in inhibition of DNA synthesis and arrest of cell growth in the G_1 phase of the cell cycle. Serum deprivation results in a negative pleiotropic response, while addition of ACTH has more specific effects. Cells arrested by the addition of ACTH have a larger mean volume and greater protein and RNA content than do cells arrested by serum deprivation. ACTH exerts its effects on an event that occurs early in the G_1 phase, as demonstrated by the fact that the ability of ACTH to inhibit serum-stimulated growth of resting cells decreases within 4 hr after the cells restart their growth. Cells arrested by addition of ACTH resemble hypertrophic adrenal cells *in vivo.* Similar observations regarding the effects of ACTH on growth of cultured bovine adrenocortical cells were reported by Gospodarowicz *et al.*[60] In addition, these workers noted that the ACTH dose–response curve for steroidogenesis and growth inhibition were nearly identical. Finally, they also reported that fibroblast growth factor is a potent mitogen for normal bovine adrenal cells. They took advantage of this observation to obtain cloned cultures of normal bovine adrenal cells. Further work is required to determine the physiological role of fibroblast growth factor in control of adrenal growth, and also to reconcile the differences in the observed effects of ACTH on adrenal growth *in vivo* and *in vitro.*

Considered together, the studies reviewed above suggest a self-consistent picture of the action of ACTH on adrenal growth. The primary effect of ACTH is to cause cellular hypertrophy and an increase in the unique differentiated functions of the adrenal gland. It seems quite possible, however, that growth factors other than ACTH play a more important role in adrenal hyperplasia.

5.5.2. Neural Regulation

Recent work by Engeland, Dallman, and their co-workers[61,62,63] indicates that neural factors may also play an important role in regulating adrenal growth. They observed that in rats undergoing unilateral adrenalectomy or simply adrenal manipulation, contralateral adrenal hypertrophy occurred, even though the animals had been previously hypophysectomized. Subsequent studies performed on rats with intact pituitaries indicated that contralateral glands remaining after unilateral adrenalectomy showed an increase not only in wet weight, but also in dry weight and DNA, RNA, and protein content, compared with glands from sham-operated controls. They further determined, by use of ^{51}Cr-labeled red cells, that the observed increases were not due to an increase in vascular space or retained blood. Finally, they noted that the time of day of operation and of subsequent sacrifice was not important in observing an increase in contralateral gland weight. Their results suggest that neural mechanisms are responsible, at least in part, for contralateral hypertrophy following unilateral adrenalectomy. In subsequent studies,[64] these workers showed that unilateral electrolytic lesions in the ventral hypothalamus or contralateral spinal cord hemisections between T_2 and T_3 prevent contralateral adrenal hypertrophy following unilateral adrenalectomy in the rat.

5.6. Abnormal Adrenal Function

5.6.1. Tests of the Hypothalamic–Pituitary–Adrenal Axis

It is frequently difficult to determine on clinical grounds alone whether hypercortisolism is present. This is particularly true in obese patients, who may have a "Cushingoid" appearance, or in patients with only minimal signs of hypercortisolism. Numerous tests have been found useful in suggesting the diagnosis of hypercortisolism, including measurement of 17-hydroxycorticosteroids or free cortisol in a 24-hr urine specimen, determination of the cortisol secretory rate, and evaluation of diurnal variations in plasma cortisol levels. For a detailed description of methods of procedure and outlines for interpreting the results of these well-established tests, the reader is referred to the recent review by Lagerquist and Tyler[65] or that by Gwinup and Johnson.[66]

Endogenous hypercortisolism usually results from a defect in normal suppressibility of the hypothalamic–pituitary–adrenal axis. The defect in regulation may occur at any level. Pituitary-dependent Cushing's syndrome—Cushing's disease—results from loss of suppression of pituitary ACTH release by normal levels of circulating cortisol, while adrenal tumors lead to loss of suppression at the level of the adrenal gland itself. Thus, the inability of low doses of dexamethasone (0.5 mg every 6 hr for 48 hr) to suppress production of glucocorticoids as judged from measurements of urinary 17-hydroxycorticosteroids is generally accepted as establishing the diagnosis of Cushing's syndrome.[67] Furthermore, administration of high doses of dexamethasone provides additional information regarding the cause of hypercortisolism. An alternative, simplified screening procedure is measurement of the plasma cortisol concentration following administration of 1 mg dexamethasone at 11:00 or 12:00 P.M. the previous night.[68] An additional screening test that requires only measurement of 11-hydroxycorticosteroids in an overnight urine sample was recently reported by Mattingly and Tyler.[69] A total of 127 women, including 29 normals, 49 obese normals, 38 hirsute women, and 11 women with Cushing's syndrome as determined by the standard dexamethasone suppression tests, were examined. Only one false-negative and no false-positive results were encountered. Further testing in larger numbers of patients and different groups of patients, including males, will be required to firmly establish the value of this test.

With prolonged suppression of pituitary ACTH release, such as occurs in patients with adrenal tumors or with ectopic ACTH production, pituitary reserve becomes diminished. The metyrapone test offers a means of assessing pituitary reserve and differentiating pituitary-dependent Cushing's syndrome from autonomous adrenal function or ectopic ACTH.[70] In normal persons, metyrapone inhibition of 11-β-hydroxylase decreases the level of circulating cortisol, which in turn stimulates ACTH release. Since metyrapone produces only a partial block in enzyme activity, enhanced ACTH levels lead to a compensatory increase in cortisol production, but only at the expense of an increase in the synthesis of 11-deoxycortisol (compound S). In the absence of pituitary reserve, no increase in the secretion of compound S is observed. In fact, when pituitary reserve is compromised, serum levels of compound S show a previously unexplained decrease, suggesting that metyrapone may have a second effect in addition to blocking 11-β-hydroxylase. Previous *in vitro* studies suggested that metyrapone might also partially block cholesterol SCC.[71] Carballeira et al.[72] examined this possibility further by comparing apparent cholesterol SCC and 11-β-hydroxylase activity *in vivo* with that of mitochondria isolated from adrenals obtained at surgery from two patients, one with bilateral adrenal hyperplasia and one with an adrenal adenoma. Apparent "activity" for adrenal cholesterol SCC *in vivo* was calculated from the sum of total urinary 17-hydroxy- and 17-ketocorticosteroids, while apparent 11-β-hydroxylase activity *in vivo* was calculated from measurements of urinary 11-oxy- and 11-deoxysteroids. In the patient with adrenal hyperplasia, metyrapone *in vivo* caused an increase in apparent cholesterol SCC, while *in vitro,* it inhibited SCC. In the patient with an adrenal adenoma, in contrast, inhibition by metyrapone was observed both *in vivo* and *in vitro.* Here, where there was no ongoing ACTH stimulation *in vivo,* metyrapone elicited no apparent *in vivo* increase in SCC activity. These results indicate that the apparent increase in SCC activity that follows metyrapone administration *in vivo* is secondary to stimulation by ACTH, while, in fact, metyrapone actually antagonizes mitochondrial SCC, producing a drop in compound S production in the absence of pituitary reserve.

Failure to respond to metyrapone with an increase in compound S production may result from a lack of pituitary ACTH reserve or a failure of the adrenal to respond to ACTH stimulation. Administration of exogenous ACTH and measurement of steroid response permits differentiation of these possibilities. Redman and Faas[73] reported the occurrence of unilateral adrenal hemorrhage following administration of ACTH to a patient with Cushing's syndrome and pointed out the potential hazards of prolonged ACTH stimulation.

The potential usefulness of measurements of intermediates in the cortisol synthetic pathway for discriminating among various causes of Cushing's syndrome was evaluated by McKenna *et al.*[74,75] They observed that both A.M. and P.M., as well as dexamethasone-suppressed, levels of plasma 17-hydroxypregnenolone were normal in patients with Cushing's disease, ectopic ACTH syndrome, and adrenal adenomas. In 4 of 6 patients with adrenal carcinomas, however, plasma 17-hydroxypregnenolone levels were elevated. They also observed that 17-hydroxypregnenolone was elevated in patients with poorly controlled congenital adrenal hyperplasia due to 21-hydroxylase deficiency. Thus, measurements of plasma 17-hydroxypregnenolone appear to be useful in two situations: differentiation of adrenal carcinomas from adenomas and management of congenital adrenal hyperplasia.

Differentiation of the various causes of Cushing's syndrome depends not only on biochemical tests, but also on morphological tests. Kehlet *et al.*[76] compared the efficiency of three procedures—ultrasound, [131I]19-iodocholesterol scintigraphy, and aortography—in localizing adrenal lesions. Of 18 consecutive patients with adrenal cortical disease taken to surgery, 9 had bilateral hyperplasia, 8 had an adrenal tumor, and 1 is reported as having unilateral adrenal hypertrophy. Excluding the latter patient, ultrasound examination resulted in no false positives and only 1 of a possible 8 false negatives. On the other hand, [131I]19-iodocholesterol provided correct identification of all lesions, while aortography resulted in 1 positive and 3 false negatives. The smallest lesion identified by ultrasound in this series measured 5 × 3 centimeters, while the only lesion missed by ultrasound measured somewhat less than 3 × 3 centimeters.

Thus, ultrasound appears to have a possible role in screening for unilateral adrenal lesions. Identification of an adrenal adenoma by ultrasound could alleviate the need for the more expensive procedures with greater risk, such as arteriography. It is hoped that additional reports concerning this technique will soon appear.

Selective venous catherization coupled with radioimmunoassay of ACTH offers a useful approach to distinguishing between Cushing's disease and the ectopic ACTH syndrome. Corrigan et al.[77] reported the successful use of this procedure in identifying the pituitary as the source of unregulated ACTH production.

5.6.2. Pituitary-Dependent Cushing's Syndrome (Cushing's Disease)

The primary pathogenetic abnormality in pituitary-dependent Cushing's syndrome may reside either in the pituitary corticotrophs or in hypothalamic regulation of corticotropic activity. In most cases, it is not yet possible to distinguish between these possibilities. About 10% of patients with Cushing's disease have a pituitary adenoma at the time of initial presentation. Some degree of normal regulation is retained, however, as indicated by high-dose dexamethasone suppression and metyrapone stimulation tests in patients with Cushing's disease, with and without adenoma. This observation has been taken to indicate that corticotropin function is normal, but that hypothalamic regulation is not. In addition, the effectiveness of cyproheptadine in suppressing ACTH release in Cushing's disease further suggests that the primary abnormality resides in CNS regulation of pituitary activity. Moreover, the abnormal increase in plasma ACTH concentration elicited by TRH in patients with untreated Cushing's disease, as reported by Krieger and Luria,[78] indicates again an abnormality of hypothalamic regulation.

On the other hand, cases such as that reported by Lagerquist et al.,[79] in which normal hypothalamic–pituitary function is regained following resection of a pituitary adenoma, argue strongly that the primary disorder in autonomous corticotroph hyperactivity. The report by Tyrrell et al.[80] of normal growth hormone response to hypoglycemia after correction of hypercortisolism, although it differs from previous observations by James,[81] does not support the concept of generalized hypothalamic dysfunction in Cushing's disease. It is therefore not yet possible to reach a definitive conclusion regarding the role of hypothalamic regulation in the pathogenesis of Cushing's disease.

It is quite clear that hypothalamic regulation of pituitary corticotroph activity is very complex. In addition to cyproheptadine, a number of hormonal and other pharmacological agents have recently been found to

affect ACTH release under various circumstances. Hsu et al.[82] examined
the effects of L-dopa on the pituitary response to metyrapone inhibition of
steroid production in monkeys. Although L-dopa alone did not alter basal
levels of compound S, the metyrapone-induced rise in serum ACTH and
compound S concentrations in animals receiving L-dopa was significantly
greater than that which occurred in corresponding controls. These
results, coupled with earlier observations on the effect of L-dopa on
ACTH release, suggest that in addition to serotonergic regulation, release
of ACTH may also be regulated by dopaminergic pathways. That it is is
further supported by the observation of Benker et al.,[83] who reported that
oral bromacryptine, a dopaminergic agent, caused suppression of ACTH
release in two patients with Cushing's disease. These workers also
observed that growth-hormone-release-inhibiting factor, somatostatin,
suppressed ACTH release in the same two patients. Thus, increasing
evidence of the complexity of hypothalamic regulation of pituitary ACTH
release is accumulating. A comprehensive picture of the factors that
regulate ACTH secretion is not yet available.

The optimal therapy for Cushing's disease has not yet been developed. Available forms of therapy include pituitary ablation or bilateral
adrenalectomy. Both surgical and radiation therapy of the pituitary have
been employed. Surgically, the use of the transsphenoidal approach for
resections of pituitary microadenomas appears to be quite promising.
Only a few scattered case reports have yet appeared,[79,84,85] but promising
results have been obtained. The advantages of this form of therapy are
clear: normal pituitary function is preserved, and there is no need for
continued maintenance of glucocorticoid therapy. If the primary lesion is
hypothalamic and pituitary adenomas are observed to recur, however,
transsphenoidal removal of the microadenoma may not be as attractive as
it currently appears to be.

Lawrence et al.[86] reported their experience with heavy-particle irradiation in the treatment of Cushing's disease. Of 32 patients treated with
8000–11,000 rads of α-particle radiation (plateau portion), 20 are
reported to have had complete, and 5 partial, remission, while 7 required
subsequent adrenalectomy. Those with complete remission were followed
for from 6 months to 16 years, while those with partial remission were
followed for up to 2 years. The mean time between treatment and
remission is not indicated, nor are precise data on the posttreatment
function of the pituitary adrenal axis given. The authors do report,
however, that of those patients available for study, none regained normal
circadian rhythm in cortisol secretion. No patients were subsequently
observed to develop Nelson's syndrome. Four patients did subsequently
require steroid-replacement therapy. This report confirms that heavy-
particle irradiation is effective in treating Cushing's disease in a large

percentage of cases. Complications of heavy-particle therapy appear to be few, although the report of Lawrence and co-workers does not indicate the status of pituitary TSH and gonadotropin function following treatment for Cushing's disease. In one instance, treatment was rapidly followed by the onset of Addisonian crisis.[87] This occurrence was attributed to radiation-induced infarction of a pituitary adenoma, a complication also reported to follow conventional radiation treatment.

Although transsphenoidal resection of pituitary adenomas currently appears to be a promising approach to treatment of Cushing's syndrome, no data from large numbers of patients are available to indicate the rate of complications.

5.6.3. Nelson's Syndrome

Enlargement of the sella turcica occurs in approximately 10% of patients with pituitary-dependent Cushing's disease who undergo bilateral adrenalectomy. Moore et al.[88] reported the experience at the Peter Bent Brigham Hospital with Nelson's syndrome in the last 120 patients with Cushing's disease. Of the 120 patients, 9 (7.5%) developed the syndrome from 6 months to 16 years after operation. The development of Nelson's syndrome in this series was not prevented by conventional pituitary irradiation at the time of adrenalectomy, since 2 of 20 such patients previously irradiated subsequently manifested pituitary tumors. The mean length of survival to date in this series of patients is 9.7 years. Only 1 of 9 patients succumbed to pituitary disease.

The pathogenesis of Nelson's syndrome is as poorly understood as that of Cushing's disease. It has been suggested that the syndrome results from postoperative hypothalamic stimulation of previously subclinical pituitary adenomas. In this regard, Krieger and Luria[89] reported that 3 of 4 patients with Nelson's syndrome responded to treatment with cyproheptadine (24 mg/day) for periods of 3–5 months with significant decreases in plasma ACTH concentration. Thus, it appears that in many cases, hypothalamic controls of pituitary function remain at least partially intact.

Treatment of Nelson's syndrome requires primarily a consideration of pituitary enlargement and its consequent neurological effects. Alternative approaches include surgical treatment and irradiation. Different forms of radiation therapy continue to be evaluated. Lawrence et al.[86] reported that 6 of 9 patients with Nelson's syndrome showed decreased pigmentation, and 3 of 9 showed arrest of increasing pigmentation, subsequent to heavy-particle irradiation. No other data were given, and although this report indicates a favorable response, little can be concluded from it without further evaluation of neurological status. Cassar et al.[90] reported the results of treatment by pituitary implantation of yttrium-90 or gold-198 in 8 patients with Nelson's syndrome. One patient had cranial nerve involvement, but 7 of the 8 had abnormal sellar radiographs. Two patients developed complications. One had a transient third-nerve palsy, while a second developed a CSF leak and diabetes insipidus. Otherwise, pituitary function appeared to remain intact without requirements for hormone replacement other than glucocorticoids. All patients had a decrease in pigmentation, and none showed further sellar changes.

ACKNOWLEDGMENT

The authors wish to acknowledge the fine assistance of Mrs. Glenda Foushee in the preparation of this chapter.

References

1. Oelofsen, W., 1975, The chemistry of the adrenocorticotropins and the melanotropins, *Pharmacol. Ther. B* **1**:459–500.
2. Felber, J. P., 1975, Immunochemistry of adrenocorticotropin, melanotropins and lipotropins, *Pharmacol. Ther. B* **1**:571–586.
3. Yalow, R. S., and Berson, S. A., 1971, Size heterogeneity of innumoreactive human ACTH in plasma and in extracts of pituitary glands and ACTH-producing thymoma, *Biochem. Biophys. Res. Commun.* **44**:439–445.
4. Gewirtz, G., Schneider, B., Krieger, D. T., and Yalow, R. S., 1974, Big ACTH: Conversion to biologically active ACTH by trypsin, *J. Clin. Endocrinol. Metab.* **38**:227–230.
5. Eipper, B. A., and Mains, R. E., 1975, High molecular weight forms of adrenocorticotropic hormone in the mouse pituitary and in a mouse pituitary tumor cell line, *Biochemistry* **14**:3836–3844.
6. Mains, R. E., and Eipper, B. A., 1976, Biosynthesis of adrenocorticotropic hormone in mouse pituitary tumor cells, *J. Biol. Chem.* **251**:4115–4120.
7. Eipper, B. A., Mains, R. E., and Guenzi, D., 1976, High molecular weight forms of adrenocorticotropic hormone are glycoproteins, *J. Biol. Chem.* **251**:4121–4126.
8. Nakanishi, S., Taii, S., Hirata, Y., Matsukura, S., Imura, H., and Numa, S., 1976, A large product of cell-free translation of messenger RNA coding for corticotropin, *Proc. Natl. Acad. Sci. U.S.A.* **73**:4319–4323.
9. Krieger, D. T., Choi, H.-S. H., and Anderson, P. J., 1976, The characterization of the ACTH produced by a primary pituitary tumour in a patient with Cushing's disease, *Clin. Endocrinol. (Oxford)* **5**:455–472.
10. Orth, D. N., and Nicholson, W., 1977, High molecular weight forms of human ACTH are glycoproteins, *J. Clin. Endocrinol. Metab.* **44**:214–217.
11. Pelletier, G., Leclerc, R., Labrie, F., Cote, J., Chretien, M., and Lis, M., 1977, Immunohistochemical localization of β-lipotropic hormone in the pituitary gland, *Endocrinology* **100**:770–776.
12. Guillemin, R., 1977, Endorphins, brain peptides that act like opiates, *N. Engl. J. Med.* **296**:226–228.

13. Baumann, G., and Felber, J.-P., 1976, Prolonged corticotropic action of synthetic human ACTH in man, *J. Clin. Endocrinol. Metab.* **42**:160–163.
14. Otsuka, H., and Inouye, L. K., 1975, Structure–activity relationships of adrenocorticotropin, *Pharmacol. Ther. B* **1**:501–527.
15. Moyle, W. R., Kong, Y. C., and Ramachandran, J., 1973, Steroidogenesis and cyclic adenosine 3′,5′-monosphosphate accumulation in rat adrenal cells, *J. Biol. Chem.* **248**:2409–2417.
16. Ramachandran, J., Kong, Y. C., and Liles, S., 1976, Effects of ACTH and its O-nitrophenyl sulphenyl derivative on adrenocortical function *in vivo*, *Acta Endocrinol.* (Copenhagen) **82**:587–599.
17. Finn, F. M., Johns, P. A., Nishi, N., and Hofmann, K., 1976, Differential response to adrenocorticotropic hormone analogs of bovine adrenal plasma membranes and cells, *J. Biol. Chem.* **251**:3576–3585.
18. Ways, D. K., Zimmerman, C. F., and Ontjes, D. A., 1976, Inhibition of adrenocorticotropic effects on adrenal cell membranes by synthetic adrenocorticotropin analogues: Correlation of binding and adenylate cyclase activation, *Mol. Pharmacol.* **12**:789–799.
19. Lowry, P. J., Rees, L. H., Tomlin, S., Gillies, G., and Landon, J., 1976, Chemical characterization of ectopic ACTH purified from a malignant thymic carcinoid tumor, *J. Clin. Endocrinol. Metab.* **43**:831–835.
20. Wolff, J., and Cook, G. H., 1977, Activation of steroidogenesis and adenylate cyclase by adenosine in adrenal and Leydig tumor cells, *J. Biol. Chem.* **252**:687–693.
21. Glossmann, H., and Gips, H., 1976, Adrenal cortex adenylate cyclase. Is Ca^{2+} involved in ACTH stimulation?, *Naunyn-Schmiedebergs Arch. Pharmakol.* **292**:199–203.
22. Haksar, A., Maudsley, D. V., Peron, F. G., and Bedigian, E., 1976, Lanthanum: Inhibition of ACTH-stimulated cyclic AMP and corticosterone synthesis in isolated rat adrenocortical cells, *J. Cell Biol.* **68**:142–153.
23. Moyle, W. R., MacDonald, G. J., and Garfink, J. E., 1976, Role of histone kinases as mediators of corticotropin-induced steroidogenesis, *Biochem. J.* **160**:1–9.
24. Riou, J., Evain, D., Perrin, F., and Saez, J. M., 1977, Adenosine 3′5′-cyclic monophosphate dependent protein kinase in human adrenocortical tumors, *J. Clin. Endocrinol. Metab.* **44**:413–419.
25. Wang, H., and Kimura, T., 1976, Purification and characterization of adrenal cortex mitochondrial cytochrome P-450 specific for cholesterol side chain cleavage activity, *J. Biol. Chem.* **251**:6068–6074.
26. Paul, D. P., Gallant, S., Orme-Johnson, N. R., Orme-Johnson, W. H., and Brownie, A. C., 1976, Temperature dependence of cholesterol binding to cytochrome P-450$_{scc}$ of the rat adrenal. Effect of adrenocorticotropic hormone and cycloheximide, *J. Biol. Chem.* **251**:7120–7126.
27. Williams-Smith, D. L., Simpson, E. R., Barlow, S. M., and Morrison, P. J., 1976, Electron paramagnetic resonance studies of cytochrome *P*-450 and adrenal ferredoxin in single whole rat adrenal glands, *Biochim. Biophys. Acta* **449**:72–83.
28. Mahaffee, D., Reitz, R. C., and Ney, R. L., 1974, The mechanism of action of adrenocorticotropic hormone: The role of mitochondrial cholesterol accumulation in the regulation of steroidogenesis, *J. Biol. Chem.* **249**:227–233.
29. Gill, G. N., 1976, ACTH regulation of the adrenal cortex, *Pharmacol. Ther. B* **2**:313–338.

30. Asano, K., and Harding, B. W., 1976, Biosynthesis of adrenodoxin in mouse adrenal tumor cells, *Endocrinology* **99**:977–987.
31. Dazord, A., Gallet, D., and Saez, J. M., 1977, ACTH-dependent stimulation of a specific peptide in adrenocortical cells in culture, *Biochem. Biophys. Res. Commun.* **76**:1238–1246.
32. Andersen, J. M., and Dietschy, J. M., 1976, Regulation of sterol synthesis in adrenal gland of the rat by both high and low density human plasma lipoproteins, *Biochem. Biophys. Res. Commun.* **72**:880–885.
33. Andersen, J. M., and Dietschy, J. M., 1977, Regulation of sterol synthesis in 16 tissues of rat. I. Effect of diurnal light cycling, fasting, stress, manipulation of enterohepatic circulation, and administration of chylomicrons and triton, *J. Biol. Chem.* **252**:3646–3651.
34. Andersen, J. M., and Dietschy, J. M., 1977, Regulation of sterol synthesis in 15 tissues of rat. II. Role of rat and human high and low density plasma lipoproteins and of rat chylomicron remnants, *J. Biol. Chem.* **252**:3652–3659.
35. Balasubramaniam, S., Goldstein, J. L., Faust, J. R., Brunschede, G. Y., and Brown, M. S., 1977, Lipoprotein-mediated regulation of 3-hydroxy-3-methylglutaryl coenzyme A reductase activity and cholesterol ester metabolism in the adrenal gland of the rat, *J. Biol. Chem.* **252**:1771–1779.
36. Balasubramaniam, S., Goldstein, J., and Brown, M., 1977, Regulation of cholesterol synthesis in rat adrenal gland through coordinate control of 3-hydroxy-3-methylglutaryl coenzyme A synthase and reductase activities, *Proc. Natl. Acad. Sci. U.S.A.* **74**:1421–1425.
37. Gwynne, J. T., Mahaffee, D., Brewer, H. B., Jr., and Ney, R. L., 1976, Adrenal cholesterol uptake from plasma lipoproteins: Regulation by corticotropin, *Proc. Natl. Acad. Sci. U.S.A.* **73**:4329–4333.
38. Gwynne, J., and Hess, B., 1977, Binding and degradation of human 125$_{I-HDL}$ by rat adrenocortical cells, *Metabolism* (in press).
39. Beckett, G. J., and Boyd, G. S., 1975, Evidence for the activation of bovine adrenal cholesterol ester hydrolase by a phosphorylation involving an adenosine 3':5'-monophosphate-dependent protein kinase, *Biochem. Soc. Trans.* **3**:892–894.
40. Pittman, R. C., and Steinberg, D., 1977, Activatable cholesterol esterase and triacylglycerol lipase activities of rat adrenal and their relationship, *Biochim. Biophys. Acta* **487**:431–444.
41. Stylianopoulou, F., and Clayton, R. B., 1976, Strain-dependent gonadal effects upon the response of adrenal cholesterol esters to ACTH in C57BL/10J and DBA/2J mice, *Endocrinology* **99**:1638–1644.
42. Beckett, G. J., and Boyd, G. S., 1975, The effect of dietary rape-seed oil on cholesterol-ester metabolism and cholesterol-ester-hydrolase activity in rat adrenal, *Eur. J. Biochem.* **53**:335–342.
43. Naghshineh, S., Treadwell, C. R., Gallo, L., and Vahouny, G. V., 1974, Activation of adrenal sterol ester hydrolase by dibutyryl cAMP and protein kinase, *Biochem. Biophys. Res. Commun.* **61**:1076–1082.
44. Falke, H. E., Degenhart, H. J., Abeln, G. J., and Visser, H., 1975, Studies on isolated rat adrenal cell metabolism of hydroxylated sterols, *Mol. Cell. Endocrinol.* **3**:375–383.
45. Falke, H. E., Degenhart, H. J., Abeln, G. J., and Visser, H., 1976, Effects of 25-hydroxycholesterol and aminoglutethimide in isolated rat adrenal cells: A model for congenital lipoid adrenal hyperplasia?, *Mol. Cell. Endocrinol.* **4**:107–114.

46. Saruta, T., and Kaplan, N. M., 1972, Adrenocortical steroidogenesis: The effects of prostaglandins, *J. Clin. Invest.* **51**:2246–2251.
47. Honn, K. V., and Chavin, W., 1976, Prostaglandin modulation of the mechanism of ACTH action in the human adrenal, *Biochem. Biophys. Res. Commun.* **73**:164–170.
48. Laychock, S. G., and Rubin, R. P., 1976, Indomethacin-induced alterations in corticosteroid and prostaglandin release by isolated adrenocortical cells of the cat, *Br. J. Pharmacol.* **57**:273–278.
49. Laychock, S. G., and Rubin, R. P., 1976, Radioimmunoassay measurement of ACTH-facilitated PGE_2 and $PGE_{2\alpha}$ release from isolated cat adrenocortical cells, *Prostaglandins* **11**:753–767.
50. Laychock, S. G., Warner, W., and Rubin, R. P., 1977, Further studies on the mechanisms controlling prostaglandin biosynthesis in the cat adrenal cortex: The role of calcium and cyclic AMP, *Endocrinology* **100**:74–81.
51. Inrie, R. C., Ramiah, T. R., Antoni, F., and Hutchinson, W. C., 1965, The effect of adrenocorticotrophin on the nucleic acid metabolism of the rat adrenal gland, *J. Endocrinol.* **32**:303–313.
52. Fuhrman, S. A., and Gill, G. N., 1974, Hormonal control of adrenal RNA polymerase activities, *Endocrinology* **94**:691–700.
53. Fuhrman, S. A., and Gill, G. N., 1975, Adrenocorticotropic hormone stimulation of adrenal RNA polymerase I and III activities. Nucleotide incorporation into internal positions and 3′ chain termini, *Biochemistry* **14**:2925–2933.
54. Fuhrman, S. A., and Gill, G. N., 1976, Adrenocorticotropic hormone regulation of adrenal RNA polymerases. Stimulation of nuclear RNA polymerase III, *Biochemistry* **15**:5520–5527.
55. Saez, J. M., Morera, A. M., and Gallet, D., 1977, Opposite effects of ACTH and glucocorticoids on adrenal DNA synthesis *in vivo*, *Endocrinology* **100**:1268–1275.
56. Ramachandran, J., and Suyama, A. T., 1975, Inhibition of replication of normal adrenocortical cells in culture by adrenocorticotropin, *Proc. Natl. Acad. Sci. U.S.A.* **72**:113–117.
57. O'Hare, J. M., and Neville, A. M., 1973, Effects of adrenocorticotrophin on steroidogenesis and proliferation by adult adrenal cells in monolayer culture, *Biochem. Soc. Trans.* **1**:1088–1091.
58. Weidman, E. R., and Gill, G. N., 1977, Differential effects of ACTH or 8-Br-cAMP on growth and replication in a functional adrenal tumor cell line, *J. Cell. Physiol.* **90**:91–103.
59. Gill, G. N., and Weidman, E. R., 1977, Hormonal regulation of initiation of DNA synthesis and of differentiated function in Y-1 adrenal cartical cells, *J. Cell Physiol.* **92**:65–76.
60. Gospodarowicz, D., III, C. R., Hornsby, P. J., and Gill, G. N., 1977, Control of bovine adrenal cortical cell proliferation by fibroblast growth factor: Lack of effect of epidermal growth factor, *Endocrinology* **100**:1080–1089.
61. Engeland, W. C., Shinsako, J., and Dallman, M. F., 1975, Corticosteroids and ACTH are not required for compensatory adrenal growth, *Am. J. Physiol.* **229**:1461–1464.
62. Engeland, W. C., and Dallman, M. F., 1975, Compensatory adrenal growth is neurally mediated, *Neoroendocrinology* **19**:352–362.
63. Dallman, M. F., Engeland, W. C., and Shinsako, J., 1976, Compensatory adrenal growth: A neurally mediated reflex, *Am. J. Physiol.* **231**:408–414.

64. Engeland, W. C., and Dallman, M. F., 1976, Neural mediation of compensatory adrenal growth, *Endocrinology* **99**:1659–1662.
65. Lagerquist, L., and Tyler, F., 1976, Diagnosis and treatment of disorders of the adrenal cortex, *Pharmacol. Ther. C* **1**:259–277.
66. Gwinup, G., and Johnson, B., 1975, Clinical testing of the hypothalamic–pituitary–adrenocortical system in states of hypo- and hypercortisolism, *Metabolism* **24**:777–791.
67. Liddle, G. W., 1960, Tests of pituitary–adrenal suppressibility in the diagnosis of Cushing's syndrome, *J. Clin. Endocrinol. Metab.* **20**:1539–1560.
68. Eddy, R. L., Jones, A. L., Gilliland, P. F., Ibarra, J. D., Jr., Thompson, J. Q., and McMurray, J. F., Jr., 1973, Cushing's syndrome: A prospective study of diagnostic methods, *Am. J. Med.* **55**:621–630.
69. Mattingly, D., and Tyler, C., 1976, Overnight urinary 11-hydroxycorticosteroid estimations in diagnosis of Cushing's syndrome, *Br. Med. J.* **2**:668–669.
70. Liddle, G. W., Estep, H. L., Kendall, J., Williams, W. C., Jr., and Townes, A. W., 1959, Clinical application of a new test of pituitary reserve, *J. Clin. Endocrinol. Metab.* **19**:875–894.
71. Cheng, S. C., Harding, B. W., and Carballeira, A., 1974, Effects of metyrapone on pregnenolone biosynthesis and on cholesterol–cytochrome P-450 interaction in the adrenal, *Endocrinology* **94**:1451–1458.
72. Carballeira, A., Fishman, L. M., and Jacobi, J. D., 1976, Dual sites of inhibition by metyrapone of human adrenal steroidogenesis: Correlation of *in vivo* and *in vitro* studies, *J. Clin. Endocrinol. Metab.* **42**:687–695.
73. Redman, J. F., and Faas, F. H., 1976, Acute unilateral adrenal hemorrhage following ACTH administration in a patient with Cushing's syndrome, *Am. J. Med.* **61**:533–536.
74. McKenna, T. J., Miller, R. B., and Liddle, G. W., 1977, Plasma pregnenolone and 17-OH-pregnenolone in patients with adrenal tumors, ACTH excess, or idiopathic hirsutism, *J. Clin. Endocrinol. Metab.* **44**:231–236.
75. McKenna, T. J., Jennings, A. S., Liddle, G. W., and Burr, I. M., 1977, Pregnenolone, 17-OH-pregnenolone, and testosterone in plasma of patients with congenital adrenal hyperplasia, *J. Clin. Endocrinol. Metab.* **42**:918–925.
76. Kohlet, H., Blichert-Toft, M., Hancke, S., Pedersen, J. F., Kristensen, J. K., Efsen, F., Dige-Petersen, H., Fogh, J., Lockwood, K., and Hasner, E., 1976, Comparative study of ultrasound, ^{131}I-19-iodocholesterol scintigraphy, and aortography in localising adrenal lesions, *Br. Med. J.* **2**:665–667.
77. Corrigan, D. F., Schaaf, M., Whaley, R. A., Czerwinski, C. L., and Earll, J. M., 1977, Selective venous sampling to differentiate ectopic ACTH secretion from pituitary Cushing's syndrome, *N. Engl. J. Med.* **296**:861–862.
78. Krieger, D. T., and Luria, M., 1977, Plasma ACTH and cortisol responses to TRF, vasopressin or hypoglycemia in Cushing's disease and Nelson's syndrome, *J. Clin. Endocrinol. Metab.* **44**:361–368.
79. Lagerquist, L. G., Meikle, A. W., West, C. D., and Tyler, F. H., 1974, Cushing's disease with cure by resection of a pituitary adenoma, *Am. J. Med.* **57**:826–830.
80. Tyrrell, J. B., Wiener-Kronish, J., Lorenzi, M., Brooks, R. M., and Forsham, P. H., 1977, Cushing's disease: Growth hormone response to hypoglycemia after correction of hypercortisolism, *J. Clin. Endocrinol. Metab.* **44**:218–221.
81. James, V. H. T., Landon, J., Wynn, V., and Greenwood, F. C., 1968, A fundamental defect in adrenocortical control in Cushing's disease, *J. Endocrinol.* **40**:15–28.
82. Hsu, T.-H., Hsu, C. K., and Gann, D. S., 1976, Potentiation of the ACTH

response to metyrapone by L-Dopa in the monkey, *Endocrinology* **99**:1115–1118.

83. Benker, G., Hackenberg, K., Hamburger, B., and Reinwein, D., 1976, Effects of growth hormone release-inhibiting hormone and bromocryptine (CB 154) in states of abnormal pituitary–adrenal function, *Clin. Endocrinol.* **5**:187–190.

84. Decker, R. E., Epstein, J. A., Carras, R., and Rosenthal, A. D., 1976, Transsphenoidal microsurgery for pituitary tumors: Experience with 45 cases, *Mt. Sinai J. Med. N.Y.* **43**:565–577.

85. Ganguly, A., Stanchfield, J., Roberts, R., West, C., and Tyler, F., 1976, Cushing's syndrome in a patient with an empty sella turcica and a microadenoma of the adenohypophysis, *Am. J. Med.* **60**:306–309.

86. Lawrence, J. H., Tobias, C. A., Linfoot, J. A., Born, J. L., and Chong, C. Y., 1976, Heavy-particle therapy in acromegaly and Cushing's disease, *J. Am. Med. Assoc.* **235**:2307–2310.

87. Cook, D. M., Jordan, R. M., Kendall, J. W., and Linfoot, J. A., 1976, Rapid appearance of transient secondary adrenocortical insufficiency after alpha-particle radiation therapy for Cushing's disease, *J. Clin. Endocrinol. Metab.* **43**:295–300.

88. Moore, T. J., Dluhy, R. G., Williams, G. H., and Cain, J. P., 1976, Nelson's syndrome: Frequency, prognosis, and effect of prior pituitary irradiation, *Ann. Intern. Med.* **85**:731–734.

89. Krieger, D. T., and Luria, M., 1976, Effectiveness of cyproheptadine in decreasing plasma ACTH concentrations in Nelson's syndrome, *J. Clin. Endocrinol. Metab.* **43**:1179–1182.

90. Cassar, J., Doyle, F. H., Lewis, P. D., Mashiter, K., Van Noorden, S., and Joplin, G. F., 1976, Treatment of Nelson's syndrome by pituitary implantation of yttrium-90 or gold-198, *Br. Med. J.* **2**:269–272.

.

Aldosterone and the Renin–Angiotensin System

Edward G. Biglieri

6.1. Introduction

Measurement of the components of the mineralocorticoid hormone pathway to aldosterone and of the renin–angiotensin system (RAS) has now been coupled with the ability to measure an effective competitive antagonist of angiotensin II, a converting enzyme inhibitor, and smaller but active fragments of angiotensin II. This combination has permitted further in-depth probes of the system. The aldosterone–renin–angiotensin system (A-RAS) not only is a major effector of pathological disorders, but also can be the marker of events or substances that are more proximate causes of a specific disorder. The effectiveness of inquiries into the A-RAS as a regulator of blood pressure, electrolyte metabolism, and regulation of aldosterone secretion is examined herein.

6.2. The Renin–Angiotensin System

6.2.1. Angiotensin and Blood Pressure

Figure 1 outlines the steps in the formation of the effector substances of the RAS. Renin, an enzyme, cleaves from renin substrate a decapep-

EDWARD G. BIGLIERI • Endocrinology Division of the Medical Service and the Clinical Study Center, San Francisco General Hospital; Department of Medicine, University of California, San Francisco, California.

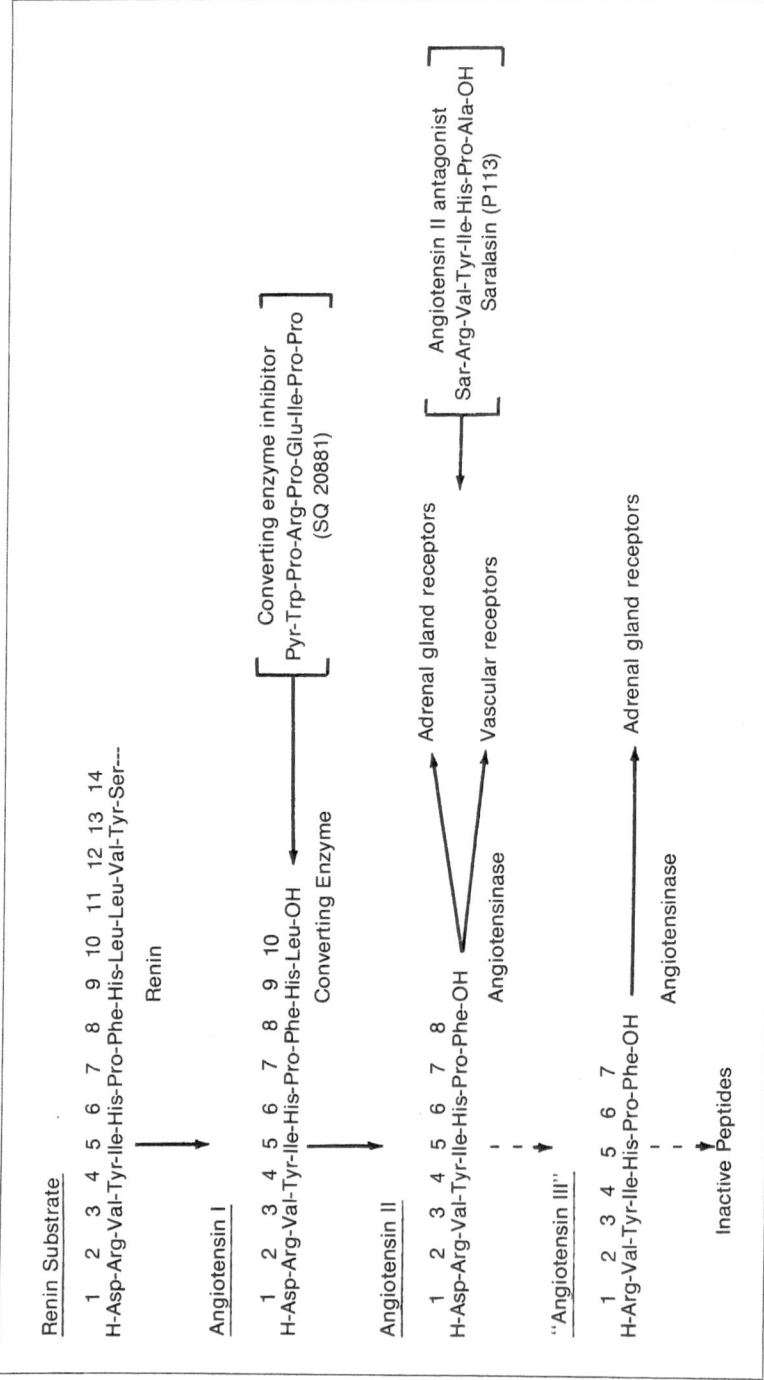

Fig. 1. The renin–angiotension system and its effector peptides and sites of blockade.

tide, angiotensin I. Through the action of converting enzyme, which is located mainly in pulmonary tissue and in vascular beds, a two-amino acid fragment is removed, resulting in the formation of the octapeptide angiotensin II. SQ 20881, a nonapeptide, inhibits this action, so that angiotensin I—which has no pressor action—accumulates, and the effects of angiotensin II on blood pressure and subsequently on aldosterone secretion are prevented. The action of angiotensin II on blood pressure and aldosterone production is also blocked by the competitive antagonist saralasin. Angiotensin II is degraded into inactive peptides by peptidases. The heptapeptide angiotensin III has interesting properties: it exists in the circulation (10–25% of angiotensin II levels) and can stimulate aldosterone secretion without a major pressor effect.

6.2.1.1. Diagnostic Use of the Angiotensin II Inhibitor Saralasin

Several varieties of evidence may suggest or indicate that angiotensin II is playing a critical role in a patient's blood pressure elevation. In hypertensive patients, elevated plasma renin activity (PRA) or, in patients with unilateral renal disease, renal venous renin ratios exceeding 1.5:1 (affected/contralateral side) indicates angiotensin II dependency, and normalization of blood pressure after correction of a renovascular lesion confirms that angiotensin II has had a major role. On the other hand, drugs that prevent renin release, such as propranolol, have not been very helpful in establishing angiotensin II as a major factor in hypertension. Saralasin, however, shows great promise in evaluating the contribution of angiotensin II to the blood pressure level, since it can rapidly establish that angiotensin II dependency is present. This highly specific antagonist of angiotensin II at the receptor level is well tolerated at doses ranging from 0.5 to 20 ug/kg body weight per min given intravenously for up to 30 min. The usual dose is 10 ug/kg body weight per min. In patients with high-renin states, such as accelerated or malignant hypertension and renovascular hypertension, a prompt and sustained decrease in blood pressure occurs within minutes. In patients with low–or normal-renin states, the response is less clear (see below), and even in other situations, the test is not entirely discriminating[1]. Designating a decrease of 10/8 (systolic/diastolic) mm Hg or more within 15 min as a positive response, Streeten et al.[2] found a positive response in only 31 of 300 unselected hypertensive patients. A total of 54 patients had high PRA levels after appropriate testing, but only 23 of the 54 had positive saralasin responses. Of the 31 positive responders, 11 (36%) had unilateral renal disease, but no detectable lesion was found in 11 other patients who had both elevated renin levels and positive saralasin responses. In a large group of patients (149) with normal PRA, only 4 had a positive saralasin response.

Other difficulties with the use of saralasin arise from the fact that in conditions in which plasma renin is suppressed, plasma volume is increased, or salt intake is high, saralasin acts as an agonist, rather than an antagonist. For this reason, an early increase in blood pressure may be seen during administration of saralasin to hypertensive patients with normal or low PRA, i.e., in patients whose RAS is suppressed.[2-4] Under these conditions, the agonist effect of saralasin is also evident in an active increase in plasma aldosterone concentration.[5] A low dose of saralasin (1 μg/kg per min) is used in these circumstances. The agonist effect of saralasin can be prevented by preparing the patient with diuretic therapy or sodium restriction,[2] but it may be difficult to establish the proper state of sodium balance necessary to probe the RAS accurately. A positive response in the sodium-depleted hypertensive patient may be more a reflection of an angiotensin II response to sodium depletion than of an angiotensin II dependency of the hypertension.[4]

The use of a converting-enzyme inhibitor (CEI) has attractive features as an investigative tool: it is devoid of agonist properties and can be administered as a slow bolus injection of 1 mg/kg body weight, and a blood pressure response occurs within 30 min. The results of one comparison of CEI (SQ 20881; see Fig. 1) and saralasin are shown in Fig. 2.[6] The key feature of the CEI maneuver is that during normal sodium intake, major differences in blood pressure response induced by CEI and saralasin occur in the low- and normal-renin groups. In the normal-renin group, saralasin produced a minimal increase in diastolic pressure (+2.0 ± 1.5%), whereas CEI effected a 10.2 ± 1.2% fall; in the low-renin group, saralasin had a pressor effect (8.5 ± 2.9%), whereas CEI had little effect (1.2±2.4%). In these studies, however, large doses of saralasin (10 mg/kg body weight per min) were used, and doses of this size are known to have agonist properties in the low-renin state. One implication of these studies is that angiotensin II could be involved in the genesis of blood pressure elevation in most hypertensive patients, but this involvement remains to be established. In addition, the modifying effect of various sodium intakes on the blood pressure response to this drug has yet to be critically evaluated.

Blood volume is the important modifier of the response to saralasin and may also be important in the response to CEI. Gavras et al.[4] demonstrated the importance of volume or state of sodium repletion or both in the response of blood pressure to saralasin and indirectly to other inhibitors of the RAS. Their studies showed that the response to saralasin could be modified by salt intake in high-, normal-, and low-renin types of hypertension. Sodium-repleted or partially repleted patients had pressor responses to saralasin accompanied by increases in plasma aldosterone. Depressor responses were seen when sodium was depleted. Low-renin

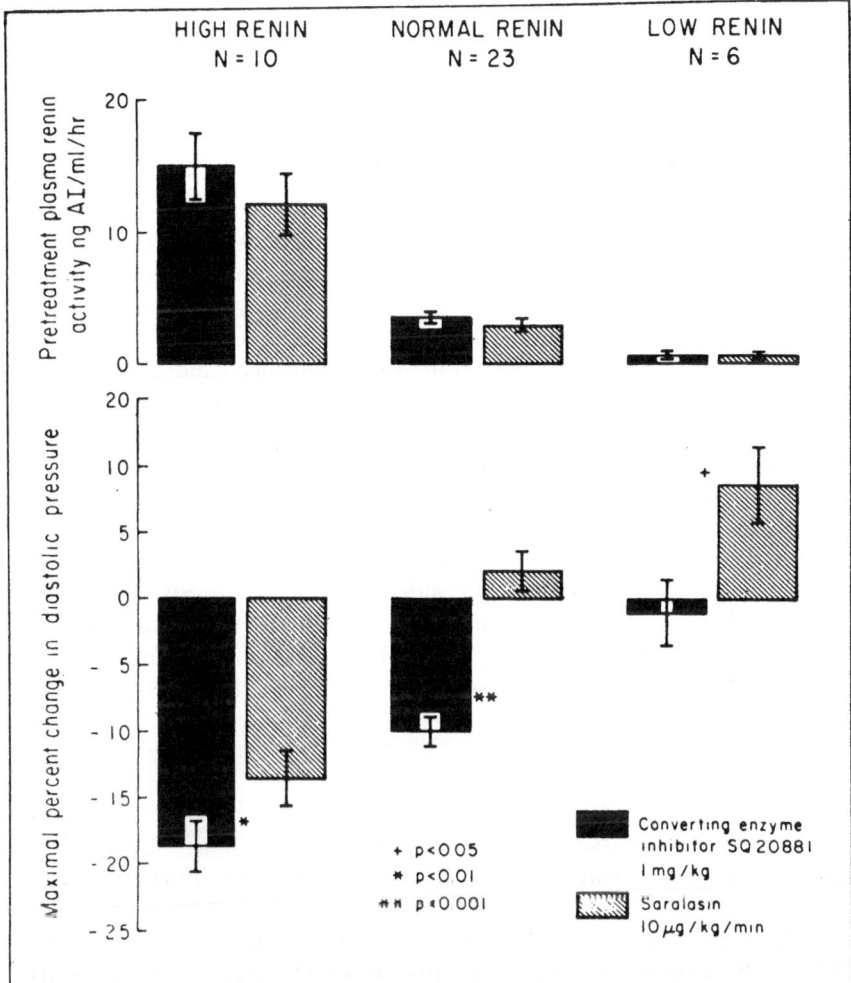

Fig. 2. Levels of PRA for each renin subgroup prior to angiotension blockage (top) and the maximal induced percentage change in diastolic pressure for each treatment group (bottom). Mean values ± standard error are shown for renin and blood pressure measurements. Reproduced from Case *et al.*[6] with permission from the authors and publisher.

hypertensive patients required more vigorous sodium depletion with diuretics to effect renin stimulation and hence a depressor response. Thus, patients with all types of hypertension respond to saralasin when renin levels are increased. The degree of sodium balance may set the responsiveness of the RAS in maintaining the elevated blood pressure.

The important fact to remember is that the response to saralasin or CEI under modified conditions of sodium balance may reduce their effectiveness in identifying the angiotensin-dependent form of hypertension.

6.2.2. Hyporeninemic Hypoaldosteronism and 'Abnormal' Renin

Although hyporeninemic hypoaldosteronism is a frequent occurrence in patients with chronic renal failure, approximately one fourth of the reported cases have had diabetes mellitus.[7,8] Day et al.[9] found "big" renin in patients with some pathological states, suggesting that big renin may be a precursor of normal renin. Big renin has a molecular weight about 50% greater than that of renin and is inactive, but it becomes activated at low pH. The finding of big renin in two patients with diabetes mellitus and low normal aldosterone excretion suggests that it may play a role in the patient with the hyporeninemic hypoaldosterone syndrome, possibly by its failure to be transformed to renin. It has been additionally proposed that patients with hyporeninemic hypoaldosteronism have an adrenal biosynthetic defect of late aldosterone biosynthesis, methyl oxidase type I (18-hydroxylation) and type II (dehydrogenation)[10] (see Section 6.3.1). While the evidence is suggestive, such biosynthetic defects are rare, and it is uncertain what role they may play in this group of patients.

6.2.3. Bartter's Syndrome

The finding in 1975 by Verberckmoes et al.[11] that indomethacin increases serum potassium concentration, decreases both elevated PRA and plasma aldosterone concentration, and restores normal pressor responses to angiotensin II in patients with Bartter's syndrome portended the role of prostaglandins (PGs) in this disorder. That overproduction of PGE by the kidneys is a "cardinal" feature of this syndrome was clearly documented by Bartter et al.[12] Increased urinary PGE_2, which mainly reflects renal synthesis of PGE, was observed in 6 patients. The PGE metabolite 16-carbon dioic acid, which serves as an index of total body production of PGE, was increased in only 1 of the 6 patients.[12] Fichman et al.[13] observed an increase in blood PGA that may represent conversion from PGE. While Verberckmoes et al.[14] did not measure urinary PGs in their patients, they did present evidence for hyperplasia of renal medullary interstitial cells, a presumed source of renal PGs. These increased levels were reduced by treatment with indomethacin, a potent inhibitor of PG synthesis (acting on the conversion of arachidonic acid to PGG_2).[12,13,15] The dependence of the hyperreninemia and aldosteronism on PGs was demonstrated by the reduction of both the PRA and the aldosterone production after application of PG synthetase inhibitors.[12] After treatment, sodium and potassium retention occur, with a rise in serum potassium concentration and a mild decrease in glomerular filtration rate.[12,13,15] Serum potassium becomes normalized,[12,13] but not in all patients. Whether or not prolonged treatment sustains both the hormonal reductions and the maintenance of a normal serum potassium concentration has yet to be established. Although an increase in renal PGs is an additional component of the syndrome, the more basic defect may still remain, namely, a defect in tubular sodium or chloride reabsorption that favors potassium secretion.

A more general inhibition of PG synthesis during treatment, rather than in the kidney alone, is suggested by the restoration of pressor sensitivity to angiotensin II. The overproduction of PGE in arteriolar walls could lead to resistance to angiotensin II. The mechanism of the sodium retention during treatment is not entirely clear. Bartter *et al.*[12] believe that the decrease in PRA is due directly to a decrease in PGE, not to sodium retention, since they found that salt loading or volume expansion did not suppress renin levels. The initial resistance to angiotensin II could be partially dependent on the on the local vascular overproduction of PGs. Urinary excretion of kallikrein is increased in patients with Bartter's syndrome, it is possible that kallikrein also participates in modifying pressor responses in this syndrome.[16]

6.3. Aldosterone and the Mineralocorticoid Hormones

6.3.1. Biosynthesis

The principal mineralocorticoid hormone secreted by the zona glomerulosa is aldosterone. The major pathway (see Fig. 3) involves progesterone, deoxycorticosterone (DOC), corticosterone (B), and 18-hydroxycorticosterone (18-OHB). The enzymatic defects in the late stages of biosynthesis are those of 18-hydroxylation (methyl oxidase type I) and dehydrogenation (methyl oxidase type II)[10] Although small quantities of B and DOC are secreted by the zona glomerulosa, the major proportion of these steroids arises from the zona fasciculata. It is here that 18-hydroxydeoxycorticosterone (18-OHDOC) is produced and secreted. The major regulatory factor for glomerulosa-produced steroids is the RAS, whereas that for steroids produced by the fasciculata is ACTH. Thus, in the salt-losing syndrome, in which methyl oxidase type II is deficient, the increase in renin stimulates the precursor steroids proximal to the site of the deficiency, and 18-OHB is elevated in the presence of aldosterone

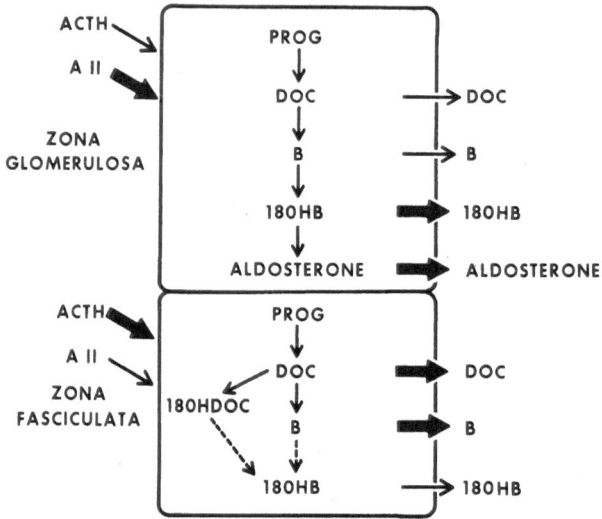

Fig. 3. Biosynthesis of the mineralocorticoid hormones. (PROG) Progesterone; (DOC) deoxycorticosterone; (B) corticosterone; (18OHB) 18-hydroxycorticosterone; (18OHDOC) 18 hydroxydeoxycorticosterone.

deficiency. In the 17-hydroxylation deficiency variant of congenital adrenal hyperplasia, the ACTH drives the increase of steroids that arise predominantly in the fasciculata, DOC and B, while the suppression of renin reduces aldosterone production in the glomerulosa.[17]

6.3.2. Measurement of Plasma Deoxycorticosterone, 18-Hydroxydeoxycorticosterone, and 18-Hydroxycorticosterone Concentrations in Man

Deoxycorticosterone is secreted primarily by the zona fasciculata under the control of ACTH. But although ACTH is the primary regulator of DOC production,[18] in its absence, the RAS plays a significant role. Maximal production in response to ACTH stimulation is achieved when sodium intake is reduced.[19] Although the levels of plasma DOC are similar to those of aldosterone (4–17 ng/dl),[20] most of the DOC is bound to corticosteroid-binding globulin. The levels of DOC required to produce significant potassium depletion and hypertension are high, 20 times the normal value,[19] and occur only in patients with the 11β- and 17α-hydroxylation deficiency syndromes.

Studies of plasma 18-OHDOC concentration[21] essentially support data obtained by measuring its urinary metabolite, tetrahydro-18-OHDC.[22] There are, however, two areas that are still controversial: (1) the response of 18-OHDOC to sodium restriction and (2) the rarity of increased 18-OHDOC production in patients with hypertension. Plasma levels of 18-OHDOC, produced in the zona fasciculata, increase briskly (up to 23-fold) in response to a brief infusion of ACTH,[21,23] Infusion of angiotensin II results in a decrease, however, and sodium restriction causes an increase, in plasma levels of 18-OHDOC. The mechanisms responsible for the last two responses are not clear at present. Whether alterations in metabolic clearance rate are responsible has yet to be established. The finding that at least 22% of hypertensive patients with normal renin levels have 18-OHDOC levels slightly greater than normal on high sodium intakes was surprising and it is still uncertain whether these plasma[22] and secretory or excretory levels[24,25] establish a role for 18-OHDOC in blood pressure regulation.

18-Hydroxycorticosterone is a steroid formed primarily in the zona glomerulosa.[10] It has virtually no mineralocorticoid activity, and its regulation is similar to that of aldosterone, but its secretory rate is $2-2\frac{1}{2}$ times greater than that of aldosterone. This steroid is a marker of the methyl oxidase type II deficiency of aldosterone biosynthesis.[10] Radioimmunoassay of 18-OHB has shown further similarities to aldosterone: mean plasma levels during normal sodium intake were 22.5 ± 9.3 ng/dl in the upright position and 9.9 ± 3.8 ng/dl in the recumbent position.[26]

6.3.3. Low-Aldosterone Hypertension and Adrenal Hypertensive Steroids Other Than Aldosterone

Using PRA and aldosterone measurements to classify hypertension, Brunner et al.[27] were able to identify a small group of patients with both low aldosterone and low renin levels. In patients within this classification, mineralocorticoid hormones other than aldosterone are present. It was within this group that patients with the 17α-hydroxylation deficiency syndrome were first defined and continue to be identified by the presence of hypertension, hypokalemia, suppressed PRA, markedly reduced aldosterone, and reduced cortisol production.[28] As discussed in Section 6.3.2.2, 18-OHDOC, a weak mineralocorticoid hormone, could in time play a role in suppressing renin and hence aldosterone secretion in these patients.

Liddle et al.[29] described patients with a familial renal disorder characterized by hypertension and hypokalemia who were resistant to treatment with both spironolactone and low-sodium diet; aldosterone excretion was negligible, and renin was reduced. Triamterene reduced blood pressure and caused a rise in serum potassium concentration in these patients, but aldosterone levels remained low. There is no evidence to date that suggests a mineralocorticoid excess in these patients. A recent case[30] suggests the existence of still another mineralocorticoid excess syndrome with reduced production of aldosterone and suppression of renin; the disorder differs from that described by Liddle and colleagues, since the patient responded to spironolactone. In another case,[31] in which hyperaldosteronism was suppressible with dexamethasone, careful studies produced convincing evidence that an ACTH-dependent steroid that produced hypertension was being secreted.[31] In this case, however, an abundant sodium intake was necessary to effect increases in blood pressure. Administration of exogenous ACTH rapidly induces hypertension and renin suppression in sheep[32]; increased amounts of 17,20-dihydroxyprogesterone were measured in these hypertensive animals, but a role for this steroid in human hypertension has not been established. Plasma 16β-hydroxydehydroepiandrosterone, an uncertain mineralocorticoid hormone, is not increased in patients with low-renin hypertension.[33] Increased mineralocorticoid activity, measured by bioassay and mineralocorticoid receptor assay, in the absence of known mineralocorticoid hormones, provides strong presumptive evidence for the presence of an unidentified steroid.[34]

6.3.4. Aldosterone Binding

A series of reports this year pointed out that the metabolic clearance rate of aldosterone is increased as a result of adrenal stimulation by ACTH.[35–38] The following mechanism has been proposed. A significant amount of aldosterone is bound to corticosteroid-binding globulin[38] or a heat-labile plasma protein fraction,[36] or both. With rising plasma cortisol concentrations, smaller amounts of aldosterone are bound tightly, thus increasing the plasma metabolic clearance rate. Up to one third of plasma aldosterone is bound to albumin, and 24–28% is bound to higher-affinity sites.[38] Although the plasma metabolic clearance rate is increased by ACTH and cortisol, the whole-blood metabolic clearance rate is unaltered.[37] The displaced aldosterone moves into the red blood cells and is removed with equal efficiency by liver cells.

6.3.5. Angiotensin III and Aldosterone Production

The heptapeptide angiotensin III (des-Asp^1-angiotensin II) is a naturally occurring metabolite of angiotensin II. This peptide has minimal pressor activity, but is as potent as angiotensin II in stimulating aldosterone secretion. In isolated adrenal cell preparations, angiotensin III is a more potent stimulator of aldosterone secretion than is angiotensin II. Angiotensin III might be an intracellular effector of aldosterone production. The circulating levels of angiotensin III are small, and its principal effect may occur intracellularly by conversion from angiotensin II.

At doses of 20 ng/kg body weight per min given for 30 min, angiotensin III increases plasma aldosterone concentration without the increase in blood pressure that occurs with comparable infusion rates of angiotensin II.[39] Infusion at higher concentrations can produce pressor effects. A competitive inhibitor of angiotensin II, similar to saralasin, sar^1-Ile^8-angiotensin II, blocks the pressor response to infused angiotensin II, but not the aldosterone increase, in the ACTH-suppressed nephrectomized dog.[40] An inhibitor of angiotensin III, des-Asp^1-Ile^8-angiotensin II, blocks the aldosterone increase but not the pressor response to a similar angiotensin II infusion.[40] These findings were not confirmed in man,[39] and confusing findings were obtained in patients with Bartter's syndrome using the angiotensin III inhibitor.[41] Since, as noted earlier (see Sections 6.2.1.1 and 6.2.1.2), antagonists (competitive inhibitors) have been shown to be agonists under proper conditions, additional information is required before any definitive statement as to the precise role of angiotensin III is made. Nevertheless, angiotensin III is a potentially exciting substance for the study of zona glomerulosa cell function.

References

1. Brunner, H. R., Gavras, H., Laragh, J. H., and Keenan, R., 1973, Angiotensin II blockade in man by Sar^1-Ala^8-angiotensin II for understanding and treatment of high blood pressure, *Lancet* **2**:1045–1048.
2. Streeten, D. H. P., Anderson, G. H., Jr., and Dalakos, T. G., 1976, Angiotensin blockade: Its clinical significance, *Am. J. Med.* **60**:817–824.
3. Case, D. B., Wallace, J. M., Keim, H. J., Sealey, J. E., and Laragh, J. H., 1976, Usefulness and limitations of saralasin, a partial competitive agonist of angiotensin II, for evaluating the renin and sodium factors in hypertensive patients, *Am. J. Med.* **60**:825–836.
4. Gavras, H., Ribeiro, A. B., Gavras, I., and Brunner, H. R., 1976, Reciprocal relation between renin dependency and sodium dependency in essential hypertension, *N. Engl. J. Med.* **295**:1278–1283.
5. Hollenberg, N. K., Williams, G. H., Burger, B., Ishikawa, I., and Adams, D. F., 1976, Blockade and stimulation of renal, adrenal, and vascular angiotensin II receptors with 1-Sar,8-Ala angiotensin II in normal man, *J. Clin. Invest.* **57**:39–46.
6. Case, D. B., Wallace, J. M., Keim, H. J., Weber, M. A., Drayer, J. I. M., White, R. P., Sealey, J. E., and Laragh, J. H., 1976, Estimating renin participation in hypertension: Superiority of converting enzyme inhibitor over saralasin, *Am. J. Med.* **61**:790–796.

 7. Christlieb, A. R., Kaldany, A., and D'Elia, J. A., 1976, Plasma renin activity and hypertension in diabetes mellitus, *Diabetes* **25**:969–974.
 8. De Leiva, A., Christlieb, A. R., Melby, J. C., Graham, C. A., Day, R. P., Luetscher, J. A., and Zager, P. G., 1976, Big renin and biosynthetic defect of aldosterone in diabetes mellitus, *N. Engl. J. Med.* **295**:639–643.
 9. Day, R. P., Luetscher, J. A., and Gonzales, C. M., 1975, Occurrence of big renin in human plasma, amniotic fluid and kidney extracts, *J. Clin. Endocrinol. Metab.* **40**:1078–1084.
10. Ulick, S., 1976, Diagnosis and nomenclature of the disorders of the terminal portion of the aldosterone biosynthetic pathway, *J. Clin. Endocrinol. Metab.* **43**:92–96.
11. Verberckmoes, R., Clement, J., Michielsen, P., and van Damme, B., 1975, Bartter's syndrome with hyperplasia of renomedullary interstitial cells: Successful treatment with indomethacin, *Proc. Int. Soc. of Nephrol.*, Abst. No. 558 (June 1975).
12. Bartter, F. C., Gill, J. R., Jr., Frolich, J. C., Bowden, R. E., Hollifield, J. W., Radfar, N., Keiser, H. R., Oates, J. A., Seyberth, H., and Taylor, A. A., 1976, Prostaglandins are overproduced by the kidneys and mediate hyperreninemia in Bartter's syndrome, *Trans. Assoc. Am. Physicians* **89**:77–91.
13. Fichman, M. P., Telfer, N., Zia, P., Speckart, P., Golub, M., and Rude, R., 1976, Role of prostaglandins in the pathogenesis of Bartter's syndrome, *Am. J. Med.* **60**:785–797.
14. Verberckmoes, R., van Damme, B., Clement, J., Amery, A., and Michielsen, P., 1976, Bartter's syndrome with hyperplasia of renomedullary cells: Successful treatment with indomethacin, *Kidney Int.* **9**:302–307.
15. Gill, J. R., Jr., Frölich, J. C., Bowden, R. E., Taylor, A. A., Keiser, H. R., Seyberth, H. W., Oates, J. A., and Bartter, F. C., 1976, Bartter's syndrome: A disorder characterized by high urinary prostaglandins and a dependence of hyperreninemia on prostaglandin synthesis, *Am. J. Med.* **61**:43–51.
16. Lechi, A., Covi, G., Lechi, C., Mantero, F., and Scuro, L. A., 1976, Urinary kallikrein excretion in Bartter's syndrome, *J. Clin. Endocrinol. Metab.* **43**:1175-1178.
17. Biglieri, E. G., 1976, A perspective on aldosterone abnormalities, *Clin. Endocrinol. (Oxford)* **5**:399–410.
18. Oddie, C. J., Coghlan, J. P., and Scoggins, B. A., 1972, Plasma desoxycorticosterone levels in man with simultaneous measurement of aldosterone, corticosterone, cortisol, and 11-deoxycortisol, *J. Clin. Endocrinol. Metab.* **34**:1039-1054.
19. Schambelan, M., and Biglieri, E. G., 1972, Deoxycorticosterone production and regulation in man, *J. Clin, Endocrinol. Metab.* **34**:695–703.
20. Biglieri, E. G., 1977, Plasma deoxycorticosterone concentrations in adrenal enzymatic deficiencies causing hypertension, *in: Juvenile Hypertension* (M. I., New and L. S. Levine, eds.), pp. 171–176, Raven Press, New York.
21. Williams, G. H., Braley, L. M., and Underwood, R. H., 1976, The regulation of plasma 18-hydroxy 11-deoxycorticosterone in man, *J. Clin. Invest.* **58**:221–229.
22. Melby, J. C., Dale, S. L., Grekin, R. J., Gaunt, R., and Wilson, T. E., 1972, 18-Hydroxy-11-deoxycorticosterone (18-OH-DOC) secretion in experimental and human hypertension, *Recent Prog. Horm. Res.* **28**:287–351.
23. Dale, S. L., Komanicky, P., Pratt, J. H., and Melby, J. C., 1976, Radioimmunoassay of 18-hydroxy-11-deoxycorticosterone in plasma, *J. Clin. Endocrinol. Metab.* **43**:803–809.

24. Genest, J., Nowaczynski, W., Kuchel, O., and Sasaki, C., 1972, Progesterone levels and 18 hydroxy-deoxycorticosterone secretion rate in benign essential hypertension in humans, *in: Hypertension 1972* (J. Genest and E. Koiw, eds.), pp. 293–298, Springer-Verlag, New York.

25. Nowaczynski, W., Kuchel, O., Genest, J., Messerli, F. H., Honda, M., Tolis, G., Seth, K., Parvin-Pande, R., Kubo, S., Grose, J., Ledoux, F., and Lebel, M., 1975, Dynamic aldosterone and 18-hydroxydeoxycorticosterone studies in labile and stable benign essential hypertension, *J. Steroid Biochem.* **6**:767–778.

26. Martin, V. I., Edwards, C. R. W., Biglieri, E. G., Vinson, G. P., and Bartter, F. C., 1975, The development and application of a radioimmunoassay for 18-hydroxy-corticosterone, *Steroids* **26**:591–604.

27. Brunner, H. R., Laragh, J. H., Baer, L., Newton, M. A., Goodwin, F. T., Krakoff, L. R., Bard, R. H., and Bühler, F. R., 1972, Essential hypertension: Renin and aldosterone, heart attack and stroke, *N. Engl. J. Med.* **286**:441–449.

28. Biglieri, E. G., Herron, M. A., and Brust, N., 1966, 17-Hydroxylation deficiency in man, *J. Clin. Invest.* **45**:1946–1954.

29. Liddle, G. W., Bledsoe, T., and Coppage, W. J., Jr., 1963, A familial renal disorder simulating primary aldosteronism but with negligible aldosterone secretion, *Trans. Assoc. Am. Physicians* **76**:199–213.

30. Sann, L., Revol, A., Zachmann, M., Legrand, J. C., and Bethenod, M., 1976, Unusual low plasma renin hypertension in a child, *J. Clin. Endocrinol. Metab.* **43**:265–271.

31. New, M. I., Peterson, R. E., Saenger, P., and Levine, L. S., 1976, Evidence for an unidentified ACTH-induced steroid hormone causing hypertension, *J. Clin. Endocrinol. Metab.* **43**:1283–1293.

32. Scoggins, B. A., Coghlan, J. P., and Denton, D. A., 1976, Mechanism of ACTH induced hypertension, *Proc. Endocrine Soc.*, 58th Meeting, No. 211.

33. Sekihara, H., Sennett, J. A. Liddle, G. W., McKenna, T. J., and Yarbro, L. R., 1976, Plasma 16β-hydroxydehydroepiandrosterone in normal and pathological conditions in man, *J. Clin. Endocrinol. Metab.* **43**:1078–1084.

34. Baxter, J. D., Schambelan, M., Matulich, D. T., Spindler, B. J., Taylor, A. A., and Bartter, F. C., 1976, Aldosterone receptors and the evaluation of plasma mineralocorticoid activity in normal and hypertensive states, *J. Clin. Invest.* **58**:579–589.

35. Pratt, J. H., Dale, S. L., and Melby, J. C., 1976, The effect of administered ACTH on aldosterone metabolism and secretion, *J. Clin. Endocrinol. Metab.* **42**:355–360.

36. Messerli, F. H., Nowaczynski, W., Honda, M. Genest, J., and Kuchel, O., 1976, Effects of ACTH on steroid metabolism, *J. Clin. Endocrinol. Metab.* **42**:1074–1080.

37. Zipser, R. D., Speckart, P. F., Zia, P. K., Edmiston, W. A., Lau, F. Y. K., and Horton, R., 1976, The effect of ACTH and cortisol on aldosterone and cortisol clearance and distribution in plasma and whole blood, *J. Clin. Endocrinol. Metab.* **43**:1101–1109.

38. Zager, P. G., Burtis, W. J., Luetscher, J. A., Dowdy, A. J., and Sood, S., 1976, Increased plasma protein binding and lower metabolic clearance rate of aldosterone in plasma of low cortisol concentration, *J. Clin. Endocrinol. Metab.* **42**:207–214.

39. Kono, T., Oseko, F., Shimpo, S., Nanno, M., and Endo, J., 1975, Biological activity of des-Asp^1-angiotensin II (angiotensin III) in man, *J. Clin. Endocrinol. Metab.* **41**:1174–1177.

40. Bravo, E. L., Khosla, M. C., and Bumpus, F. M., 1975, Action of (1-des (aspartic acid) 8-isoleucine) angiotensin II upon the pressor and steroidogenic activity of angiotensin II, *J. Clin. Endocrinol. Metab.* **40**:530–533.

41. Kono, T., Oseko, F., Ikeda, F., Nanno, M., and Endo, J., 1976, Biological activity of des-Asp^1,Ileu^8-angiotensin II (Ileu^8-angiotensin III) in man, *J. Clin. Endocrinol. Metab.* **43**:940–943.

Vasopressin and Water Metabolism

Gary L. Robertson

7.1. Introduction

The antidiuretic hormone, arginine vasopressin, is known to play a major role in the complex homeostatic system by which man and other mammals regulate salt and water balance. Efforts to define its function in normal as well as abnormal states of water metabolism have long been hampered by the lack of a suitable assay method. Recently, several laboratories have succeeded in developing radioimmunoassay techniques that permit vasopressin to be measured easily and accurately at physiological concentrations in small volumes of plasma or other body fluids. These methodological advances have stimulated a new investigative interest in the hormone that is the source of an increasing volume of information about its physiology, pharmacology, and pathophysiology. These findings have clarified some long-standing controversies about vasopressin function and are beginning to provide a much more detailed and comprehensive picture of how the various parts of the system act and interact to regulate

GARY L. ROBERTSON • Professor of Medicine, Indiana University School of Medicine; Chief, Endocrinology and Metabolism Section, Medical Service, Veterans Administration Hospital.

water balance in health and disease. There have also been a few surprises that reveal some previously unrecognized effects of vasopressin function and challenge conventional views about the importance of certain others.

The purpose of this chapter will be to review selectively these new findings, putting special emphasis on those that relate most directly to clinical medicine. The history of these developments will be summarized only briefly, but selected reviews and papers from the older literature will also be cited for those who would like more background information. The technical aspects of the radioimmunoassays on which many of the new findings are based will not be discussed, since they were recently reviewed elsewhere.[1]

7.2. Physiology

7.2.1. Osmoregulation

Blood osmolality has long been recognized to be an important variable in the regulation of vasopressin secretion.[2] In recent years, considerable progress has been made in defining the anatomical relationship of the osmoreceptor to the neurohypophysis and its other regulatory afferents (Fig. 1). By systematically ligating different branches of the internal carotid artery in dogs and determining the effect on the response to hypertonic saline, Jewell and Verney[3] first localized the osmoreceptor to the anterior hypothalamus and concluded that it was probably very near or synonymous with the cell bodies of the neurohypophysis. Recent animal studies have confirmed these findings and established for the first time that the osmoreceptor function is not performed by the neurosecretory cell itself. Thus, in rats[4] or cats[5] with cannulas chronically implanted at different places in the anterior hypothalamus, the injection of small volumes of hypertonic sucrose or saline consistently evoked an antidiuretic response only at sites some distance from the supraoptic nucleus. Conversely, the vasopressin response to prolonged fluid deprivation can be prevented in rats by producing small lesions in the medial preoptic area of the hypothalamus that do not involve the neurohypophysis.[6]

These conclusions are further supported by studies performed about the same time in several patients with hypothalamic pathology and the rare clinical syndrome of adipsic hypernatremia. As originally suggested by indirect studies,[7] and confirmed recently by direct assay of plasma vasopressin,[8,9] some of these patients have a total lack of osmotically mediated vasopressin secretion, but continue to exhibit a normal response to hemodynamic stimuli. These unique experiments of nature confirm that the osmoreceptor in man also must be totally separate from the neurosecretory cells and indicate further that it is not an integral part of

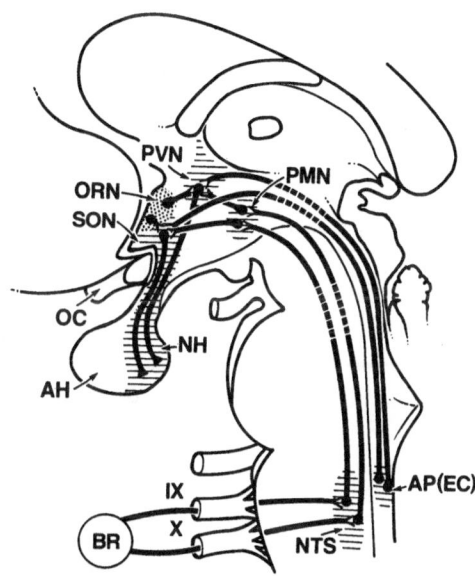

Fig. 1. Schematic representation of the neurohypophysis and its principal regulatory afferents. (AH), Adenohpophysis; (NH), neurohypophysis; (OC), optic chiasm; (SON), supraoptic nucleus; (PVN), paraventricular nucleus; (PMN), posteromedial nucleus; (ORN), osmoreceptor neurons; (BR), baroreceptors; (NTS), nucleus tractus solitarius; [AP (EC)], area postrema (emetic center).

neuronal pathways by which hemodynamic variables influence vasopressin secretion (Fig. 1).

It has also been possible to define more fully the functional properties of this osmoregulatory system. Immunoassay studies in man and animals have shown that the osmostat behaves like a threshold receptor the set point, sensitivity, and precision of which can be characterized by analyzing the relationship between plasma vasopressin and osmolality.[10-14] In healthy adults, the osmostat appears to be "set" so that vasopressin secretion is suppressed to low or undetectable levels whenever plasma osmolality falls to 280 mOsm/kg or below (Fig. 2). Under these conditions, the urine becomes maximally dilute and urine flow normally rises to a rate that can keep pace with any but the most excessive rates of water ingestion. For practical purposes, therefore, the lower limit to which plasma osmolality can be reduced in a healthy person is generally determined by the osmotic threshold for vasopressin release. Above this threshold, vasopressin secretion rises steeply in direct proportion to osmolality, reaching a level sufficient to effect maximum antidiuresis at a plasma osmolality around 295 mOsm/kg.[10] At about this level, thirst begins,[1,15] and a further

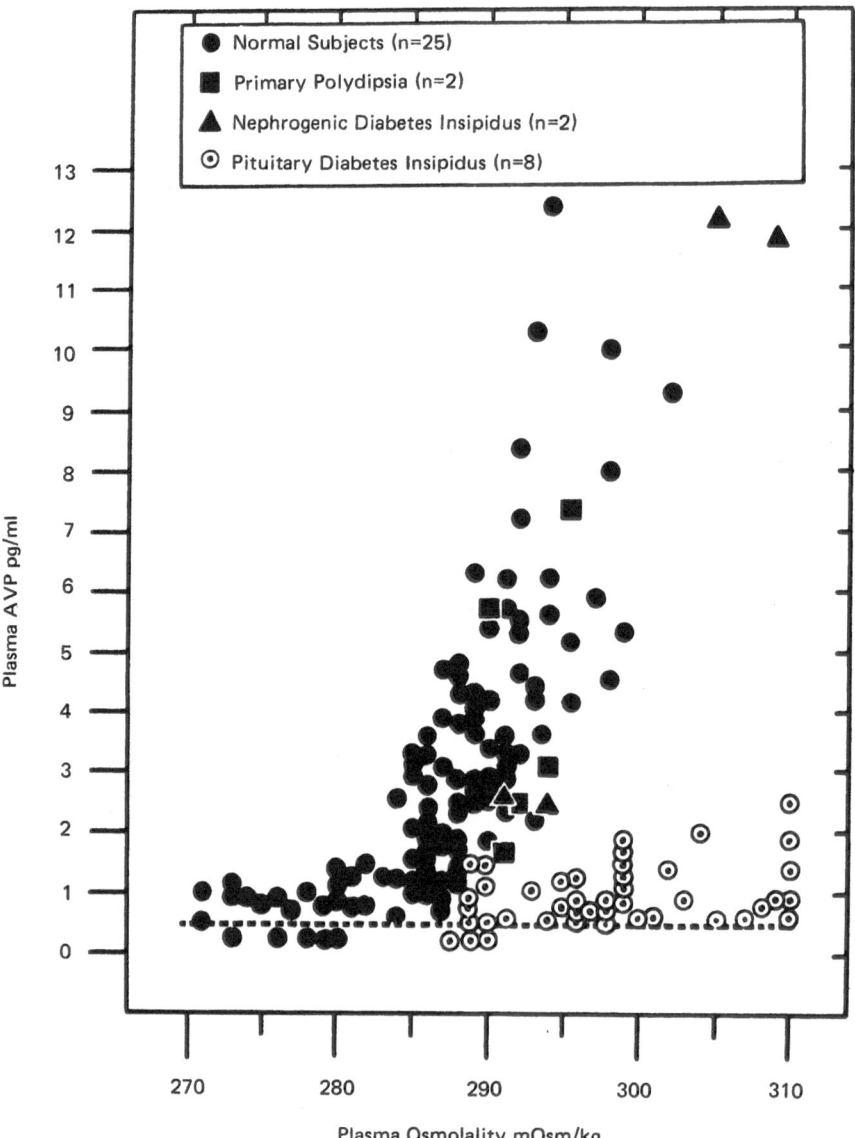

Fig. 2. Relationship between plasma vasopressin concentration and plasma osmolality in healthy adults and patients with polyuria of diverse etiologies. (Reproduced from Robertson *et al.*[10])

rise in plasma osmolality is normally prevented by the ingestion of water. Between these limits imposed by the osmotic thresholds for thirst and vasopressin, tonicity may be regulated even more precisely by osmoreceptor-mediated adjustments in water excretion. As indicated by the slope of the regression line, changes in plasma osmolality as small as 1% will increase or decrease plasma vasopressin by an average of 1 pg/ml, an amount sufficient to produce pronounced changes in urinary concentration and flow.[10] This extraordinary sensitivity makes the osmoreceptor well suited to effect the kind of precise regulation of free water balance that is so characteristic of healthy adults and points to the need for unusually accurate and precise measurements of plasma osmolality or its principal determinant, plasma sodium, when studying any aspect of antidiuretic function.

Application of the same method of regression analysis to individual subjects has shown that the relatively wide scatter that characterizes the relationship between plasma osmolality and vasopressin in a healthy adult population (Fig. 2) is due largely to individual differences in the set or sensitivity or both of the osmoreceptor mechanism, rather than to instability or imprecision in its response characteristics.[16] The individual variations in osmoreceptor function seem to be associated with discernible differences in the regulation of water balance[1] that must be taken into account when assessing antidiuretic function in clinical disorders such as diabetes insipidus. The factors responsible for these physiological variations in osmoreceptor function have not been determined. Aging appears to be associated with an increase in the slope or sensitivity of the vasopressin response,[17] but this property must be subject to other influences as well, since it varies markedly even in adults of comparable age.[16] A sex difference in osmoreceptor sensitivity was observed in one study that measured vasopressin excretion,[18] but not in another that measured the hormone in plasma.[16] Further study is needed to determine whether this discrepancy relates to differences in the renal handling of vasopressin or to some other unrecognized influence on hormone secretion. The extent to which individual differences in the volume of distribution or rate of metabolism of the hormone, or both, are responsible for normal variations in the relationship between plasma vasopressin and osmolality has not been determined.

The specificity of the osmoreceptor is another property the complexity and importance of which are now beginning to be more fully understood. More than 95% of the osmotic activity of plasma is normally contributed by sodium and its anions, a solute shown by Verney[2] to be particularly potent in eliciting an antidiuretic response. He also found, however, that the injection of hypertonic sucrose, but not urea or glucose, could induce an antidiuresis, and concluded that the control mechanism functioned like an osmoreceptor with a specificity for certain solutes. Recent immunoassay studies have fully confirmed these conclusions and established for the first time the relative potency of different blood solutes in effecting vasopressin release. In man, for example, mannitol was shown to be just as potent, particle for particle, as sodium chloride,[16] whereas urea has less than 1/3 the activity (R. Zerbe, R. Shelton, and G. Robertson, unpublished). More significantly, these immunoassay studies have also revealed that a rise in blood glucose acutely suppresses plasma vasopressin.[16] This paradoxical effect, which could not have been appreciated under the water-loaded conditions employed in Verney's studies, has not yet been explained, but may be related to the way acute hyperglycemia alters the hydroosmotic gradient across either the blood–brain barrier or some other selectively permeable membrane associated with the osmoreceptor.[19]

Whatever its functional or anatomical basis, the existence of this kind of osmoreceptor specifically has some practical implications. In immediate terms, it means that neither plasma osmolality nor sodium concentration can be relied on to provide a universally valid reference point for assessing vasopressin function. The kind of nomogram exemplified by Fig. 1 is useful only when blood glucose and urea are within the normal range. Measurements of plasma sodium may not provide a totally satisfactory solution either, because it has not been determined whether other naturally occurring solutes such as glycerol can affect vasopressin secretion. This uncertainty and the extraordinary sensitivity of the osmoreceptor necessitate special precautions in the design and interpretation of any mechanistic study of antidiuretic function.

In the future, it may also be useful to consider the possibility that the specificity of the osmoreceptor is, like its other properties, subject to physiological or pathological alterations. Such a condition, which might result from a change in the permeability characteristics of the blood–brain barrier or osmoreceptor neurons or both, could be distinguished from other causes of vasopressin dysfunction only by systematically determining the hormonal response to a variety of different solutes.

7.2.2. Baroregulation

It has also been known for many years that changes in blood volume and pressure affect vasopressin secretion.[2] Evidence accumulated during the 1960's established that these hemodynamic influences are exerted, at least in part, via neurogenic afferents that originate in pressure-sensitive receptors in the left atrium, aortic arch, and carotid sinus and reach the brainstem through the vagal and glossopharyngeal nerves[20] (see Fig. 1). The central pathways by which these signals are integrated and transmitted to the neurohypophysis have not yet been defined, but probably involve a primary synapse in the nucleus tractus solitarius,[21] with a secondary relay in the posteromedial nucleus of the hypothalamus.[22]

In recent years, the functional properties of this hemodynamic control system have come under closer scrutiny. Early studies based on bioassay or indirect methods led to a widely held view that hypovolemia was a particularly potent stimulus to vasopressin secretion and probably was at least as important as osmolality in mediating the hormonal response to changes in water balance.[23] Recently, however, this concept has been challenged by more detailed immunoassay studies of the vasopressin response to small to moderate reductions in blood volume. As demonstrated first in rats, these two variables appear to be related by an exponential rather than a linear function.[11] Thus, significant increases in plasma vasopressin are not detected until blood volume is reduced by more than 8%. In man, the characteristics of this system have not been so thoroughly defined, but seem to be similar qualitatively, if not quantitatively, to those in the rat. Both bioassay[24] and immunoassay[25] studies indicate that reducing blood volume 6–9% by phlebotomy has no effect on plasma vasopressin in recumbent adults. Orthostasis, which probably reduces central blood volume by 10–15%, produces a small and inconstant increase in plasma vasopressin,[13,26,27] while the combined hypovolemic stimulus of phlebotomy plus orthostasis results in much larger and more consistent hormonal responses in association with variable reductions in arterial pressure.[25] Taken as a whole, these results strongly suggest that the relationship between vasopressin secretion and blood volume in man follows an exponential pattern similar to that in the rat; i.e., the response is imperceptibly small until blood volume declines by 10–15%, but then increases rapidly as the hypovolemia progresses to larger, more unphysiological proportions. The levels of vasopressin achieved under these conditions greatly exceed those required to effect maximum antidiuresis,[10,25] and are probably in the range within which they exert significant pressor effects on certain vascular beds.[28]

The relative insensitivity of vasopressin secretion to small changes in total blood volume has not yet been explained, but may be due to the effectiveness with which other compensatory mechanisms maintain central blood volume constant in the face of a variety of stresses.[29] If this explanation is valid, then anything that interferes with these compensatory reflexes might "sensitize" vasopressin to hypovolemic stimuli. There are some unpublished data[20] suggesting that general anesthesia, which is known to impair many cardiovascular reflexes,[30] may have such an effect. Whether there are other pharmacological or physiological conditions that alter the sensitivity of vasopressin to hemodynamic influences is unknown.

By permitting direct comparison with the functional properties of the osmoreceptor, these studies of the volumetric control of vasopressin secretion provide a better basis for understanding the role of each system in normal and disordered states of water balance. It is clear, for example, that the vasopressin response normally evoked by changes in water intake must be mediated largely, if not exclusively, by the osmoreceptor mechanism, since pertubations of this type usually do not alter body water by more than 2–3%, an amount far short of that required to affect the relatively insensitive volume-control system. This concept is consistent with other findings that patients in whom osmoreceptor function has been destroyed exhibit a markedly deficient vasopressin response to dehydration even though their neurohypophysis and its baroregulatory afferents remain totally intact.[7–9] It also explains an older observation that sodium depletion produced by sweating does not result in a significant reduction in the tonicity of body water until extracellular fluid falls by more than 10%,[31] the point at which the volume-control system might be expected to begin to exert an increasingly important influence on vasopressin secretion. A clinically applicable corollary of these observations is that hypovolemia of a degree sufficient to induce osmotically inappropriate antidiuresis should be detectable in most cases by certain simple bedside tests such as an orthostatic fall in blood pressure. The ability to reliably differentiate hypovolemic hyponatremia from that due to more basic defects in vasopressin regulation (cf. Section 7.3.2) would help to clarify the diverse pathophysiological mechanisms involved in this common electrolyte disorder.

The same kind of quantitative considerations suggest that the influence of blood pressure on vasopressin secretion may be more important than previously recognized. Stimulus–response studies recently performed in both man[25] and animals[1] showed that there is also an exponential relationship between plasma vasopressin and the degree of hypotension produced. This response appears to be quantitatively similar for several different kinds of hypotensive stimuli and, in healthy young adults, can usually be demonstrated following a reduction in mean arterial pressure as small as 5%.[25] This "threshold" approximates the precision with which arterial pressure can be measured by indirect methods and is considerably less than the spontaneous fluctuations known to occur in healthy adults in the course of a normal day.[32]

These findings raise the possibility that many instances of nonosmotic secretion of vasopressin could be due to changes in blood pressure too small or too transient to be detected except by close and careful monitoring. This possiblity is particularly relevant to certain unexplained aspects of vasopressin physiology, such as the episodic bursts of secretion observed in some people during normal activity[33] or the nocturnal rise in plasma vasopressin that has been observed in recumbent man.[34] It has already been shown that a number of drugs and hormones known to affect water balance do so, at least in part, via baroreceptor-mediated changes in vasopressin secretion. Isoproterenol,[35,36] norepinephrine,[37,38] prostaglandin,[39] and even nicotine[40] have all been implicated in this regard, and it is probable that many other vasoactive agents act similarly.

7.2.3. Hormonoregulation

The renin–angiotensin system may be one important exception to the way in which vasoactive substances affect vasopressin. Unlike other pressor agents, which seem to suppress secretion, the infusion of angiotensin II has been reported to elevate plasma vasopressin both in animals[41] and in man.[42] The pathway for this effect has not been established, but may involve a direct action on one or more portions of the CNS, since similar or even greater increases in vasopressin have been reported when angiotensin is injected directly into brain ventricles or the cranial arteries.[43,44]

These observations have attracted considerable interest because they fit so aptly with others indicating that the renin–angiotensin system also stimulates thirst[45] and, in a manner appropriate to a negative-feedback control system, is itself suppressed by infusions of vasopressin.[46] Although this concept of a direct link between the two hormonal systems responsible for regulating salt and water balance has obvious teleological appeal, its physiological relevance is still open to question. The dose–response characteristics of these relationships have not yet been adequately defined, but in all the studies reported to date, angiotensin has been infused in relatively large pressor doses, and there is some evidence that more physiological increases achieved by stimulating endogenous renin activity have little or no effect on plasma vasopressin.[27] Similar questions have been raised recently concerning the physiological importance of the renin–angiotensin system in regulating thirst.[47] These considerations do not exclude the possibility that pathological increases in the activity of the renin–angiotensin system might stimulate both thirst and vasopressin secretion. But even if they did, this effect alone might not be sufficient to produce clinically significant abnormalities in free-water balance, since there is some evidence from studies in goats[48] and anesthetized dogs[49,50] that even large doses of angiotensin II do not effect vasopressin secretion in the absence of a concurrent osmotic stimulus. Further studies defining the dose–response characteristics and the interaction between angiotensin and osmotic stimuli in conscious man are needed to clarify this potentially important issue.

7.2.4. Interaction of Osmotic and Hemodynamic Stimuli

The ability of physiological changes in blood pressure and, to a lesser extent, blood volume to stimulate vasopressin secretion raises the obvious question of how these hemodynamic variables affect the operation of the osmoregulatory system. Early studies based on indirect or bioassay methods indicated that moderate hypovolemia could counteract suppression[51] or augment stimulation[52] of vasopressin by blood osmolality. They did not resolve, however, the fundamentally more important issue whether these two systems act in an independent or integrated manner. Evidence for the latter has now been provided by immunoassay studies in rats, which show that moderate reductions in blood volume or pressure do not interfere in any way with *either* the stimulatory *or* the inhibitory effects of blood osmolality on vasopressin secretion.[11,19] Instead, hemodynamic stimuli appear to influence the hormone by lowering the threshold or "set" of the osmoregulatory system. This shift appears to be accompanied by a similar reduction in the osmotic threshold for thirst.[15] In man, the characteristics of this interaction have not been so well defined, but appear to be similar qualitatively, if not quantitatively, to those in the rat. Thus, the relationship between plasma vasopressin and osmolality is shifted to the left by upright posture, which reduces intrathoracic or "effective" blood volume,[13] and is displaced to the right when volume is expanded with infusions of saline or dextran.[13,53,54]

These adjustments in the set of the osmoregulatory system would be expected to alter free-water balance in such a way as to counteract the hemodynamic disturbances with which they are associated. This correction would appear to be only partial, however, since reducing blood volume by 15% in the rat lowers the osmotic threshold for vasopressin release from 290 to 286 mOsm/kg, an amount sufficient to increase free-water balance by less than 2%.[19] This buffering action, which seems to be characteristic of man as well,[13] may confer a homeostatic advantage by enabling the antidiuretic system to strike an appropriate balance between competing needs to preserve both the tonicity and the volume of body water. For example, it might explain why the capacity of healthy adults to regulate free-water balance precisely is not more obviously compromised by the relatively large fluctuations in central blood volume or pressure that accompany normal activity.

This kind of interaction between the osmotic and hemodynamic control of vasopressin could also account for some of the peculiar abnormalities in osmoregulatory function that have been observed with more pathological derangements in blood volume. For example, isolated mineralocorticoid deficiency has been shown to result in hypovolemia, hyponatremia, and inappropriately high plasma vasopressin levels that suppress normally on water-loading.[55] Resetting of the osmoregulatory system ot abnormally low levels has also been observed in hepatic[56] and cardiac[57] failure, conditions in which either total or effective blood volume may be significantly reduced. Whether other causes of hypovolemic hyponatremia such as diuretic abuse exhibit similar changes remains to be determined.

The mechanism by which osmotic and hemodynamic stimuli interact to control vasopressin secretion is still unknown. It is clear, however, that afferents from the two types of receptors must converge at some point and exert their effects on the same population of neurosecretory neurons (see Fig. 1). Such convergence could take place at the level of the neurohypophysis itself, or more proximally at an intermediate neuron chain. The latter hypothesis is consistent with electrophysiological studies that have shown that there are scattered throughout the lateral and anterior hypothalamus neurons the firing rate of which can be altered by both osmotic and volume stimuli.[58]

7.2.5. Nociceptive Influences

Due largely to the original work of Rydin and Verney,[59] it has come to be widely believed that emotion, pain, and other types of noxious stress are potent stimuli for vasopressin release. Recent evidence suggests, however, that this belief may be incorrect, or at least a misleading oversimplification. Immunoassay studies from two laboratories have now shown that a variety of stresses, such as pain, etherization, centrifugation, or water immersion, uniformly fail to increase plasma vasopressin in conscious rats.[1,60] This unresponsiveness stands in contrast to the pronounced effects of the same stresses on corticosterone secretion and the consistency with which osmotic or other kinds of stimuli elicit readily discernible increases in plasma vasopressin in this species.

Limited as they are to rats, these results cannot totally exclude the existence of a nociceptive influence on vasopressin secretion. They do indicate, however, a need to critically reevaluate the entire concept, with a view to determining precisely which stresses are active in this regard and in which species. In so doing, it will be important to distinguish between effects that are a direct result of the stress *per se* and those that are secondary to changes in blood pressure or other recognized stimuli to vasopressin secretion. Vasovagal hypotension can result from pain or intense emotion of almost any cause[61] and, given the potency of this variable, could be the mechanism by which many noxious stimuli affect vasopressin secretion. Clarification of this question is essential for separating the role of nonspecific stress from the other possible causes of the abnormal vasopressin function that occurs with so many acute and chronic illnesses.

These studies also shed some light on the hypothetical role of vasopressin in mediating or facilitating the effect of stress on the pituitary–adrenal axis. This idea, which was first advanced 10–15 years ago,[62,63] has been revived of late by the deomonstration that hypophyseal portal blood from monkeys undergoing surgical stress contains extremely high concentrations of vasopressin.[64] Studies in conscious rats have now shown, however, not only that stressful stimuli increase corticosterone without affecting vasopressin, but also that osmotic stimuli that increase vasopressin have no discernible effect on corticosterone.[1,60] This dissociation means either that vasopressin plays little or no role in pituitary–adrenal activation, as previously suggested by studies in Brattleboro rats,[65,66] or that if it does act as a releasing factor, it must be secreted from neurosecretory cells with functional and anatomical characteristics quite different from those that are involved in regulating water balance. These hypothetical cells would be distinguished by the fact that they do not respond to osmotic stimuli and, when stimulated by nociceptor afferents, release vasopressin at a site from which it does not gain access in perceptible amounts to the peripheral circulation. Neurons containing vasopressin can be identified in several areas of the hypothalamus outside the supraoptic and paraventricular nuclei[67,68] but it has not yet been established whether any exhibit the properties predicted for those with ACTH-releasing functions.

7.2.6. Other Stimuli

There is now good evidence that at least three variables other than blood osmolality, volume, and pressure can have significant effects on neurohypophyseal function.

Serendipitous observations made while studying the effects of ethanol in aging man first suggested that nausea or vomiting or both might be a potent stimulus for vasopressin secretion.[17] More systematic studies using apomorphine as the emetic agent confirmed this impression and showed that the rise in vasopressin was more closely related to nausea than to vomiting and could not be accounted for by changes in blood osmolality or pressure.[1] Further evidence that this response was mediated via the medullary emetic center (see Fig. 1) rather than via other dopaminergic pathways was provided by the observation that apomorphine has little or no effect on vasopressin secretion in rats, a species known to lack a complete emetic reflex. In animals that, like man, are able to vomit, a link between the emetic center and vasopressin secretion could serve a useful homeostatic purpose by minimizing water excretion whenever it is apt to be lost excessively from the GI tract. It should also be noted, however, that the rise in plasma vasopressin induced by emesis in man is 50- to 100-fold greater than that required to achieve maximum antidiuresis,[10] and is well within a concentration range expected to influence many aspects of GI function.[69-71] It is possible, therefore, that vasopressin secretion also plays a more integral and active role in the emetic reflex of man. Further studies of this system are needed to determine how it interacts with other stimuli and whether it is the pathway by which certain drugs and illnesses cause abnormal water retention.

It is interesting that these studies are not the first to note a relationship between the GI tract and vasopressin secretion. In anesthetized dogs, traction on the intestines has been shown to produce large increases in the antidiuretic activity of plasma.[72] This effect, which also could not be accounted for by changes in blood pressure and could be abolished by cervical cordotomy but not vagatomy, has been widely interpreted as an example of general nociceptive stimulation of vasopressin secretion. In view of the paucity of evidence demonstrating such an effect for other noxious stimuli (cf. Section 7.2.5), however, an alternate interpretation may be that manipulation of the intestines stimulates vasopressin release via spinal afferents that act on the emetic center in a manner analogous to apomorphine. If this is the case, an antiemetic such as fluphenazine, which abolishes the vasopressin response to apomorphine,[73] might also be useful in controlling the inappropriate antidiuresis often observed after abdominal surgery.

Acute hypoxia also appears to be an effective stimulus to vasopressin release. Studies using direct[74] as well as indirect[75] methods in anesthetized dogs and cats showed that an acute reduction in arterial pO_2 to 40 mm Hg or below increases antidiuretic activity. This effect appears to be mediated largely via chemoreceptors in the carotid sinus, since it cannot be accounted for by changes in blood osmolality or pressure and occurs independently of changes in pCO_2.[75] Acute hypercapnea alone may also stimulate vasopressin release by an undefined mechanism.[74] Although neither effect has yet been demonstrated in conscious animals or man, they seem to occur at blood gas pressures commonly observed clinically in pneumonia or other causes of acute respiratory impairment, and may be one of the mechanisms by which these disorders so frequently cause the syndrome of inappropriate antidiuresis (cf. Section 7.3.2). They do not seem to be responsible, however, for the impaired water excretion seen in *chronic* pulmonary disease, since the latter appears to be due to the retention of sodium and is not associated with any demonstrable abnormality in either vasopressin secretion or urinary dilution.[76,77]

7.2.7. Neurophysin

It has been known for many years that vasopressin is stored in the neurophypophysis in association with a larger binding protein that is one of a group generally referred to as *neurophysins*. Early work was concerned principally with separating the various neurophysins and defining their physical and chemical characteristics.[78,79] These achievements paved the way for the development of specific radioimmunoassays,[80–82] which have now made it possible to study the distribution, secretion, and metabolism of the neurophysins in greater detail.[68] Recent studies have shown that one neurophysin is secreted in response to nicotine, a stimulus known to release vasopressin, while the other is stimulated more markedly by estrogen and is presumed to be associated with oxytocin.[81] This specificity and the good correlation with plasma vasopressin after nicotine stimulation[83] suggested that the assay of plasma neurophysin might be used as an alternative to vasopressin assays to assess neurohypophyseal function. So far, however, this approach has proved to be of limited utility because some assays are too insensitive to measure neurophysin in plasma under physiological conditions, while others, which can measure basal levels, are unable to detect changes in response to stimuli, such as hypertonic saline infusion, that consistently elicit increases in plasma vasopressin.[82] This problem is complicated by the fact that in plasma, the molar concentration of neurophysin greatly exceeds that of vasopressin,[81–83] while in the hypothalamus and pituitary, the molar ratio of the two substances more closely approximates unity.[84] This discrepancy suggests that vasopressin and neurophysin either are secreted in disproportionate amounts or are distributed and metabolized in different ways. Whichever mechanism is responsible, it would seem effectively to preclude the use of assays for one substance to reliably assess changes in the other.

It has not yet been determined whether plasma neurophysin is merely an incidental by-product of vasopressin secretion or serves some physiological purpose of its own. Although it probably complexes with vasopressin in storage granules of the neurohypophysis, it is unlikely to act as a carrier protein for the hormone in plasma because its binding constant is relatively low at physiological pH.[85] Rats with a hereditary inability to make vasopressin but not oxytocin also appear to lack one of the neurophysins,[86,87] indicating strongly that the synthesis of the two substances is closely related, perhaps through a common precursor or prohormone.[88]

7.3. Pathology

7.3.1. Diabetes Insipidus

Radioimmunoassays of plasma[10,14,89-91] and urine[18,92] from patients with clinical diabetes insipidus have confirmed that the disorder is associated with a marked deficiency of vasopressin secretion. At least in the acquired type of disease, this deficiency is rarely if ever complete, since some hormone can usually be detected in plasma and urine when the intake of water is restricted or other potent stimuli are applied.[10,92] Although the concentrations of vasopressin achieved under these conditions sometimes approximate those found in healthy adults, they are always subnormal relative to the degree of hypertonic dehydration present (see Fig. 2). Thus, when plotted in relation to concurrent plasma osmolality, they can be readily distinguished from the values found in normal subjects or patients with other types of polyuria.[10,89] In patients with primary polydipsia and neurogenic diabetes insipidus, the relationship between plasma vasopressin and osmolality is completely normal (Fig. 2), while that between urine osmolality and plasma vasopressin is not.[10] These observations confirm the pathogenesis of the urinary concentrating defects previously described for these disorders, and also indicate that unlike many other endocrine organs, the neurohypophysis does not undergo significant atrophy or hypertrophy of function in response to long-term suppression or stimulation. This characteristic greatly simplifies the use of vasopressin assays for differentiating among these three types of polyuria.

The vasopressin deficiency in acquired diabetes insipidus behaves as though it were due to a marked reduction or gain or sensitivity of the osmoregulatory system. Thus, analysis of the relationship between plasma vasopressin and osmolality in these patients yields a regression function with a correlation coefficient and intercept similar to those in healthy persons, but a slope less than $1/10$ the mean normal value (Fig. 2).[10,16] This result indicates that the secretory capacity of the neurohypophysis must be reduced by about 90% before the disorder becomes clinically manifest. It also serves as a reminder that anything that affects plasma osmolality in these patients might also be expected to produce small but significant changes in vasopressin secretion. Damage to the thirst mechanism is particularly important in this regard, since, by allowing the development of hypertonic dehydration, it may sometimes promote the release of vasopressin in amounts sufficient to reduce or even abolish spontaneous polyuria.[16,93]

The vasopressin response to dehydration can be lost or impaired in at least two ways. Probably the most common and widely recognized cause is destruction of the neurohypophysis, such as is produced by tumor or surgery, or by unknown causes. As might be expected, such cases exhibit quantitatively similar reductions in their vasopressin response to osmotic and nonosmotic stimuli. Less commonly, deficiencies of vasopressin secretion can also result from a lesion that damages the osmoreceptor mechanism without involving the neurohypophysis.[7,9] In these cases, plasma vasopressin rises to normal or supranormal levels following nonosmotic stimuli, but shows little or no response to hypertonicity. Clinically, these patients have all been distinguished by the presence of hypodipsia, chronic hypernatremia, and a lack of polyuria under basal conditions. It is important to note, however, that these findings may not be invariable, since there is some evidence from animal studies that the osmoreceptors for thirst and vasopressin secretion are not precisely the same.[4,94] Whether selective loss of the vasopressin osmoreceptor ever results in clinical diabetes insipidus in man has not been established.

Remarkable advances have also been made recently in the treatment of diabetes insipidus. About ten years ago, it was discovered by accident that the oral sulfonylurea chlorpropamide had a significant antidiuretic effect in patients with diabetes insipidus.[95] These observations were quickly confirmed,[96] and the drug has since come to be widely used in the treatment of this disorder.[97] There is still disagreement, however, as to precisely how chlorpropamide produces its antidiuretic effect. It is clear that some mechanism related to the antidiuretic hormone must be involved, since, like vasopressin, chlorpropamide is ineffective in nephogenic diabetes insipidus. *In vitro* studies with the toad bladder were the first to suggest that chlorpropamide acts by potentiating the effects of small amounts of endogenous vasopressin.[98,99] Evidence supporting such a mechanism was obtained shortly thereafter in the Brattleboro rat,[100,101] and clinical studies employing indirect methods were also interpreted as being consistent with this view.[102] Immunoassay studies showing that chlorpropamide causes a slight increase in vasopressin excretion in normal subjects suggested, however, that the drug might also act by stimulating vasopressin secretion in diabetes insipidus.[103] Unfortunately, this effect could not be confirmed with an immunoassay for plasma vasopressin.[104] In fact, the antidiuresis produced by chlorpropamide was associated with a significant fall in plasma vasopressin from low to undetectable levels. This paradoxical effect, which may have been secondary to the improved hydration permitted by the antidiuresis, is fully consistent with the original view that the major therapeutic action of chlorpropamide is at the renal level. These findings do not exclude, however, the possibility that chlorpropamide also causes a subtle stimulation of vasopressin secretion, since such an effect could easily have been obscured by the associated fall in plasma osmolality. Further studies in which hydration is held constant will be needed to resolve this question.

Similar uncertainty exists concerning the mechanism of action of clofibrate and carbamazepine, two other drugs discovered to be almost as effective as chlorpropamide in producing antidiuresis in diabetes insipidus.[105,106] Clofibrate, which is used more commonly to treat hyperlipidemia, has been reported to increase the urinary excretion of vasopressin.[107] It does not seem to have any discernible effect on plasma vasopressin,[108] however, and has been reported to potentiate the antidiuretic effects of a synthetic analogue of vasopressin.[109] Carbamazepine, which is usually used to treat tic douloureux and epilepsy, was reported by two laboratories to increase the bioassayable antidiuretic activity of plasma,[110,111] but immunoassay studies find that it causes a fall in plasma vasopressin much like that seen with chlorpropamide.[112] This consistent but unexplained lack of agreement between the plasma immunoassays, on one hand, and the urinary immunoassays and plasma bioassays, on the other, precludes any final conclusions about whether these drugs act primarily by increasing the secretion, delaying the metabolism, or potentiating the effects of endogenous vasopressin. Moreover, none of these mechanisms fully explains the paradoxical but widely observed phenomenon that these drugs have more potent antidiuretic effects in patients with diabetes insipidus than in healthy adults.[103] In this context, the recent observation that maximum doses of lysine vasopressin transiently impair the antidiuretic response to subsequent treatment with any of the oral agents is particularly interesting, since it suggests that all three drugs may have a common mechanism of action that involves some kind of enhanced renal responsiveness endangered by a deficiency of circulating vasopressin.[108]

Another alternative for treating diabetes insipidus that has become available recently is 1-deamino-8-D-arginine vasopressin (DDAVP), a synthetic analogue of vasopressin with reduced pressor and enhanced antidiuretic properties.[113] This compound is also more resistant to degradation than the native molecule[114] and, as a consequence, requires less frequent administration. When taken 2 or 3 times daily by nasal insufflation, it provides complete and sustained relief of polyuria in most patients with diabetes insipidus,[115,116] and appears to be particularly useful in children,[117] who are less tolerant than adults of the oral agents and injections of Pitressin. In some cases, its duration of action may be lengthened by

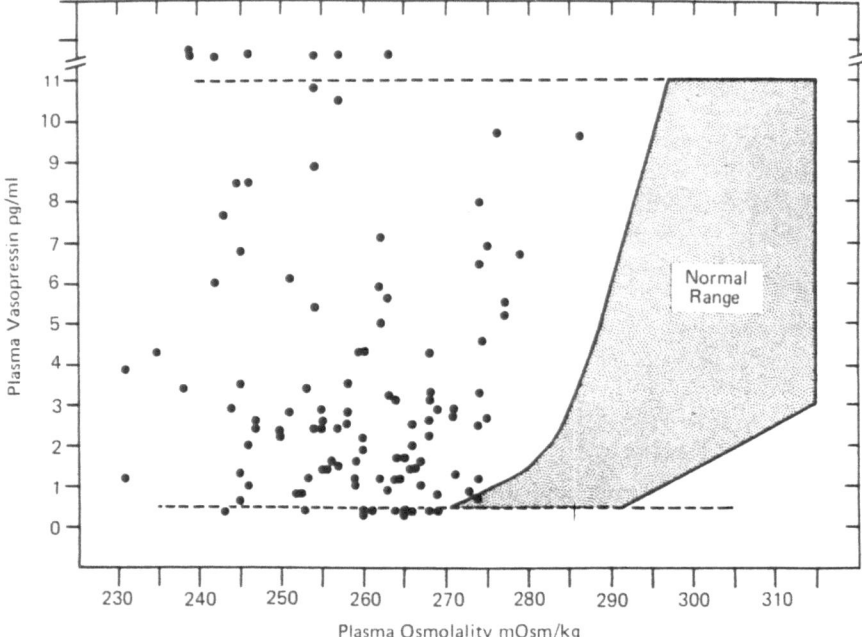

Fig. 3. Relationship between plasma vasopressin and plasma osmolality in 106 patients with SIAD. (Reproduced from Robertson.[1])

simultaneous administration of small doses of clofibrate.[109] Clinical experience with DDAVP in the United States is limited[118] because it has not yet been approved for general distribution.

7.3.2. Syndrome of Inappropriate Antidiuresis

Since its initial description almost 20 years ago,[119] the syndrome of inappropriate antidiuresis (SIAD) has been recognized with increasing frequency in a great variety of malignant and nonmalignant diseases.[120] The original supposition that the cause of the disorder is an inability to suppress vasopressin normally in response to water-loading has now been abundantly confirmed by both bioassay[121] and immunoassay[14,18,91,92,122–125] measurements. In one study comprising more than 100 patients,[1] 90% of the plasma vasopressin values showed clear evidence of inadequate suppression (Fig. 3). Although elevated sufficiently to account for the impaired urinary dilution,[10] most of the plasma vasopressin values were less than 10 pg/ml, the upper limit for normally hydrated healthy adults,[10,13] and could be recognized as abnormal only in relation to the presence of hypotonicity. Just as in the polyuric disorders, therefore, measurements of plasma vasopressin are of little diagnostic value unless they are obtained while the patient is abnormally hydrated and expressed in relation to the simultaneous plasma osmolality.

The same studies have also shown that SIAD is a heterogenous disorder in terms of the underlying osmoregulatory defect, and thus should not be expected to exhibit completely uniform clinical or laboratory characteristics.[126] One type of defect is of particular interest because it seems to result from resetting of the osmoreceptor to abnormally low levels. These patients might be expected to differ significantly from those with other types of SIAD because water-loading should eventually suppress vasopressin to a level that permits maximum urinary dilution and a rate of urine flow sufficient to prevent further overhydration. Several patients who exhibit exactly these characteristics were recently described.[127,128] The mechanism by which resetting of the osmostat occurs is unknown, but in view of its frequency and the diversity of clinical settings with which it is associated, it may be the final common expression of several different pathogenetic processes.[16]

Recent studies of the renin–angiotensin system and plasma aldosterone in patients with SIAD have also provided some useful insights into the pathophysiology of this disorder.[129] In most cases, plasma renin activity is suppressed, a finding consistent with the modest expansion of body water that is responsible for the hyponatremia. Hence, this measurement might provide a simple and effective way of differentiating "true" SIAD from other causes of hyponatremia, such as severe volume depletion or other disorders associated with increased plasma renin activity. Plasma aldosterone does not seem to be suppressed in SIAD, indicating that the sodium wasting that characterizes the disorder is due predominantly to decreased readsorption in the proximal nephron.

Until recently, water restriction or hypertonic saline infusion or both were the only uniformly effective ways of correcting the electrolyte abnormalities in SIAD. Chance observations that patients treated with lithium or demeclocycline develop a kind of reversible nephrogenic diabetes insipidus[130,131] prompted efforts to use these drugs to treat patients with SIAD.[132,133] The mechanism by which these drugs inhibit the effect of vasopressin on the kidney has not been fully defined, but seems to involve a step distal to the formation of AMP.[131,134] Although both have been used successfully for this purpose, at tolerable doses, lithium seems to be effective in a relatively small proportion of people[134] and has frequent and sometimes disturbing side effects.

Demeclomycine, which has a more consistent action and fewer side effects, appears at present to be the best alternative to water restriction for treating patients with chronic SIAD.

References

1. Robertson, G. L., 1977, Vasopressin function in health and disease, *Recent Prog. Horm. Res.* **33:**333–385.
2. Verney, E. B., 1947, The antidiuretic hormone and the factors which determine its release, *Proc. R. Soc. London Ser. B* **135:**25–106.
3. Jewell, P. A., and Verney, E. B., 1957, An experimental attempt to determine the site of the neurohypophysial osmoreceptors in the dog, *Philos. Trans. R. Soc. London Ser. B* **240:**197–324.
4. Peck, J. W., and Blass, E. M., 1975, Localization of thirst and antidiuretic osmoreceptors by intracranial injections in rats, *Am. J. Physiol.* **228:**1501–1509.
5. Bennett, C. T., and Pert, A., 1974, Antidiuresis produced by injections of histamine into the cat supraoptic nucleus, *Brain Res.* **78:**151–156.
6. VanGemert, M., Miller, M., Carey, R. J., and Moses, A. M., 1975, Polyuria and impaired ADH release following medial preoptic lesioning in the rat, *Am. J. Physiol.* **228:**1293–1297.
7. DeRubertis, F. R., Michelis, M. F., and Davis, B. B., 1974, "Essential" hypernatremia: Report of three cases and review of the literature, *Arch. Intern. Med.* **134:**889–895.
8. Halter, J. B., Goldberg, A. P., Robertson, G. L., and Porte, D., Jr., 1977, Selective osmoreceptor dysfunction in the syndrome of chronic hypernatremia, *J. Clin. Endocrinol. Metab.* **44:**609–616.
9. Shelton, R., and Robertson, G., 1976, Selective loss of vasopressin secretion and thirst due to osmoreceptor dysfunction, *Clin. Res.* **24:**278A (abstract).
10. Robertson, G. L., Mahr, E. A., Athar, S., and Sinha, T., 1973, Development and clinical application of a new method for the radioimmunoassay of arginine vasopressin in human plasma, *J. Clin. Invest.* **52:**2340–2352.
11. Dunn, F. L., Brennan, T. J., Nelson, A. E., and Robertson, G. L., 1973, The role of blood osmolality and volume in regulating vasopressin secretion in the rat, *J. Clin. Invest.* **52:**3212–3219.
12. Hayward, J. N., Pavasuthipaisit, K., Perez-Lopez, F. R., and Sofroniew, M. V., 1976, Radioimmunoassay of arginine vasopressin in rhesus monkey plasma, *Endocrinology* **98:**975–981.
13. Robertson, G. L., and Athar, S., 1976, The interaction of blood osmolality and blood volume in regulating plasma vasopressin in man, *J. Clin. Endocrinol. Metab.* **42:**613–620.
14. Shimamoto, K., Murase, T., and Yamaji, T., 1976, A heterologous radioimmunoassay for arginine vasopressin, *J. Lab. Clin. Med.* **87:**338–344.
15. Fitzsimons, J. T., 1972, Thirst, *Physiol. Rev.* **52:**468–561.
16. Robertson, G. L., Shelton, R. L., and Athar, S., 1976, The osmoregulation of vasopressin, *Kidney Int.* **10:**25–37.
17. Helderman, J. H., Vestal, R. E., Rowe, J. W., Tobin, J. D., Andres, R., and Robertson, G. L., 1977, The response of arginine vasopressin to intravenous ethanol and hypertonic saline in man: The impact of aging, *J. Gerontol.* (in press).
18. Merkelbach, U., Czernichow, P., Gaillard, R. C., and Vallotton, M. B., 1975, Radioimmunoassay of [8-arginine]-vasopressin. II. Application to determination of antidiuretic hormone in urine, *Acta Endocrinol. (Copenhagen)* **80:**453–464.
19. Robertson, G. L., Athar, S., and Shelton, R. L., 1977, Osmotic control of vasopressin function, in: *Disturbances in Body Fluid Osmolality* (T. E. Andreoli,

J. J. Grantham, and R. C. Rector, Jr., eds.), pp. 125–148, The American Physiological Society, Bethesda, Maryland.

20. Share, L., 1969, Extracellular fluid volume and vasopressin secretion, in: *Frontiers in Neuroendocrinology* (W. F. Ganong and L. Martini, eds.), pp. 183–210, Oxford University Press, New York.

21. Kirchheim, H. R., 1976, Systemic arterial baroreceptor reflexes, *Physiol. Rev.* **56:**100–177.

22. Calaresu, F. R., and Thomas, M. R., 1975, Electrophysiological connections in the brain stem involved in cardiovascular regulation, *Brain Res.* **87:**335–338.

23. Gauer, O. H., 1968, Osmocontrol versus volume control, *Fed. Proc. Fed. Am. Soc. Exp. Biol.* **27:**1132–1136.

24. Goetz, K. L., Bond, G. C., and Smith, W. E., 1974, Effect of moderate hemorrhage in humans on plasma ADH and renin, *Proc. Soc. Exp. Biol. Med.* **145:**277–280.

25. Robertson, G. L., 1977, The role of osmotic and hemodynamic variables in regulating vasopressin secretion, in: *Proceedings of the Fifth International Congress of Endocrinology*, Hamburg, July 1976, Vol. 1, *Excerpta Med. Int. Congr. Ser.*, No. 402 (V. H. T. James, ed.), pp. 126–130, Excerpta Medica, Amsterdam.

26. Segar, W. E., and Moore, W. W., 1968, The regulation of antidiuretic hormone release in man. I. Effects of change in position and ambient temperature on blood ADH levels, *J. Clin. Invest.* **47:**2143–2151.

27. Share, L., Claybaugh, J. R., Hatch, F. E., Jr., Johnson, J. G., Lee, S., Muirhead, E. E., and Shaw, P., 1972, Effects of change in posture and of sodium depletion on plasma levels of vasopressin and renin in normal human subjects, *J. Clin. Endocrinol. Metab.* **35:**171–174.

28. Schmid, P. G., Abboud, F. M., Wendling, M. G., Ramberg, E. S., Mark, A. L., Heistad, D. D., and Eckstein, J. W., 1974, Regional vascular effects of vasopressin: Plasma levels and circulatory responses, *Am. J. Physiol.* **227:**998–1004.

29. Gauer, O. H. Henry, J. P., and Behn, C., 1970, The regulation of extracellular fluid volume, *Annu. Rev. Physiol.* **32:**547–595.

30. Vatner, S. F., and Braunwald, E., 1975, Cardiovascular control mechanisms in the conscious state, *N. Engl. J. Med.* **293:**970–976.

31. McCance, R. A., 1936, Experimental sodium chloride deficiency in man, *Proc. R. Soc. London Ser. B* **119:**245–268.

32. Bevan, A. T., Honour, A. J., and Stott, F. H., 1969, Direct arterial pressure recording in unrestricted man, *Clin. Sci.* **36:**329–344.

33. Katz, F. H., Loeffel, D. E., Roper, E. F., Lock, J. P., and Husain, M., 1976, Circadian variation of plasma vasopressin in normal active humans, in: *Proceedings of the 58th Annual Meeting of the Endocrine Society*, San Francisco, California, June 1976, published as a supplement to *Endocrinology* **98**(322).

34. George, C. P. L., Messerli, F. H., Genest, J., Nowaczynski, W., Boucher, R., Kuchel, O., and Rojo-Ortega, M., 1975, Diurnal variation of plasma vasopressin in man, *J. Clin. Endocrinol. Metab.* **41:**332–338.

35. Berl, T., Cadnapaphornchai, P., Harbottle, J. A., and Schrier, R. W., 1974, Mechanism of stimulation of vasopressin release during beta adrenergic stimulation with isoproterenol, *J. Clin. Invest.* **53:**857–867.

36. Robertson, G. L., Kinney, R. A., and Nelson, A. E., 1974, The effect of isoproterenol on vasopressin secretion, *Proceedings of the 56th Annual Meeting of the Endocrine Society*, Atlanta, Georgia, June 1974, published as a supplement to *Endocrinology* **94**(217).

37. Berl, T., Cadnapaphornchai, P., Harbottle, J. A., and Schrier, R. W., 1974, Mechanism of suppression of vasopressin during alpha-adrenergic stimulation with norepinephrine, *J. Clin. Invest.* **53**:219–227.
38. Shimamoto, K., and Miyahara, M., 1976, Effect of norepinephrine infusion on plasma vasopressin levels in normal human subjects, *J. Clin. Endocrinol. Metab.* **43**:201–204.
39. Berl, T., and Schrier, R. W., 1973, Mechanism of effect of prostaglandin E_1 on renal water excretion, *J. Clin. Invest.* **52**:463–471.
40. Cadnapaphornchai, P., Boykin, J. L., Berl, T., McDonald, K. M., and Schrier, R. W., 1974, Mechanism of effect of nicotine on renal water excretion, *Am. J. Physiol.* **227**:1216–1220.
41. Bonjour, J. P., and Malvin, R. L., 1970, Stimulation of ADH release by the renin angiotensin system, *Am. J. Physiol.* **218**:1555–1559.
42. Uhlich, E., Weber, P., Eigler, J., and Gröschel-Stewart, U., 1975, Angiotensin stimulated AVP-release in humans, *Klin. Wochenschr.* **53**:177–180.
43. Mouw, D., Bonjour, J. P., Malvin, R. L., and Vander, A., 1971, Central action of angiotension in stimulating ADH release, *Am. J. Physiol.* **220**:239–242.
44. Keil, L. C., Summy-Long, J., and Severs, W. B., 1975, Release of vasopressin by angiotensin II, *Endocrinology* **96**:1063–1065.
45. Fitzsimons, J. T., 1976, The physiological basis of thirst, *Kidney Int.* **10**:3–11.
46. Tagawa, H., Vander, A. J., Bonjour, J. P., and Malvin, R. L., 1971, Inhibition of renin secretion by vasopressin in unanesthetized sodium-deprived dogs, *Am. J. Physiol.* **220**:949–951.
47. Stricker, E. M., Bradshaw, W. G., and McDonald, R. H., Jr., 1976, The renin–angiotensin system and thirst: A reevaluation, *Science* **194**:1169–1171.
48. Andersson, B., and Westbye, O., 1970, Synergistic action of sodium and angiotensin on brain mechanisms controlling fluid balance, *Life Sci.* **9**:601–608.
49. Shimizu, K., Share, L., and Claybaugh, J. R., 1973, Potentiation by angiotensin II of the vasopressin response to an increasing plasma osmolality, *Endocrinology* **93**:42–50.
50. Cadnapaphornchai, P., Boykin, J., Harbottle, J. A., McDonald, K. M., and Schrier, R. W., 1975, Effect of angiotensin II on renal water excretion, *Am. J. Physiol.* **228**:155–159.
51. Arndt, J. O., 1965, Diuresis induced by water infusion into the carotid loop and its inhibition by small hemorrhage, *Pfluegers Arch.* **282**:313–322.
52. Johnson, J. A., Zehr, J. E., and Moore, W. W., 1970, Effects of separate and concurrent osmotic and volume stimuli on plasma ADH in sheep, *Am. J. Physiol.* **218**:1273–1280.
53. Moses, A. M., Miller, M., and Streeten, D. H. P., 1967, Quantitative influence of blood volume expansion on the osmotic threshold for vasopressin release, *J. Clin. Endocrinol. Metab.* **27**:655–662.
54. Moses, A. M., and Miller, M., 1971, Osmotic threshold for vasopressin release as determined by saline infusion and by dehydration, *Neuroendocrinology* **7**:219–226.
55. Boykin, J., McCool, A., Robertson, G., McDonald, K., and Schrier, R., 1975, Mechanism of impaired water excretion in mineralocorticoid deficient dogs, American Federation for Clinical Research, Atlantic City, New Jersey, May 1975, *Clin. Res.* **23**:233A (abstract).
56. Earley, L. E., and Sanders, C. A., 1959, The effect of changing serum osmolality on the release of antidiuretic hormone in certain patients with

decompensated cirrhosis of the liver and low serum osmolality, *J. Clin. Invest.* **38:**545–550.

57. Takasu, T., Lasker, N., and Shalhoub, R. J., 1961, Mechanisms of hyponatremia in chronic congestive heart failure, *Ann. Intern. Med.* **55:**368–383.

58. Menninger, R. P., and Frazier, D. T., 1972, Effects of blood volume and atrial stretch on hypothalamic single-unit activity, *Am. J. Physiol.* **223:**288–293.

59. Rydin, H., and Verney, E. B., 1938, The inhibition of water-diuresis by emotional stress and by muscular exercise, *Q. J. Exp Physiol.* **27:**343–374.

60. Keil, L. C., and Severs, W. B., 1977, Reduction in plasma vasopressin levels of dehydrated rats following acute stress, *Endocrinology* **100:**30–38.

61. Weissler, A. M., and Warren, J. V., 1959, Vasodepressor syncope, *Am. Heart J.* **57:**786–794.

62. Nichols, B. L., Jr., 1961, The role of antidiuretic hormone in corticotrophin release, *Yale J. Biol. Med.* **33:**415–434.

63. Yates, F. E., 1967, Physiological control of adrenal cortical hormone secretion, in: *The Adrenal Cortex* (A. B. Eisenstein, ed.), pp. 133–183, Little, Brown and Company, Boston.

64. Zimmerman, E. A., Carmel, P. W., Husain, M. K., Ferrin, M., Tannenbaum, M., Frantz, A. G., and Robinson, A. G., 1973, Vasopressin and neurophysin: High concentrations in monkey hypophyseal portal blood, *Science* **182:**925–927.

65. McCann, S. M., Antunes-Rodrigues, J., Nallar, R., and Valtin, H., 1966, Pituitary–adrenal function in the absence of vasopressin, *Endocrinology* **79:**1058–1064.

66. Arimura, A., Saito, T., Bowers, C. Y., and Schally, A. V., 1967, Pituitary–adrenal activation in rats with hereditary hypothalamic diabetes insipidus, *Acta Endocrinol.* **54:**155–165.

67. George, J. M., and Jacobowitz, D. M., 1975, Localization of vasopressin in discrete areas of the rat hypothalamus, *Brain Res.* **93:**363–366.

68. Zimmerman, E. A., and Robinson, A. G., 1976, Hypothalamic neurons secreting vasopressin and neurophysin, *Kidney Int.* **10:**12–24.

69. Schapiro, H., and Britt, L. G., 1972, The action of vasopressin on the gastrointestinal tract, *Am. J. Dig. Dis.* **17:**649–667.

70. Barr, J. W., Lakin, R. C., and Rosch, J., 1975, Similarity of arterial and intravenous vasopressin on portal and systemic hemodynamics, *Gastroenterology* **69:**13–19.

71. Schapiro, H., 1975, Inhibitory action of antidiuretic hormone on canine pancreatic exocrine flow, *Am. J. Dig. Dis.* **20:**853–857.

72. Ukai, M., Moran, W. H., and Zimmerman, B., 1968, The role of visceral afferent pathways on vasopressin secretion and urinary excretory patterns during surgical stress, *Ann. Surg.* **168:**16–28.

73. Shelton, R. L., Kinney, R. M., and Robertson, G. L., 1977, Emesis: A species specific stimulus for vasopressin (VP) release, *Clin. Res.* **25:**301A (abstract).

74. Forsling, M. L., and Rees, M., 1975, Effects of hypoxia and hypercapnia on plasma vasopressin concentration, *J. Endocrinol.* **67:**62P–63P.

75. Pluss, R. G., Anderson, R. J., and Schrier, R. W., 1977, Effect of hypoxia on renal water excretion, *Clin. Res.* **25:**139A (abstract).

76. Farber, M. O., Bright, T. P., Strawbridge, R. A., Robertson, G. L., and Manfredi, F., 1975, Impaired water handling in chronic obstructive lung disease, *J. Lab. Clin. Med.* **85:**41–49.

77. Farber, M. O., Kiblawi, S., Strawbridge, R. A., Robertson, G. L., Weinberger,

M. H., and Manfredi, F., 1977, Studies on ADH and renin–angiotensin-aldosterone system in chronic obstructive lung disease, *J. Lab. Clin. Med.* (in press).

78. Acher, R., 1968, Neurophysin and neurohypophysial hormones, *Proc. R. Soc. London Ser. B* **170:**7–16.
79. Hope, D. B., and Hollenberg, M. D., 1968, Crystallization of complexes of neurophysins with vasopressin and oxytocin, *Proc. R. Soc. London Ser. B* **170:**37–47.
80. Cheng, K. W., and Friesen, H. G., 1971, A radioimmunoassay for vasopressin binding proteins—neurophysin, *Endocrinology* **88:**608–619.
81. Robinson, A. G., 1975, Isolation, assay, and secretion of individual human neurophysins, *J. Clin. Invest.* **55:**360–367.
82. Tissot-Berthet, M. C., Reinharz, A. C., and Vallotton, M. B., 1975, Radioimmunoassay of neurophysin I and II in human plasma, *Ann. N. Y. Acad. Sci.* **248:**257–271.
83. Husain, M. K., Frantz, A. G., Ciarochi, F., and Robinson, A. G., 1975, Nicotine-stimulated release of neurophysin and vasopressin in humans, *J. Clin. Endocrinol. Metab.* **41:**1113–1117.
84. Zimmerman, E. A., Robinson, A. G., Husain, M. K., Acosta, M., Frantz, A. G., and Sawyer, W. H., 1974, Neurohypophysial peptides in the bovine hypothalamus: The relationship of neurophysin I to oxytocin, and neurophysin II to vasopressin in supraoptic and paraventricular regions, *Endocrinology* **95:**931–936.
85. Breslow, E., and Walter, R., 1972, Binding properties of bovine neurophysins I and II: An equilibrium dialysis study, *Mol. Pharmacol.* **8:**75–81.
86. Burford, G. D., Jones, C. W., and Pickering, B. T., 1971, Tentative identification of a vasopressin-neurophysin and an oxytocin-neurophysin in the rat, *Biochem. J.* **124:**809–813.
87. Sunde, D., and Sokol, H. W., 1975, Quantification of rat neurophysins by polyacrylamide gel electrophoresis (PAGE): Applications to the rat with hereditary hypothalamic diabetes insipidus, *Ann. N.Y. Acad. Sci.* **248:**345–364.
88. Gainer, H., Sarne, Y., and Brownstein, M. J., 1977, Neurophysin biosynthesis: Conversion of a putative precursor during axonal transport, *Science* **195:**1354–1356.
89. Robertson, G. L., Klein, L. A., Roth, J., and Gorden, P., 1970, Immunoassay of plasma vasopressin in man, *Proc. Natl. Acad. Sci. U.S.A.* **66:**1298–1305.
90. Husain, M. K., Fernando, N., Shapiro, M., Kagan, A., and Glick, S. M., 1973, Radioimmunoassay of arginine vasopressin in human plasma, *J. Clin. Endocrinol. Metab.* **37:**616–625.
91. Skowsky, W. R., Rosenbloom, A. A., and Fisher, D. A., 1974, Radioimmunoassay measurement of arginine vasopressin in serum: Development and application, *J. Clin. Endocrinol. Metab.* **38:**278–287.
92. Miller, M., and Moses, A. M., 1972, Urinary antidiuretic hormone in polyuric disorders and in inappropriate ADH syndrome, *Ann. Intern. Med.* **77:**715–721.
93. Shelton, R., Athar, S., and Robertson, G., 1976, Vasopressin (VP) deficiency without polyuria: A syndrome due to severe hypodipsia and hypernatremia, *Clin. Res.* **24:**101A (abstract).
94. Andersson, B., 1971, Thirst—and brain control of water balance, *Amer. Sci.* **59:**408–415.

95. Arduino, F., Ferraz, F. P. J., and Rodrigues, J., 1966, Antidiuretic action of chlorpropamide in idiopathic diabetes insipidus, *J. Clin. Endocrinol. Metab.* **26:**1325–1328.
96. Meinders, A. E., Touber, J. L., and deVries, L. A., 1967, Chlorpropamide treatment in diabetes insipidus, *Lancet* **2:**544–546.
97. Miller, M., and Moses, A. M., 1976, Drug-induced states of impaired water excretion, *Kidney Int.* **10:**96–103.
98. Ingelfinger, J. R., and Hayes, R. M., 1969, Evidence that chlorpropamide and vasopressin share a common site of action, *J. Clin. Endocrinol. Metab.* **29:**738–740.
99. Mendoza, S., 1970, Effect of chlorpropamide on the permeability of urinary bladder of the toad and the response to vasopressin, adenosine 3′,5′-monophosphate and theophylline, *Endocrinology* **86:**1028–1032.
100. Miller, M., and Moses, A. M., 1970, Potentiating of vasopressin action by chlorpropamide *in vivo, Endocrinology* **86:**1024–1027.
101. Berndt, W. O., Miller, M., Kettyle, W. M., and Valtin, H., 1970, Potentiation of the antidiuretic effect of vasopressin by chlorpropamide, *Endocrinology* **86:**1028–1032.
102. Miller, M., and Moses, A. M., 1970, Mechanism of chlorpropamide action in diabetes insipidus, *J. Clin. Endocrinol. Metab.* **30:**488–496.
103. Moses, A. M., Numann, P., and Miller, M., 1973, Mechanism of chlorpropamide-induced antidiuresis in man: Evidence for release of ADH and enhancement of peripheral action, *Metabolism* **22:**59–66.
104. Robertson, G. L., and Mahr, E., 1971, The mechanism of chlorpropamide antidiuresis in diabetes insipidus: Studies with a new radioimmunoassay for plasma vasopressin, *Endocrinology* **88:**125.
105. de Gennes, J.-L., Bertrand, C., Bigorie, B., and Truffert, J., 1970, Études préliminaires de l'action antidiurétique du clofibrate (ou atromid S) dans le diabéte insipide pitressosensible, *Ann. Endocrinol.* **31:**300–308.
106. Tietze, H. U., and Finkenwirth, H., 1970, Beeinflussung des Diabetes insipidus durch Tegretal, *Monatsschr. Kinderheilkd.* **118:**237–238.
107. Moses, A. M., Howanitz, J., van Gemert, M., and Miller, M., 1973, Clofibrate-induced antidiuresis, *J. Clin. Invest.* **52:**535–542.
108. Meinders, A. E., Van Leeuwen, A. M., Borst, J. G. G., and Cejka, V., 1975, Paradoxical diuresis after vasopressin administration to patients with neurohypophyseal diabetes insipidus treated with chlorpropamide, carbamazepine or clofibrate, *Clin. Sci. Mol. Med.* **49:**283–290.
109. Rado, J. P., and Marosi, J., 1975, Prolongation of duration of action of 1-deamino-8-D-arginine vasopressin (DDAVP) by ineffective doses of clofibrate in diabetes insipidus, *Horm. Metab.* **7:**527–528.
110. Frahn, H., Šmejkal, E., and Kratzenstein, R., 1969, Antidiuretic effect of an anticonvulsant drug [5-carbamyl-5H-dibenzo(B,F)azepin = Tegretal] associated with measureable increase of ADH activity in serum of patients suffering from diabetes insipidus and of patients with polyuria and polydipsia following hypophysectomy, *Acta Endocrinol. (Copenhagen)* **138**(Suppl.):240.
111. Kimura, T., Matsui, K., Sato, T., and Yoshinaga, K., 1974, Mechanism of carbamazepine (Tegretol)-induced antidiuresis: Evidence for release of antidiuretic hormone and impaired excretion of a water load, *J. Clin. Endocrinol. Metab.* **38:**356–362.
112. Meinders, A. E., Cejka, V., and Robertson, G. L., 1974, The antidiuretic action of carbamazepine in man, *Clin. Sci. Mol. Med.* **47:**289–299.

113. Vávra, L., Machová, A., Holeček, V., Cort, J. H., Zaoral, M., and Šorm. F., 1968, Effect of a synthetic analogue of vasopressin in animals and in patients with diabetes insipidus, *Lancet* **1**:948–952.
114. Edwards, C. R. W., Kitau, M. J., Chard, T., and Besser, G. M., 1973, Vasopressin analogue DDAVP in diabetes insipidus: Clinical and laboratory studies, *Br. Med. J.* **3**:375–378.
115. Andersson, K.-E., and Arner, B., 1972, Effects of DDAVP, a synthetic analogue of vasopressin, in patients with cranial diabetes insipidus, *Acta. Med. Scand.* **192**:21–27.
116. Ward, M. K., and Fraser, T. R., 1974, DDAVP in treatment of vasopressin-sensitive diabetes insipidus, *Br. Med. J.* **3**:86–89.
117. Aronson, A. S., Andersson, K.-E., Bergstrand, C. G., and Mulder, J. L., 1973, Treatment of diabetes insipidus in children with DDAVP, a synthetic analogue of vasopressin, *Acta Paediatr. Scand.* **62**:133–140.
118. Robinson, A. G., 1976, DDAVP in the treatment of central diabetes insipidus, *N. Engl. J. Med.* **294**:507–511.
119. Schwartz, W. B., Bennett, W., Curelop, S., and Bartter, F. C., 1957, A syndrome of renal sodium loss and hyponatremia probably resulting from inappropriate secretion of antidiuretic hormone, *Am. J. Med.* **23**:529–542.
120. Bartter, F. C., 1973, The syndrome of inappropriate secretion of antidiuretic hormone (SIADH), *Dis. Mon.* November, pp. 1–47.
121. Baumann, G., Lopez-Amor, E., and Dingman, J. F., 1972, Plasma arginine vasopressin in the syndrome of inappropriate antidiuretic hormone secretion, *Am. J. Med.* **52**:19–24.
122. Robertson, G. L., Bhoopalam, N., and Zelkowitz, L. J., 1973, Vincristine neurotoxicity and abnormal secretion of antidiuretic hormone, *Arch. Intern. Med.* **132**:717–720.
123. DeFronzo, R. A., Colvin, O. M., Braine, H., Robertson, G. L., and Davis, P. J., 1974, Cyclophosphamide and the kidney, *Cancer* **33**:483–491.
124. Zimbler, H., Robertson, G. L., Bartter, F. C., Delea, C. S., and Pomerov. T., 1975, Ewing's sarcoma as a cause of the syndrome of inappropriate secretion of antidiuretic hormone, *J. Clin. Endocrinol. Metab.* **41**:390–391.
125. Beardwell, C. G., 1971, Radioimmunoassay of arginine vasopressin in human plasma, *J. Clin. Endocrinol. Metab.* **33**:254–260.
126. Shelton, R., Athar, S., and Robertson, G., 1976, Heterogeneity of vasopressin (VP) dysfunction in the syndrome of inappropriate antidiuresis (SIAD), *Proceedings of the 58th Annual Meeting of the Endocrine Society*, San Francisco, California, June 1976, published as a supplement to *Endocrinology* **98**(323).
127. DeFronzo, R. A., Goldberg, M., and Agus, Z. S., 1976, Normal diluting capacity in hyponatremic patients: Reset osmostat or a variant of the syndrome of inappropriate antidiuretic hormone secretion, *Ann. Intern. Med.* **84**:538–542.
128. Michelis, M. F., Fusco, R. D., Bragdon. R. W., and Davis, B. B., 1974, Reset of osmoreceptors in association with normovolemic hyponatremia, *Am. J. Med. Sci.* **267**:267–273.
129. Fichman, M. P., Michelakis, A. M., and Horton, R., 1974, Regulation of aldosterone in the syndrome of inappropriate antidiuretic hormone secretion (SIADH), *J. Clin. Endocrinol. Metab.* **39**:136–144.
130. Lee, R. V., Jampol, L. M., and Brown, W. V., 1971, Nephrogenic diabetes insipidus and lithium intoxication—complications of lithium carbonate therapy, *N. Engl. J. Med.* **284**:93–94.

131. Singer, I., and Rotenberg, D., 1973, Demeclocycline-induced nephrogenic diabetes insipidus, *Ann. Intern. Med.* **79:**679–683.
132. White, M. G., and Fetner, C. D., 1975, Treatment of the syndrome of inappropriate secretion of antidiuretic hormone with lithium carbonate, *N. Engl. J. Med.* **292:**390–392.
133. Cherrill, D. A., Stote, R. M., Birge, J. R., and Singer, I., 1975, Demeclocycline treatment in the syndrome of inappropriate antidiuretic hormone secretion, *Ann. Intern. Med.* **83:**654–656.
134. Forrest, J. N., Jr., Cohen, A. D., Torretti, J., Himmelhoch, J. M., and Epstein, F. H., 1974, On the mechanism of lithium-induced diabetes insipidus in man and the rat, *J. Clin. Invest.* **53:**1115–1123.

The Ovary

Mortimer B. Lipsett and Griff T. Ross

8.1. Secondary Amenorrhea

Over the years, considerable effort has been devoted to defining the subsets of the population of women with secondary amenorrhea. It has long been recognized that some of these women had ample evidence of estrogen secretion, whereas others could be categorized, by vaginal smear and urinary estrogen determinations, as belonging to a low-estrogen group. Systematic studies of women with secondary amenorrhea have now revealed the interrelationships between serum estrogen concentrations and other diagnostic tests.

Kletzky *et al.*[1] examined 90 women with secondary amenorrhea of over 6 months' duration. Excluding those patients with premature menopause or polycystic ovarian disease, the remaining 57 patients could be divided into two groups on the basis of serum estrogen concentrations and progesterone withdrawal bleeding. Of these women, 42 had a mean serum estradiol level of 60 pg/ml, a value comparable to that of the late follicular phase, and had progesterone-induced withdrawal bleeding. By contrast, the mean serum estradiol concentration in the 15 women who did not bleed in response to progesterone was only 18 pg/ml. Thus, progesterone withdrawal bleeding, as expected, defined the adequacy of estrogen stimulation of the endometrium and thereby the blood estrogen level. These two groups of patients could not be distinguished on the basis

MORTIMER B. LIPSETT and GRIFF T. ROSS • National Institutes of Health, Bethesda, Maryland.

of plasma LH or FSH concentrations, although the patients with polycystic ovarian disease were separable on the basis of high LH levels, and those patients with premature menopause were denoted by high FSH levels.

In an extension of this work, Kletzky et al.[2] measured plasma estradiol, FSH, and LH at 15-min intervals for 4 hr in 15 patients with hypothalamic–pituitary amenorrhea. In those patients who did not have progesterone-induced withdrawal bleeding, the low or low normal levels of LH, FSH, and estradiol showed little variation. These patients were characterized as hypothalamic–pituitary failure. In the progesterone-responsive group (hypothalamic–pituitary dysfunction), FSH, LH, and estradiol had the normal oscillations of peak height and frequency. These latter patients secreted the same total amount of LH during the 4-hr period as did normal women. The total amount of gonadotropin secreted by the women with hypothalamic–pituitary failure was significantly lower than that of normal women, and accounts for the low estradiol secretion. Of this latter group, 6 patients had some evidence of a pituitary lesion, and 4 had high prolactin secretion (see below).

These data correlate well with those obtained by Vaitukaitis et al.,[3] who studied clomiphene and GnRH responsiveness of women with secondary amenorrhea. In those patients who did not respond to clomiphene by a doubling of plasma LH and FSH, basal gonadotropin levels were low, serum estradiol was generally below 20 pg/ml, and the integrated response of LH to GnRH was the same as that of women in the early follicular phase. Interestingly, FSH responsiveness was greater than normal, a response reminiscent of that of the prepubertal girl. When the response to clomiphene was normal, the response to GnRH was the same as that of luteal-phase women. Since clomiphene is an antiestrogen, both theory and study indicate that it is effective only when estrogen concentrations are adequate, and it is undoubtedly the estrogen concentration that defines the response to GnRH. Another and similar study[4] confirmed, in large part, the results reported by the previous authors. In both series, there were women with hypothalamic–pituitary failure who had no evidence of pituitary tumor, so that there is almost certainly a group of women who have selective depression of LH secretion with a variable decrease in FSH. Kistner[5] had shown earlier that an ovulatory response to clomiphene is more frequent in those women who have withdrawal bleeding following progesterone.

The data of Goldenberg et al.[6] are also pertinent. They found that those women with secondary amenorrhea who had progesterone withdrawal bleeding had a subsequent preovulatory surge of LH. They interpreted this as demonstrating the capacity of the hypothalamic–pituitary axis to respond to changes in steroid concentrations and would thereby support the subsequent appellation of hypothalamo–pituitary dysfunction.

8.2. Hyperprolactinemic Amenorrhea

8.2.1. Etiology

In 1953, Argonz and del Castillo[7] described the syndrome of secondary amenorrhea, decreased estrogens, and low urinary gonadotropins. These data were obtained with difficulty and imprecision because bioassays were required for all the determinations. When a radioimmunoassay for prolactin was added to those for the other hormones, it became possible to explore this syndrome definitively. It is now apparent that it is considerably more common than was recognized and is susceptible to successful therapy.

Franks et al.[8] measured serum prolactin in 105 women with amenorrhea. Prolactin was increased in 8 of the 40 women classified as functional secondary amenorrhea (this excludes the amenorrhea either following cessation of oral contraceptive therapy or occurring with weight loss). Only 3 of these patients had galactorrhea. Similar patients examined by the same group were shown to have low plasma estrogens.[9] The prolactin concentration tended to be only moderately increased, about 6 times normal, whereas it is generally greatly increased in those women with the syndrome of amenorrhea and galactorrhea associated with pituitary tumor.[10,11] The clinical and endocrine features of 35 women with hyperprolactinemic amenorrhea were examined in detail by Jacobs et al.[10] Of the 35 patients, 17 had no evidence of pituitary tumor. These patients had a subnormal response to TRH, in contrast to the heightened response of TSH to TRH in states of hypothyroidism. Plasma estrogens were low, and as a result, there was no progesterone withdrawal bleeding, and the response to clomiphene was usually anovulatory. Bohnet et al.[12] continued the delineation of this syndrome by showing that basal LH levels were low and showed little of the characteristic spiking. They commented that the longer the duration of the amenorrhea, the poorer was the response to GnRH.

Of interest in a somewhat different context was their note that the two patients who ovulated in response to clomiphene had short luteal phases and low plasma progesterone levels, thereby defining an inadequate corpus luteum. Jewelewicz et al.[13] had reported earlier that the lowest luteal-phase progesterone concentrations occurred in women with the highest prolactin levels, and Corenblum et al.[14] associated luteal-phase defects with prolactin hypersecretion. These findings are possibly the clinical counterpart of the studies of McNatty et al.[15] who found that high concentrations of prolactin depressed progesterone secretion by isolated granulosa cells, and showed later[16] that prolactin and progesterone concentrations in follicular fluid are negatively correlated. Despite these impressive studies, del Pozo et al.[17] showed that there was no alteration of the normal menstrual cycle in women whose prolactin levels were decreased from 10 to 2 ng/ml by bromocryptine. A possible synthesis of these apparently conflicting data is that normal prolactin concentrations have little effect, but as the concentration increases, suppression of steroid secretion by the luteinized granulosa cell occurs.

Although there is this direct effect of prolactin on ovarian progesterone secretion, there must be a central effect as well, since plasma LH concentrations are either low or low normal despite decreased plasma estrogen concentrations. As noted above, the response to GnRH was abnormal, again implicating the pituitary–hypothalamic axis. Glass et al.[18] reported, however, that basal plasma estradiol concentrations and the amount of FSH and LH released by GnRH were negatively correlated, in contrast to the positive correlation noted during the normal menstrual cycle. Since the effects of GnRH depend critically on the plasma estrogen concentration, on the duration of the state of low LH secretion, and on other as yet undefined factors, some disagreement about response to GnRH is to be expected. Aono et al.[19] obtained normal or somewhat increased responses of FSH and LH to GnRH, but also showed that the positive-feedback effect of estrogens was absent in these patients. Patients with secondary amenorrhea, but without elevated plasma prolactins, had a partial response to the estrogen.

8.2.2. Postpartum Amenorrhea

It had been suggested by Zaraté et al.[20] that the ovary in the postpartum period was refractory to hMG, and that this was pertinent to hyperprolactinemic amenorrhea. The same group,[21] however, noted the same refractoriness after suppressing prolactin with bromocryptine and concluded that the lack of response was not mediated by prolactin. Others[22] obtained a response to hMG during the postpartum period with early and significant increases in plasma estrogens. The response to GnRH in some of these patients was inadequate,[23] again placing the effect of prolactin at a central site. Mroueh and Siler-Khodr[24] reported that the ovaries of women with inappropriate lactation were refractory to hMG. In the nonpregnant women with hyperprolactinemic amenorrhea, however, higher doses of hMG and hCG produced the expected increase in estrogens and ovulation.[25] Some of the conflicting data may also be due to small variations in the time of study. For example, Keye and Jaffe[26] found a decreased responsiveness to GnRH in the early puerperium, but this had increased to normal by the 5th to 8th week.

8.2.3. Treatment

The response of women with hyperprolactinemic amenorrhea to bromocryptine has been well documented. Bromocryptine restored the cycle to normal in all patients in one report[10] and in 8 of 14 in another.[27] The former group made the observation that an increase of gonadotropins following GnRH predicted the response to bromocryptine.

Other therapies of the hyperprolactinemic amenorrhea syndrome have been reported. McIntosh[28] treated 5 women for 1–3 months with 200–600 mg pyridoxine. Three women developed regular ovulatory menses. He pointed out that pyridoxine-5-phosphate is a cofactor in the decarboxylation of DOPA to dopamine, the presumptive prolactin-inhibiting factor, and in the decarboxylation of 5-hydroxytryptophan to serotonin. Prompted by the previously noted association of psychological disturbance and secondary amenorrhea, Zacur et al.[29] noted briefly that psychological counseling of three women with this syndrome could reduce prolactin levels and result in menses.

Since bromocryptine had proved so successful in the treatment of hyperprolactinemic amenorrhea, attempts have been made to use this drug in euprolactinemic amenorrhea. Tolis and Naftolin[30] studied 3 such women in detail. Pulsatile gonadotropin secretion was decreased and plasma estrogen concentrations were below normal follicular phase levels. With bromocryptine, there was amplification of gonadotropin secretion and 2 women ovulated. Seppala et al.[27] reported that 9 of 18 such women had restoration of ovulatory menstrual cycles in response to bromocryptine. This group[31] also found that plasma estradiol levels increased from 60 to 180 pg/ml without significant change in FSH or LH. They commented that in subsequent studies they noted that the LH reponse to GnRH may be enhanced by bromocryptine. At any rate, the mechanism or mechanisms by which bromocryptine induces ovulation seem to be the same in euprolactinemic as in hyperprolactinemic amenorrhea.

8.2.4. Androgens

Of some interest is the study of plasma androgens in women with hyperprolactinemic amenorrhea. Bassi *et al.*[32] measured plasma and urinary androgens and proandrogens and showed that the plasma concentrations of dehydroepiandrosterone and dehydroepiandrosterone sulfate, as well as the urinary excretion of the latter, were increased in women with hyperprolactinemic amenorrhea. This did not occur in other women with secondary amenorrhea. Possibly relevant is the finding of Boyns *et al.*[33] that prolactin promoted androgen synthesis by human adrenal cortex *in vivo*. Seppala *et al.*[34] also noted that bromocryptine did not alter the plasma concentrations of testosterone or dihydrotestosterone in women with hyperprolactinemic amenorrhea.

8.3. Post-Pill Amenorrhea

Patients with amenorrhea following discontinuation of oral contraceptives have varying causes for the amenorrhea. Marshall *et al.*[35] identified underlying conditions to account for the post-pill amenorrhea in 14 of 24 patients. These were pregnancy, premature ovarian failure, polycystic ovarian disease, and pituitary tumor (6 of 24). Similarly, Gómez *et al.*[36] found that 30% of women presenting with post-pill galactorrhea and hyperprolactinemia had evidence of pituitary tumors.

The patients with post-pill normoprolactinemic amenorrhea were not a homogeneous group.[35] Of 9 patients, 6 had a normal response to clomiphene, indicating that both negative- and positive-feedback systems were intact. Two patients treated with clomiphene had a normal increase in plasma estradiol, but there was no secondary LH peak. Thus, in these patients, one might postulate failure of positive feedback. One patient was unresponsive to clomiphene despite a normal plasma estradiol and a normal response to GnRH. This suggests that negative feedback was abnormal and that hypothalamic dysfunction was causative. Euprolactinemic patients with secondary amenorrhea responded to bromocryptine at the same rate as did those with hyperprolactinemia.[27] Thus, treatment with a dopamine agonist will permit normal prolactin levels.

8.4. Polycystic Ovary Syndrome

8.4.1. Characterization

The polycystic ovary syndrome (PCO) has also been the subject of recent careful study. Although it has been known that patients of many types were included within this syndrome, precise hormonal characterization was not previously possible. The finding of theca cell luteinization and the high androgen secretion suggested excessive LH stimulation, and bioassay data were in accord. When LH was measured by radioimmunoassay, it was elevated in all of 16 patients with PCO.[37] In a subsequent study, however, Gambrell et al.[38] reported that about one-third of their patients with PCO had elevated serum LH and one-third had low levels.

Berger et al.[39] and Patton et al.[40] were able to divide their patients with PCO into two groups, those who had normal or only slightly enlarged ovaries and those who had ovaries 2–4 times normal size. Plasma LH concentrations were normal in the former and high in the latter, although there were differences neither in clinical presentation nor in androgen patterns between the groups. In addition, Patton et al.[40] found that patients with high LH had a greater absolute response to GnRH than did those in the other group, and that this occurred in the setting of higher plasma estrogen concentrations and was similar to responses seen in normal women shortly before ovulation. The role of estrogen levels in predicting (determining?) the response to GnRH was noted by Nillius and Wide,[41] who correlated estrogen excretion with the LH response to GnRH in women with secondary amenorrhea.

Givens et al.[42] compared the clinical and hormonal features and ovarian pathology of women with PCO who were divided into two groups on the basis of either high or normal LH concentration. In contrast to the findings in previous studies, neither ovarian size nor stromal thecal luteinization differed between the groups. Plasma testosterone concentrations were the same in both groups, but plasma androstenedione levels were almost twice as high in the high-LH group (517 vs. 286 ng/dl; normal, 176). Both groups of patients were then studied during administration of dexamethasone, 2 mg/day for 4 days; dexamethasone, 2 mg/day for 4 days, plus ethinyl estradiol, 0.5 mg/day; and finally, dexamethasone plus 5000 IU hCG/day for 3 days. During dexamethasone administration, urinary and plasma LH increased in the normal LH group and there was a concomitant increase in androstenedione and testosterone. In the high-LH group, the direction of change of these hormones was opposite. When ethinyl estradiol was added, LH increased in both groups. In the low-LH group, hCG caused a 5 mg/day increase in urinary 17-ketosteroid excretion, but only an insignificant increase in the high-LH group. Similarly, the increase in plasma testosterone and androstenedione was greater in the low-LH group.

Although the biochemical differences of these two groups were clear, interpretation of the data and of those of the previous studies is difficult. The groups appear to differ both at the hypothalamic–pituitary level and at the ovarian compartment. Which is primary is uncertain. Nevertheless, continued dissection of the PCO syndrome will doubtless uncover the pathogenetic abnormalities in the near future.

In a series of papers dealing with the hypothalamic–pituitary axis in the PCO syndrome, the Birmingham group examined several aspects of the regulatory mechanisms. Shaw *et al.*[43] reported that 1 mg estradiol benzoate elicited an increase of LH in plasma of 23 mIU/ml in 15 of 19 women with PCO. This was accompanied by smaller increases in plasma FSH. Thus, the positive estrogen feedback that causes the midcycle LH surge is generally intact in PCO syndrome, and any gonadotropin abnormalities must occur at a time when they affect follicular maturation. They also confirmed an earlier report of their own that the estrogen-induced LH surge predicted response to clomiphene. They then examined the response to GnRH[44] and noted that the LH response was of the same magnitude as that of normal women during the luteal phase. It should be noted that their 18 patients had normal basal LH levels. There was a high negative correlation ($\eta = -0.86$) between plasma LH and testosterone that was interpreted by the authors as being related to the suppression of the ovulatory surge of LH. When estradiol or progesterone was given prior to administration of GnRH,[45] women with PCO behaved as normal women, showing again that positive feedback is intact in the PCO syndrome. There were some quantitative changes however. Estradiol augmentation of GnRH release of LH was less than normal in PCO, and the effect of progesterone was greater. Katz and Carr[46] also compared the effects of GnRH in women with PCO or functional secondary amenorrhea. In this group, basal LH was increased, as was plasma estrogen, but the peak LH response was the same in both groups. It is clear that the patients with PCO studied here differed from those studied in the previous three papers. Lawrence *et al.*[47] incriminated androgens as the cause of another abnormality seen in PCO. Using clomiphene or hMG, they induced ovulation in women with either PCO or secondary amenorrhea and found that the pregnancy rate was only 21% in PCO, where the androgens were increased, but it was 75% in women with secondary amenorrhea and normal androgens.

8.4.2. Wedge Resection

Judd *et al.*[48] followed the course of women with PCO subjected to wedge resection because they did not ovulate in response to clomiphene. Both plasma testosterone and androstenedione concentrations fell for the 3 days following resection, and androstenedione, but not testosterone, concentration increased promptly thereafter. The pattern was the same in the 5 patients who ovulated and the 3 who did not. The authors speculate that decreases in intraovarian androgens are responsible for the ovulation, since circulating gonadotropins did not differ between the two groups until the ovulatory LH surge. This difference may be expressed via estrogen secretion, since only those patients who ovulated had a preovulatory estrogen increase.

8.4.3. Ovarian Enzymes

A variety of enzymatic abnormalities have been postulated to exist in PCO, but without much substantiation. Cox and Shearman[49] reported some years ago, however, that some patients with PCO excrete pregnene-triolone ($3\alpha,17\alpha,20\alpha$-trihydroxy-$5\beta$-pregnan-11-one). Maschler *et al.*[50] have now shown that in such patients, the ovary contains an 11β-hydroxylase capable of 11-hydroxylating C-21-deoxysteroids, but not C-21-hydroxysteroids. Although this finding apparently does not contribute to our understanding of the pathogenesis of the syndrome, it does indicate that the ovaries of some patients with PCO differ qualitatively as well as quantitatively from those of the normal population.

8.5. Menstrual Cycle Progesterone

Although the normal human menstrual cycle has been studied intensively, there remain a few features that have not been clarified. Progesterone levels in venous blood from the ovary containing the dominant follicle and in antral fluid of large preovulatory follicles rise prior to the LH surge. Yussman and Taymor,[51] however, were unable to demonstrate that plasma progesterone increased prior to the LH peak, and more recently, Thorneycroft *et al.*[52] found that plasma progesterone began to increase coincident with the LH peak. However, Abraham *et al.*[53] and now Laborde *et al.*[54] have found that plasma progesterone increases just before the LH peak. In all these studies, frequent sampling was necessary. The opposing views are of interest because they bear on the question of regulation of steroid secretion during the periovulatory period. If progesterone does increase coincident with the LH surge, this could be interpreted as indicating that early luteinization begins prior to ovulation. An increase in progesterone without a concomitant increase in LH should direct attention to intrinsic follicular activity just prior to ovulation, and increased LH levels in antral fluid from large follicles are consistent with this alternative. Chattoraj *et al.*[55] showed that urinary progesterone excretion increased from 0.2 μg/24 hr during the follicular phase to 1.4 μg/24 hr during the luteal phase.

8.6. Estrogens and the Adrenal

The role of estrogens in adrenal maturation has received renewed attention. Sobrinho *et al.*[56] administered stilbestrol to 5 untreated patients with gonadal dysgenesis. Although steroid excretion did not increase, the ratio of pregnenetriol to pregnanediol increased, and this was interpreted as a decrease in activity of adrenal 3β-hydroxysteroid dehydrogenase. Abraham and Maroulis[57] gave either stilbestrol or conjugated estrogens to postmenopausal women for 2 months and reported increases in plasma pregnenolone, as well as dehydroepiandrosterone and its sulfate, although androgens and cortisol were unchanged. Anderson and Yen,[58] however, could not verify these reports during either acute or chronic administration of estrogen with or without ACTH. They measured the plasma Δ^5-steroids, pregnenolone, 17-hydroxypregnenolone, dehydroepiandrosterone and its sulfate, and androstenedione, testosterone, and cortisol. All behaved similarily. Thus, they were unable to show any effect of estrone on the adrenal 3β-hydroxysteroid dehydrogenase.

8.7. Human Chorionic Gonadotropin

In 1976, there were several major advances in the correlation of the structure of hCG with its function and in the use of hCG and its subunits in diagnosing and treating reproductive disorders. Fifty years ago, Ascheim and Zondek[59] discovered that the urine from pregnant women contained gonadotropic activity, subsequently shown to be hCG secreted by the trophoblast. Since this hormone is so intimately involved with pregnancy, it seems appropriate to discuss it here, although present knowledge takes the discussion into several apparently unrelated fields.

8.7.1. Structural Properties

Human CG is a glycoprotein, consisting of two dissimilar, noncovalently linked polypeptide subunits with attached carbohydrate side chains.[60,61] The subunits, designated as α and β in accord with the convention used for other human and nonhuman glycoprotein hormones, have been dissociated, isolated, and purified, and primary structures have been proposed for both.[62,63] The α-subunits of all human glycoprotein hormones, including hCG, consist of 89–92 amino acid residues in identical sequences, but the carbohydrate side chains differ significantly.[64,65] In contrast to the α-subunits, β-subunits have similar but distinctive amino acid contents and sequences. Current proposals for the structure of hCGβ reveal that the subunit consists of 145 amino acid residues. Among the first 115 aminoterminal amino acid residues, 80% are identical to those of HLHβ, but the 30 carboxyterminal residues are unique to hCGβ.[65–67]

Purified hCG α- and β-subunits, natural or desialylated (see below), can be reassociated with each other or with complementary subunits from other human or nonhuman glycoprotein hormones.[68,69] Rates of recombination and of changes in conformation have been monitored by a variety of physical techniques, such as ANS fluorescence, ultraviolet absorption spectroscopy, circular dichroism, and ultracentrifugation, coupled with *in vitro* and *in vivo* assays. The kinetics of reassociation have been consistent with a rapid initial subunit pairing followed by a slower, rate-limiting refolding, leading to recovery of biological activity and receptor binding. The biological activity of hCG depends on reversible tertiary structural configurations of the subunits in the molecule, and the carbohydrate moiety of these does not appear to be obligatory for either formation or maintenance of this property.

Purified hCG preparations have interstitial-cell-stimulating, follicle-stimulating, and thyroid-stimulating activities, and the relative proportions of these biological activities remain constant during purification of the hormone.[70] Moreover, dissociation of the molecule into subunits results in loss, and recombination results in recovery, of all three activities in the same proportions.[71,72] Similar rates of recombination of heterologous complementary subunits with widely varying carbohydrate contents have led to the conclusion that the carbohydrate moiety is not required for the folding and unfolding of the molecule.

8.7.2. Sialic Acid

The role of the terminal carbohydrate, sialic acid, has been examined intensively, since it has been shown to determine the fate of other glycoproteins. Progressive removal of sialic acid from hCG resulted in faster clearance from plasma[73,74] and a proportionate reduction in biological activity as measured by bioassay.

The rapid clearance of desialylated hCG seems to depend on hepatic clearance, since Birken and Canfield[75] found 86% of the injected dose taken up by the liver, approximately 10% by the kidney, and less than 1% by other tissues following injection of ^{131}I-labeled asialo-hCG preparations by tail vein into female rats. Although crude extracts of urine from pregnant women contain variable amounts of desialylated hCG,[76] there is no direct experimental evidence that desialylation plays any significant role in catabolism of the hormone in humans.

Moyle *et al.*[77] examined effects of removing variable amounts of individual monosaccharides from the carbohydrate side chains on the potency of hCG in receptor assays and in biological assays *in vitro* based on cAMP production and secretion of testosterone by suspensions of rat Leydig cells. Although the modified molecule competed actively with hCG for receptor sites on Leydig cell membranes, there were discrepancies in the relative potencies based on secretion of testosterone and stimulation of cAMP production. From these studies, it is clear that the carbohydrate moiety of the molecule is not required for receptor activity, but may be a determinant of biological effects once the ligand is bound to the receptor. These data also demonstrate the dangers of equating receptor binding and biological activity.

Both α- and β-subunits, and natural fragments thereof, are immunogenic and antigenic. Furthermore, synthetic carbohydrate-free replicas of β-subunit fragments have been shown to be immunogenic. These preparations have been used to produce conformation- or sequence-specific reagents for studying the structural determinants of the immunological and biological properties of the hormone. A widely distributed antiserum, produced by Vaitukaitis et al.[78] who immunized rabbits with the entire β-subunit of hCG, has been shown to recognize tertiary structural properties that, although unique to the β-subunit of hCG, do not depend on its unique carboxyterminal amino acid sequence. Antisera produced by immunizing rabbits with a natural carboxyterminal peptide isolated following tryptic digestion of desialylated S-carboxymethylated hCG β-subunits recognize the carboxyterminal 15 amino acid residues, and S-carboxymethylated hCGβ and hCG are equipotent antigenically in assays using this antiserum.[79]

8.7.3. Human Chorionic Gonadotropin in Pregnancy

While there is no evidence that hCG dissociates into subunits *in vivo*, substances with physical and antigenic properties of free α-subunit have been identified in fractions recovered by gel filtration of serum and urine from pregnant women.[80,81] Quantities of these substances in placental extracts, serum, and urine changed progressively during normal gestation, with ratios of hCGα to native hCG changing as much as 10-fold in placental extracts. Very little or no free hCGβ has been found in either placental extracts or serum from pregnant women.[81] hCG and hCGα have been identified in fetal umbilical artery and vein blood collected at the time of delivery and in fetal blood recovered earlier in gestation.[82,83] No significant differences between umbilical artery and vein blood with respect to concentrations of either hCG or its subunits were noted. It is not clear yet what biological significance can be attributed to this unbalanced production of subunits or whether it can be exploited diagnostically.

8.7.4. Trophoblastic Neoplasms

Gel filtration and specific immunoassays have been used to examine extracts of tumor tissue, serum, and urine from women with metastatic gestational trophoblastic neoplasms.[84] In serum or urine from 18 such women who responded to chemotherapy, intact hCG but no free subunits were detected. In contrast, tumor extracts, urine, and plasma from women with tumors unresponsive to chemotherapy contained variable proportions of free α- and β-subunits and intact hCG.[84] These studies provide a rational explanation for discrepancies noted in ratios of biological to immunological activities of hCG secreted by normal and neoplastic trophoblast.[85] It is perhaps paradoxical that only in women with trophoblastic cancer is the production of α- and β-subunits balanced, whereas in normal pregnancy, there is unbalanced synthesis of the subunits.

8.7.5. Other Cancers

Vaitukaitis *et al.*[85] used an anti-hCGβ serum to assay specimens collected randomly from men, women, and children with various nongestational trophoblastic and nontrophoblastic neoplasms and showed that many of these specimens contained hCG or hCGβ. This observation has been generalized with the use of sensitive immunofluorescent methods to show that cell membranes of many tumor cells appear to contain substances immunologically similar to hCGβ.[86-88] Weintraub and Rosen[89,90] identified free α- and β-subunits following gel filtration of tumor extracts from patients with nontrophoblastic neoplasms and showed "isolated" secretion of hCG subunits. These observations emphasize the importance of using immunoassays that distinguish subunits from native hormone for following this marker in the diagnosis and treatment of cancer.

hCG and hCGβ levels have been shown to be sensitive markers of metastatic disease among men with nonseminomatous testicular tumors.[91,92] Subunit levels were found to be reflective or predictive (by up to 5 months) of recurrent disease in patients with these tumors undergoing chemotherapy or radiation therapy. Kahn *et al.*[93] found elevated plasma levels of hCG or one of its subunits in serum from 17 of 27 patients with malignant functioning islet cell tumors of the pancreas. In contrast, none of 43 patients with benign tumors or 6 patients with nonfunctioning malignant tumors was found to have measurable levels of these markers in their serum. Free α-subunits have been found in serum from some women with ovarian and cervical neoplasms[91] and HeLa strains CCL 2, 2.1, and 2.2, obtained from the American Tissue Culture Collection, have been shown to secrete a substance antigenically similar to, but physically different from, hCG α-subunits.[94]

The demonstration of free subunits in human serum, urine, and tumor extracts suggests independent genetic regulation of subunit synthesis by normal and abnormal trophoblast and by other neoplastic cells. Identification of labeled substances with the physical and antigenic properties of hCG and its α- and β-subunits in tissue and medium following incubation of intact placental tissue[95] or monolayer cultures of human tumor cells[96] with labeled precursors provides evidence consistent with the secretion of free subunits *in vivo*. Moreover, identification of substances with antigenic properties similar to but physical and chemical properties different from those of subunits isolated following dissociation of purified hCG is consistent with the concept that synthesis of the definitively secreted forms of hCG and its subunits may proceed by way of "precursors" or "prohormones." Purification of hCG α-subunits secreted by cloned and uncloned cultures of cells from a bronchogenic carcinoma have been characterized by SDS–gel electrophoresis, by amino acid analysis, and by attempts to recombine this α-subunit with β-subunits isolated from purified hCG from pregnancy urine. Results indicate that while this substance was antigenically similar to hCGα from pregnancy urine, it had distinctive physical properties and amino acid composition. Furthermore, the recombinant with authentic β was not biologically active.[97]

8.7.6. Universality of Human Chorionic Gonadotropin Production

Knowledge of the primary structures and conformational properties of human glycoprotein hormones has made it possible to develop reagents for performing highly specific assays. Recently, these assays have been used to adduce evidence suggesting that hCG may not be a unique secretory product of trophoblast or neoplasms. Several microorganisms have been shown to secrete substances with antigenic and biological activities similar to those of hCG,[98,99] and similar substances have been identified in extracts of human pituitary,[79] testis,[100] and liver and colon.[101] The demonstration that tissues other than trophoblast contain hCG raises questions about the safety of attempts to control fertility by immunizing women with fragments of the β-subunit for hCG.[102,103]

8.7.7. Human Chorionic Gonadotropin and Fertility Control

Since secretion of hCG by the blastocyst is necessary to maintain corpus luteum function at the time of the first missed menstrual period, attempts are being made to immunize women against hCG. The specificity of antisera to the β-subunit should ensure that LH and FSH secretion and effect will not be altered.

In women with limited reproductive potential, injections of hCG or hCGβ subunits coupled to carriers to enhance immunogenicity produced measurable titers of neutralizing antibodies.[104–106] Persistence of presumed ovulatory menstrual cycles despite elevated antibody titers has been regarded as indirect evidence for the specificity of the immune response in some studies,[105] but significant cross-reactivity of antibodies with hLH has been associated with interruption of menstrual cycles in others.[103]

Because of inadequate quantities of homologous chorionic gonadotropins, studies in animal model systems have been limited to the use of heterologous immunogens. However, in these model systems, which have included marmosets,[106] rhesus monkeys,[107] and baboons,[108] presumed ovulatory cycles were infertile when the anti-hCG titer was high, but subsequent cycles were fertile when the anti-hCG titers declined. The few term infants born to mothers who became pregnant after the titers had declined have been normal.[107]

While no untoward effects have been reported to date, it is important to note that follow-up is limited to periods of 1–3 years only.[105,109,110] Problems that might result from maintaining immunity over most of the reproductive life of the woman remain unexplored, emphasizing the need for continuing study of animal models prior to large-scale human application.

References

1. Kletzky, O. A., Jr., Davajan, V., Nakamura, R. M., Thorneycroft, I. H., and Mishell, D. R., 1975, Clinical categorization of patients with secondary amenorrhea using progesterone-induced uterine bleeding and measurement of serum gonadotropin levels, *Am. J. Obstet. Gynecol.* **121:**695–703.
2. Kletzky, O. A., Davajan, V., Nakamura, R. M., and Mishell, D. R., Jr., 1975, Classification of secondary amenorrhea based on distinct hormonal patterns, *J. Clin. Endocrinol. Metab.* **41:**660–668.
3. Vaitukaitis, J., Becker, R., Hansen, J., and Mecklenburg, R., 1974, Altered LRF responsiveness in amenorrheic women, *J. Clin. Endocrinol. Metab.* **39:**1005–1011.
4. Morley, J. E., Distiller, L. A., Sagel, J., and Oxenham, E., 1975, The diagnostic application of clomiphene citrate and luteinizing hormone-releasing hormone in patients with amenorrhoea and oligomenorrhoea, *Int. J. Fertil.* **20:**225–227.
5. Kistner, R. W., 1975, Induction of ovulation with clomiphene citrate, in: *Progress in Infertility*, 2nd Ed. (S. J. Behrman and R. W. Kistner, eds.), pp. 509–536, Little, Brown and Co., Boston.
6. Goldenberg, R. L., Grodin, J. M., Vaitukaitis, J. L., and Ross, G. T., 1973, Withdrawal bleeding and luteinizing hormone secretion following progesterone in women with amenorrhea, *Am. J. Obstet. Gynecol.* **115:**193–196.
7. Argonz, J., and del Castillo, E. B., 1953, A syndrome characterized by estrogenic insufficiency, galactorrhea and decreased urinary gonadotropin, *J. Clin. Endocrinol. Metab.* **13:**79–87.
8. Franks, S., Murray, M. A. F., Jequier, A. M., Steele, S. J., Nabarro, J. D. N., and Jacobs, H. S., 1975, Incidence and significance of hyperprolactinaemia in women with amenorrhoea, *Clin. Endocrinol.* **4:**597–607.

9. Hull, M. G. R., Murray, M. A. F., Franks, S., Lieberman, B. A., and Jacobs, H. S., 1976, Female hypogonadism—therapy oriented diagnosis of secondary amenorrhoea, in: *Endocrine Function of the Human Ovary* (M. Serio and V. H. T. James, eds.), pp. 245–259, Academic Press, London.
10. Jacobs, H. S., Franks, S., Murray, M. A. F., Hull, M. G. R., Steele, S. J., and Nabarro, J. D. N., 1976, Clinical and endocrine features of hyperprolactinaemic amenorrhoea, *Clin. Endocrinol.* **5:**439–454.
11. Kleinberg, D. L., Noel, G. L., and Frantz, A. G., 1977, Galactorrhea: A study of 235 cases, including 48 with pituitary tumors, *N. Engl. J. Med.* **296:**589–600.
12. Bohnet, H. G., Dahlén, H. G., Wuttke, W., and Schneider, H. P. G., 1976, Hyperprolactinemic anovulatory snydrome, *J. Clin. Endocrinol. Metab.* **43:**132–143.
13. Jewelewicz, R., Dyrenfurth, I., Warren, M., Frantz, A. G., and Vande Wiele, R. L., 1974, Effect of thyrotropin-releasing hormone (TRH) upon the menstrual cycle in women, *J. Clin. Endocrinol. Metab.* **39:**387–390.
14. Corenblum, B., Pairaudeau, N., and Shewchuk, A. B., 1976, Prolactin hypersecretion and short luteal phase defects, *Obstet. Gynecol.* **47:**486–488.
15. McNatty, K. P., Sawers, R. S., and McNeilly, A. S., 1974, A possible role for prolactin in control of steroid secretion by the human Graafian follicle, *Nature (London)* **250:**653–655.
16. McNatty, K. P., Hunter, W. M., McNeilly, A. S., and Sawers, R. S., 1975, Changes in the concentration of pituitary and steroid hormones in the follicular fluid of human Graffian follicles through the menstrual cycle, *J. Endocrinol.* **64:**555–571.
17. del Pozo, E., Goldstein, M., Friesen, H., Brun del Re, R., and Eppenberger, V., 1975, Lack of action of prolactin suppression on the regulation of the human menstrual cycle, *Am. J. Obstet. Gynecol.* **123:**719–723.
18. Glass, M. R., Shaw, R. W., Williams, J. W., Butt, W. R., Logan-Edwards, R., and London, D. R., 1976, The control of gonadotrophin release in women with hyperprolactinaemic amenorrhoea: Effect of oestrogen and progesterone on the LH and FSH response to LHRH, *Clin. Endocrinol.* **5:**521–530.
19. Aono, T., Miyake, A., Shioji, T., Kinugasa, T., Onishi, T., and Kurachi, K., 1976, Impaired LH release following exogenous estrogen administration in patients with amenorrhea–galactorrhea syndrome, *J. Clin. Endocrinol. Metab.* **42:**696–702.
20. Zaraté, A., Canales, E. S., Soria, J., Leon, C., Garrido, J., and Fonseca, E., 1974, Refactory postpartum ovarian response to gonadal stimulation in nonlactating women, *Obstet. Gynecol.* **44:**819–822.
21. Canales, E. S., Zárate, A., Soria, J., González, J., Levinson, G., and Fonesca, E., 1976, Further observations on postpartum ovarian refractoriness: Effect of gonadal stimulation in women receiving bromocryptine, *Clin. Endocrinol.* **5:**127–130.
22. Nakano, R., Mori, A., Kayashima, F., Washio, M., and Tojo, S., 1975, Ovarian response to exogenously administered human gonadotropins during the postpartum period, *Am. J. Obstet. Gynecol.* **121:**187–192.
23. Andreassen, B., and Tyson, J. E., 1974, Role of the hypothalamic–pituitary–ovarian axis in puerperal infertility, *J. Clin. Endocrinol. Metab.* **42:**1114–1122.
24. Mroueh, A. M., and Siler-Khodr, T. M., 1976, Ovarian refractoriness to gonadotropins in cases of inappropriate lactation: Restoration of ovarian function with bromocryptine, *J. Clin. Endocrinol. Metab.* **43:**1398–1401.
25. Archer, D. F., and Josimovich, J. B., 1976, Ovarian response to exogenous

gonadotropins in women with elevated serum prolactin, *Obstet. Gynecol.* **48:**155–157.

26. Keye, W. R., Jr., and Jaffe, R. B., 1976, Changing patterns of FSH and LH response to gonadotropin-releasing hormone in the puerperium, *J. Clin. Endocrinol. Metab.* **42:**1133–1138.

27. Seppälä, M., Hirvonen, E., and Ranta, T., 1976, Bromocriptine treatment of secondary amenorrhoea, *Lancet* **1:**1154–1159.

28. McIntosh, E. N., 1976, Treatment of women with the galactorrhea–amenorrhea syndrome with pyridoxine (vitamin B_6), *J. Clin. Endocrinol. Metab.* **42:**1192–1195.

29. Zacur, H. A., Chapanis, N. P., Lake, C. R., Ziegler, M., and Tyson, J. E., 1976, Galactorrhea–amenorrhea: Psychological interaction with neuroendocrine function, *Am. J. Obstet. Gynecol.* **125:**859–862.

30. Tolis, G., and Naftolin, F., 1976, Induction of menstruation with bromocryptine in patients with euprolactinemic amenorrhea, *Am. J. Obstet. Gynecol.* **126:**428–429.

31. Seppälä, M., Unnérus, H.-A., Hirvonen, E., and Ranta, T., 1976, Bromocriptine increases plasma estradiol-17β concentration in amenorrhea patients with normal serum prolactin, *J. Clin. Endocrinol. Metab.* **43:**474–477.

32. Bassi, F., Giusti, G., Borsi, L., Cattaneo, S., Giannotti, P., Forti, G., Pazzagli, M., Vigiani, C., and Serro, M., 1977, Plasma androgens in women with hyperprolactinemic amenorrhoea, *Clin. Endocrinol.* **6:**5–10.

33. Boyns, A. R., Cole, E. N., Golder, M. P., Danutra, V., Harper, M. E., Bromnsey, B., Cowley, T., Jones, G. E., and Griffiths, K., 1972, Prolactin studies with the prostate, in: *Prolactin and Carcinogensis* (A. R. Boyns and K. Griffiths, eds.), pp. 207–216. Alpha Omega Alpha, Cardiff, Wales.

34. Seppälä, M., Hirvonen, E., Unnérus, H.-A., Ranta, T., and Laatikainin, T., 1976, Prolactin and testosterone: Independent circulating levels in hyperprolactinemic and normoprolactinemic amenorrhea. The effect of prolactin suppression by bromocriptine, *J. Clin. Endocrinol. Metab.* **43:**198–200.

35. Marshall, J. C., Reed, P. I., and Gordon, H., 1976, Luteinizing hormone secretion in patients presenting with post-oral contraceptive amenorrhoea: Evidence for a hypothalamic feedback abnormality, *Clin. Endocrinol.* **5:**131–143.

36. Gómez, F., Reyes, F. I., and Faiman, C., 1977, Nonpuerperal galactorrhea and hyperprolactinemia, *Am. J. Med.* **62:**648–660.

37. Yen, S. S. C., Vela, P., and Rankin, J., 1970, Inappropriate secretion of follicle-stimulating hormone and luteinizing hormone in polycystic ovarian disease, *J. Clin. Endocrinol. Metab.* **30:**435–442.

38. Gambrell, R. D., Jr., Greenblatt, R. B., and Mahesh, V. B., 1973, Inappropriate secretion of LH in Stein–Leventhal syndrome, *Obstet. Gynecol.* **42:**429–440.

39. Berger, M. J., Taymor, M. L., and Patton, W. C., 1975, Gonadotropin levels and secretory patterns in patients with typical and atypical polycystic ovarian disease, *Fertil. Steril.* **26:**619–626.

40. Patton, W. C., Berger, M. J., Thompson, I. E., Chong, A. P., Grimes, E. M., and Taymor, M. L., 1975, Pituitary gonadotropin responses to synthetic luteinizing hormone-releasing hormone in patients with typical and atypical polycystic ovary disease, *Am. J. Obstet. Gynecol.* **121:**382–386.

41. Nillius, S. J., and Wide, L., 1971, Induction of a midcycle-like peak of luteinizing hormone in young women by exogenous oestradiol-17β, *J. Obstet. Gynaecol. Br. Commonw.* **78:**822–827.

42. Givens, J. R., Andersen, R. N., Umstot, E. S., and Wiser, W. L., 1976, Clinical findings and hormonal responses in patients with polycystic ovarian disease with normal versus elevated LH levels, *Obstet. Gynecol.* **47**:388–394.
43. Shaw, R. W., Duignan, N. M., Butt, W. R., Logan-Edwards, R., and London, D. R., 1975, Hypothalamic–pituitary relationships in the polycystic ovary syndrome. Serum gonadotrophin levels following injection of oestradiol benzoate, *Br. J. Obstet. Gynaecol.* **82**:952–957.
44. Duignan, N. M., Shaw, R. W., Rudd, B. T., Holder, G., Williams, J. W., Butt, W. R., Logan-Edwards, R., and London, D. R., 1975, Sex hormone levels and gonadotrophin release in the polycystic ovary syndrome, *Clin. Endocrinol.* **4**:287–295.
45. Shaw, R. W., Duignan, N. M., Butt, W. R., Logan-Edwards, R., and London, D. R., 1976, Modification by sex steroids of LHRH response in the polycystic ovary syndrome, *Clin. Endocrinol.* **5**:495–502.
46. Katz, M., and Carr, P. J., 1976, Abnormal luteinizing hormone response patterns to synthetic gonadotrophin-releasing hormone in patients with polycystic ovarian syndrome, *J. Endocrinol.* **70**:163–171.
47. Lawrence, D. M., McGarrigle, H. H. G., Radwanska, E., and Swyer, G. I. M., 1976, Plasma testosterone and androstenedione levels during monitored induction of ovulation in infertile women with "simple" amenorrhoea and with the polycystic ovary syndrome, *Clin. Endocrinol.* **5**:609–618.
48. Judd, H. L., Rigg, L. A., Anderson, D. C., and Yen, S. S. C., 1976, The effects of ovarian wedge resection on circulating gonadotropin and ovarian steroid levels in patients with polycystic ovary syndrome, *J. Clin. Endocrinol. Metab.* **43**:347–355.
49. Cox, R. I., and Shearman, R. P., 1961, Abnormal excretion of pregnanetriolone Δ^5-pregnenetriol in the Stein–Leventhal syndrome, *J. Clin. Endocrinol. Metab.* **21**:586–590.
50. Maschler, I., Salzberger, M., and Finkelstein, M., 1975, 11β-Hydroxylase with affinity to C-21-deoxysteroids from ovaries of patients with polycystic ovary syndrome, *J. Clin. Endocrinol. Metab.* **41**:999–1002.
51. Yussman, M. A., and Taymor, M. L., 1970, Serum levels of follicle stimulating hormone and luteinizing hormone and of plasma progesterone related to ovulation by corpus luteum biopsy, *J. Clin. Endocrinol. Metab.* **30**:396–399.
52. Thorneycroft, I. H., Sribyatta, B., Tom, W. K., Nakamura, R. M., and Mishell, D. R., Jr. 1974, Measurement of serum LH, FSH, progesterone, 17-hydroxyprogesterone and estradiol-17β levels at 4-hour intervals during the periovulatory phase of the menstrual cycle, *J. Clin. Endocrinol. Metab.* **39**:754–758.
53. Abraham, G. E., Odell, W. D., Swerdloff, R. S., and Hopper, K., 1972, Simultaneous radioimmunoassay of plasma FSH, LH, progesterone, 17-hydroxyprogesterone and estradiol-17β during the menstrual cycle, *J. Clin. Endocrinol. Metab.* **34**:312–318.
54. Laborde, N., Carril, M., Cheviakoff, S., Croxatto, H. D., Pedroza, E., and Rosner, J. M., 1976, The secretion of progesterone during the periovulatory period in women with certified ovulation, *J. Clin. Endocrinol. Metab.* **43**:1157–1163.
55. Chattoraj, S. C., Rankin, J. C., Turner, A. K., and Lowe, E. W., 1976, Urinary progesterone as an index of ovulation and corpus luteal function, *J. Clin. Endocrinol. Metab.* **43**:1402–1405.
56. Sobrinho, L. G., Kase, N. G., and Grunt, J. A., 1972, Changes in adrenocortical function of patients with gonadal dysgenesis after treatment with estrogen, *J. Clin. Endocrinol. Metab.* **33**:110–114.

57. Abraham, G. E., and Maroulis, G. B., 1975, Effect of exogenous estrogen on serum pregnenolone, cortisol and androgens in post-ménopausal women, *Obstet. Gynecol.* **45:**271–274.
58. Anderson, D. C., and Yen, S. S. C., 1976, Effects of estrogens on adrenal 3β-hydroxysteroid dehydrogenase in ovariectomized women, *J. Clin. Endocrinol. Metab.* **43:**561–570.
59. Ascheim, S., and Zondek, B., 1927, Hypophysenvorderlappenhormon und Ovarialhormon im Harn von Schwangeren, *Klin. Wochenschr.* **6:**1322.
60. Canfield, R. E., Agosto, G. M., and Bell, J. J., 1970, Studies of the chemistry of human chorionic gonadotrophin, in: *Gonadotropins and Ovarian Development* (W. R. Butt, A. C. Crooke, and M. Ryle, eds.), pp. 161–170, E. & S. Livingstone, Edinburgh.
61. Morgan, F. J., and Canfield, R. E., 1971, Nature of the subunits of human chorionic gonadotropin, *Endocrinology* **88:**1045–1053.
62. Bellisario, R., Carlsen, R. B., and Bahl, O. P., 1973, Human chorionic gonadotropin. Linear amino acid sequence of the α subunit, *J. Biol. Chem.* **248:**6796–6809.
63. Morgan, F. J., Birken, S., and Canfield, R. E., 1975, The amino acid sequence of human chorionic gonadotropin. The α subunit and β subunit, *J. Biol. Chem.* **250:**5247–5258.
64. Shome, B., and Parlow, A. F., 1974, Human follicle stimulating hormone (hFSH): First proposal for the amino acid sequence of the α-subunit (hFSHα) and first demonstration of its identity with the α-subunit of human luteinizing hormone (hLHα), *J. Clin. Endocrinol. Metab.* **39:**199–202.
65. Shome, B., and Parlow, A. F., 1973, The primary structure of the hormone-specific, beta subunit of human pituitary luteinizing hormone (hLH), *J. Clin. Endocrinol. Metab.* **36:**618–621.
66. Closset, J., Hennen, G., and Lequin, R. M., 1973, Human luteinizing hormone. The amino acid sequence of the β subunit, *FEBS Lett.* **29:**97–100.
67. Shome, B., and Parlow, A. F., 1974, Human follicle stimulating hormone: First proposal for the amino acid sequence of the hormone-specific, β subunit (hFSHβ), *J. Clin. Endocrinol. Metab.* **39:**203–205.
68. Morgan, F. J., Kammerman, S., and Canfield, R. E., 1972, Studies in the structure and activity of HCG, in: *Gonadotropins* (B. B. Saxena, C. G. Beling, and H. M. Gandy, eds.) p. 211, Wiley-Interscience, New York.
69. Morgan, F. J., Canfield, R. E., Vaitukaitis, J. L., and Ross, G. T., 1974, Properties of the subunits of human chorionic gonadotropin, *Endocrinology* **94:**1601–1606.
70. Canfield, R. E., and Ross, G. T., 1976, A new reference preparation of human chorionic gonadotropin and its subunits, *Bull. W.H.O.* **54:**463–470.
71. Louvet, J.-P., Harman, S. M., Nisula, B. C., Ross, G. T., Birken, S., and Canfield, R., 1976, Follicle stimulating activity of human chorionic gonadotropin: Effect of dissociation and recombination of subunits, *Endocrinology* **99:**1126–1128.
72. Nisula, B. C., Morgan, F. J., and Canfield, R. E., 1974, Evidence that chorionic gonadotropin has intrinsic thyrotropic activity, *Biochem. Biophys, Res. Commun.* **59:**86–91.
73. Van Hall, E. V., Vaitukaitis, J. L., Ross, G. T., Hickman, J. W., and Ashwell, G., 1971, Immunological and biological activity of HCG following progressive desialylation, *Endocrinology* **88:**456–464.
74. Van Hall, E. V., Vaitukaitis, J. L., Ross, G. T., Hickman, J. W., and Ashwell, G., 1971, Effects of progressive desialylation on the rate of disappearance of immunoreactive HCG from plasma in rats, *Endocrinology* **89:**11–15.

75. Birken, S., and Canfield, R. E., 1974, Labelled asialo-human chorionic gonadotropin as a liver-scanning agent, *J. Nucl. Med.* **15:**1176–1178.
76. Goverde, B. C., Veenkamp, F. J. N., and Homan, J. D. H., 1968, Studies on human chorionic gonadotrophin. II. Chemical composition and its relation to biological activity, *Acta Endocrinol. (Copenhagen)* **59:**105–119.
77. Moyle, W. R., Bahl, O. P., and März, L.., 1975, Role of the carbohydrate of human chorionic gonadotropin in the mechanism of hormone action, *J. Biol. Chem.* **250:**9163–9169.
78. Vaitukaitis, J. L., Braunstein, G. D., and Ross, G. T., 1972, A radioimmunoassay which specifically measures human chorionic gonadotropin in the presence of human luteinizing hormone, *Am. J. Obstet. Gynecol.* **113:**751–758.
79. Chen, H.-C., Hodgen, G. D., Matsuura, S., Lin, L. J., Gross, E., Reichert, L. E., Jr., Birken, S., Canfield, R. E., and Ross, G. T., 1976, Evidence for a gonadotropin from nonpregnant subjects that has physical, immunological, and biological similarities to human chorionic gonadotropin, *Proc. Natl. Acad. Sci. U.S.A.* **73:**2885–2889.
80. Franchimont, P., and Reuter, A., 1972, Evidence of α- and β-subunits of HCG in serum and urines of pregnant women, in: *Structure–activity Relationship of Protein and Polypeptide Hormones* (M. Margoulies and F. C. Greenwood, eds.), pp. 381–387, Excerpta Media, The Netherlands.
81. Vaitukaitis, J. L., 1974, Changing placental concentrations of human chorionic gonadotropin and its subunits during gestation. *J. Clin. Endocrinol. Metab.* **38:**755–760.
82. Hagen, C., and McNeilly, A. S., 1975, The gonadotropic hormones and their subunits in human maternal and fetal circulation at delivery, *Am. J. Obstet. Gynecol.* **121:**926–930.
83. Kaplan, S. L., Grumbach, M. M., and Aubert, M. L., 1976, α and β glycoprotein hormone subunits (hLH, hFSH, hCG) in the serum and pituitary of the human fetus, *J. Clin. Endocrinol. Metab.* **42:**995–998.
84. Vaitukaitis, J. L., and Ebersole, E. R., 1976, Evidence for altered synthesis of human chorionic gonadotropin in gestational trophoblastic tumors, *J. Clin. Endocrinol. Metab.* **42:**1048–1055.
85. Vaitukaitis, J. L., Ross, G. T., Braunstein, G. D., and Rayford, P. L., 1976, Gonadotropins and their subunits: Basic and clinical studies, *Recent Prog. Horm. Res.* **32:**289–331.
86. Acevedo, H. F., Shlifkin, M., Pouchet, G. R., and Rackshan, M., 1977, Human chorionic gonadotropin in cancer cells. I. Identification in *in vitro* and *in vivo* cancers, in: *Proceedings of the Third International Symposium on Detection and Prevention of Cancer* (H. E. Niebert, ed.), Marcel Dekker, New York.
87. Shlifkin, M., Acevedo, H. F., Pardo, M., Pouchet, G. R., and Rackshan, M., 1977, Human chorionic gonadotropin in cancer cells. II. Ultrastructural localization, in: *Proceedings of the Third International Symposium on Detection and Prevention of Cancer* (H. E. Niebert, ed.), Marcell Dekker, New York.
88. Naughton, M. A., Merrill, D. A., McManus, L. M., Fink, L. N., Berman, E., White, M. J., and Martinez-Hernandez, A., 1975, ·Localization of the β chain of human chorionic gonadotropin on human tumor cells and placental cells, *Cancer Res.* **35:**1887–1890.
89. Weintraub, B. D., and Rosen, S. W., 1973, Ectopic production of the isolated beta subunit of human chorionic gonadotropin, *J. Clin. Invest.* **52:**3135–3142.
90. Rosen, S. W., and Weintraub, B. D., 1974, Ectopic production of the isolated

alpha subunit of the glycoprotein hormones. A quantitative marker in certain cases of cancer, *N. Engl. J. Med.* **290:**1441–1447.

91. Lange, P. H., McIntire, K. R., Waldmann, T. A., Hakala, T. R., and Fraley, E. E., 1976, Serum alpha feto-protein and human chorionic gonadotropin in the diagnosis and management of nonseminomatous germ-cell testicular cancer, *N. Engl. J. Med.* **295:**1237–1240.

92. Newlands, E. S., Dent, J., Kardana, A., Searle, F., and Bagshawe, K. D., 1976, Serum α_1-fetoprotein and HCG in patients with testicular tumors, *Lancet* **2:**744–745.

93. Kahn, C. R., Rosen, S. W., Weintraub, B. D., Fajans, S. S., and Gorden, P., 1977, Ectopic production of chorionic gonadotropin and its subunits by islet cell tumors: A specific marker for malignancy, *N. Engl. J. Med.* **297:**565–569.

94. Lieblich, J. M., Weintraub, B. D., Rosen, S. W., Chou, J. Y., and Robinson, J. C., 1976, HeLa cells secrete α subunit of glycoprotein tropic hormones, *Nature (London)* **260:**530–532.

95. Maruo, T., 1976, Studies on *in vitro* synthesis and secretion of human chorionic gonadotropin and its subunits, *Endocrinol. Jpn.* **23:**119–128.

96. Tashjian, A. H., Jr., Weintraub, B. D., Barowsky, N. J., Rabson, A. S., and Rosen, S. W., 1973, Subunits of human chorionic gonadotropin: Unbalanced synthesis and secretion by clonal cell strains derived from a bronchogenic carcinoma, *Proc. Natl. Acad. Sci. U.S.A.* **70:**1419–1422.

97. Weintraub, B. D., Krauth, G., Rosen, S. W., and Rabson, A. S., 1975, Differences between purified ectopic and normal alpha subunits of human glycoprotein hormones, *J. Clin. Invest.* **56:**1043–1052.

98. Livingston, V. W.-C., and Livingston, A. M., 1974, Some cultural immunological and biochemical properties of *Progenitor cryptocides*, *Trans. N.Y. Acad. Sci.* **36:**569–582.

99. Cohen, H., and Strampp, A., 1976, Bacterial synthesis of substance similar to human chorionic gonadotrophin, *Proc. Soc. Exp. Biol. Med.* **152:**408–410.

100. Braunstein, G. D., Rasor, J., and Wade, M. E., 1975, Presence in normal human testes of a chorionic-gonadotropin-like substance distinct from human luteinizing hormone, *N. Engl. J. Med.* **293:**1339–1343.

101. Yoshimoto, Y., Wolfsen, A. R., and Odell, W. D., 1977, HCG-like substance in normal human tissues, *Science* **197:**575–577.

102. Talwar, G. P., Sharma, N. C., Dubey, S. K., Salahuddin, M., Das, C., Ramakrishnan, S., Kumar, S., and Hingorani, V., 1976, Isoimmunization against human chorionic gonadotropin with conjugates of processed β-subunit of the hormone and tetanus toxoid, *Proc. Natl. Acad. Sci. U.S.A.* **73:**218–222.

103. Stevens, V. C., and Crystle, C. D., 1973, Effects of immunization with hapten-coupled HCG on the human menstrual cycle, *Obstet. Gynecol.* **43:**485–495.

104. Talwar, G. P., Dubey, S. K., Salahuddin, M., Das, C., Hingorani, V., and Kumar, S., 1976, Antibody response to Pr-β-HCG-TT vaccine in human subjects, *Contraception* **13:**237–243.

105. Pala, A., Ermini, M., Carenza, L., and Benagiano, G., 1976, Immunization with hapten-coupled hCG-β subunit and its effect on the menstrual cycle, *Contraception* **14:**579–593.

106. Hearn, J. P., Short, R. V., and Lunn, S. F., 1976, The effects of immunising marmoset monkeys against the β-subunits of HCG, in: *Physiological Effects of Immunity Against Reproductive Hormones* (R. G. Edwards and M. H. Johnson, eds.), pp. 229–247, Cambridge University Press, London.

107. Sundaram, K., Chang, C. C., Laurence, K. A., Brinson, A. O., Atkinson, L. E., Segal, S. J., and Ward, D. N., 1976, The effectiveness in rhesus monkeys of an antifertility vaccine based on neutralization of chorionic gonadotropin, *Contraception* **14:**639–653.
108. Stevens, V. C., 1975, Female contraception by immunization with HCG— prospects' status, in: *Immunization with Hormones in Reproduction Research* (E. Nieschlag, ed.), pp. 217–231, North-Holland Publishing Co., Amsterdam.
109. Kumar, S., Sharma, N. C., Bajaj, J. S., Talwar, G. P., and Hingorani, V., 1976, Clinical profile and toxicology studies on four women immunized with Pr-β-HCG-TT, *Contraception* **13:**253–268.
110. Nath, I., Wittingham, S., Lambert, P. H., and Talwar, G. P., 1976, Screening for autoantibodies in human subjects immunized with Pr-β-HCG-TT, *Contraception* **13:**225–230.

The Testis

Daniel D. Federman

9.1. Introduction

This chapter on the testis uses the same headings as last year's. The citations should stand on their own, but reference to last year's volume may occasionally be useful. A new section on the H-Y antigen is included at the end.

9.2. Intrauterine and Neonatal Function

9.2.1. Embryonic Sex Differentiation

9.2.1.1. Normal Controls

Testicular organization begins when the male embryo is about 5 weeks old; the appearance of seminiferous tubules is correlated with the production of the Mullerian regression factor (MRF), which inhibits development of the Mullerian ducts in the male. Josso's group is the major source of new information about this compound, and their current research shows that the substance is nondialyzable and is destroyed by heat and by 0.5 M iodoacetic acid (which blocks sulfhydryl groups).[1] In cultures of calf fetal testis, cycloheximide significantly reduced MRF

DANIEL D. FEDERMAN • Harvard Medical School, Boston, Massachusetts activity, indicating that *de novo* protein synthesis is involved in its production. These and other data from this group support the interpretation that MRF is a macromolecule, probably a protein, with a molecular weight somewhere between 100,000 and 200,000 daltons.[2] On the assumption that a protein of this size would require a second messenger to have an intracellular effect, Picon[3] studied the effect of dibutyryl cAMP; to her surprise, she found that Mullerian regression was not stimulated by this compound, but rather that the effect of MRF was blunted when both were added to Mullerian anlagen *in vitro*.

The second step in genital differentiation, stimulation of the Wolffian ducts to develop into the vas, seminal vesicle, and epididymis, is regulated by testosterone (T), and there is further evidence that chorionic gonadotropin, rather than fetal pituitary luteinizing hormone (LH), is responsible for stimulation of the Leydig cells of the fetus. Past assays, in which human CG (hCG) and LH cross-reacted, were unable to settle the point, but Clements *et al.,*[4] using the immunologically specific β-subunit assay, have reexamined the problem. They had previously shown that testosterone levels in the fetus are highest between 11 and 17 weeks.[5] In the new work, they showed that hCG is measurable in the fetus before LH is, the latter beginning to rise only after the 12th week. Although LH is measureable and slowly rising during the time when T levels and effects are at peak, hCG levels are significantly higher—perhaps 6-fold as high. Since hCG is, if anything, more potent than LH in stimulating the Leydig cells of the fetus, it is clear that hCG rather than LH regulates fetal testosterone secretion. The same authors showed a striking difference between females and males with respect to follicle-stimulating hormone (FSH) levels in midtrimester, the value in females being much higher. They also showed excellent correlation among fetal pituitary, fetal serum, and amniotic fluid levels of gonadotropins, indicating that amniotic fluid concentrations could be used as an indication of the levels in the other two sites.

The influence of T on the developing nervous system is still a moot topic in man, but Schindler showed the enzymatic capability to convert androstenedione to estrone,[6] and T to dihydrotestosterone (DHT)[7] in a number of sites in the brain. Thus, the capacity for hormones to "organize" the brain is present early in fetal development.

The dynamics of pituitary gonadotropin function in the fetus are just beginning to be investigated. Few data are available, but it appears that (1) little LH or FSH is present in the pituitary by the end of the first trimester[4] and (2) fetal pituitaries will release gonadotropins in response to gonadotropin-releasing hormone (LHRH) *in vitro* beginning at a fetal age of 20 weeks,[8,9] but (3) *in vivo* injections of 10 μg LHRH produced no rise in serum FSH or LH in fetuses of 20 weeks age.[10]

9.2.1.2. Defects in Testicular Function *in Utero*

Following testicular differentiation, masculinization of the male embryo requires both MRF and T. Several papers have shed light on the failure of Mullerian suppression in the genetic male, a syndrome called *hernia uteri inguinale* because Mullerian structures are usually discovered during hernia repair.[11] Some patients also have Wolffian duct derivatives in continuity with the testis and are fertile;[12] others show little Wolffian differentiation. It is possible, therefore, that two mechanisms are at work. A paper by Sloan and Walsh[13] described affected half-brothers with the same mother, but different fathers. This restricts the genetic control to a sex- (X-)linked trait or an autosomal dominant with expression only in the male. Linkage studies that might illuminate this point are not yet at hand.

Aimakhu *et al.*[14] reported a male pseudohermaphrodite with bilateral testes, well-formed Mullerian structures, and ambiguous external genitalia. Cytogenetic analysis of lymphocytes revealed only 45,X cells, but no other tissue was studied; the report that this is a "unique case" because of the association of a 45,X karyotype with testicular differentiation seems a bit overstated.

Several excellent reviews of male gonadal function, emphasizing embryonic differentiation, have appeared. Allen[15] has summarized much relevant literature and made valuable suggestions for approaching the diagnosis in the newborn with ambiguous genitalia. The review by Odell and Swerdloff[16] is useful in that it concerns embryological aspects, but is even more so for its excellent discussion of normal and abnormal gonadal physiology in later years. Park *et al.*[17] reviewed male pseudohermaphroditism, providing a number of new and important cases that illustrate special features. They suggest that incomplete virilization in the genetic male can be due to defects in the fetal CNS or pituitary. But since external virilization is complete before fetal gonadotropin levels are significant, i.e., while chorionic gonadotropin is responsible for fetal testicular stimulation, it is difficult to see how this explanation can be correct. Further work from this group, documenting their interpretation, will be most important. Incidentally, in the discussion of this paper, Morris suggested that the term "male pseudohermaphroditism" be abandoned; he argued that the patient's increasing "right to know" will lead to discovery of the contents of hospital records, and that except for the patient with truly hermaphroditic external genitalia, the term male pseudohermaphrodite (as used, for example, in cases of testicular feminization) should be jettisoned.

Imperato-McGinley and Peterson[18] and Peterson *et al.*[19] elaborated on the syndrome of 5 α-reductase deficiency, a disorder characterized by defective conversion of T to DHT (see *The Year in Endocrinology, 1975–*

1976, Chapter 5). The new information includes the findings that (1) the defect in the female, even when homozygous, is of no apparent clinical significance; and (2) affected prepubertal males have an abnormally low ratio of urinary $5\alpha{:}\beta$ metabolites. Peterson points out that screening of newborn male pseudohermaphrodites for this ratio could be valuable in identifying patients with the disorder. Since they masculinize effectively at puberty, they should be recognized early and not, as their external genitalia may suggest should be done, be raised as females. Finally, such patients illustrate that during *in utero* development, T controls Wolffian development and DHT external masculinization, but that at puberty, T stimulates growth of the male genitalia. Since breast development does not occur in these patients at puberty, the syndrome also reveals that T, rather than DHT, must suppress the breast anlage in the fetus.

A particularly valuable review of Pinsky[20] considered disorders of male sexual developmental as models of monogenic teratogenesis. There are few areas of embyology in which the biochemistry is as well worked out, the involved structures can be observed postnatally, and a later phase of development (puberty) highlights function in the same tissues that were involved in the fetal errors. While this paper is somewhat specialized, its thoughtful presentation and extensive bibliography reward study.

The clinical implications of androgen deficiency in the male and of androgen excess in the female are reviewed in a number of papers on the management of newborns with genital ambiguity. Of these papers, that of Canty[21] provides the best discussion of surgical techniques, while that of Dewhurst[22] distills the experience of one of the outstanding British authorities (but lacks endocrine sophistication and omits some of the newer syndromes). The reader's attention is directed to a review by Donahoe and Hendren[23] and to the superlative earlier paper of Hendren and Crawford.[24]

Several papers have described additional XX males, but except for the studies with H-Y antigen (see Section 9.7), no advance in understanding has emerged. One interesting patient was Xg^a- and was born to a putative Xg^a+ father and an Xg^a- mother.[25] Although such a case could throw light on the pathogenesis of XX males, on further thought, it is frustrating. Either both X's are maternal, which requires nondisjunction in the mother plus nondisjunction and a viable 22-chromosome sperm in the father, or there was transfer of the Y-linked testis-determining locus to the X *and* loss of the Xg^a positivity in the father. In other words, both mechanisms require two very rare events. Nonpaternity cannot be excluded, however, and would require only one not so rare event.

A new syndrome of considerable theoretical importance was described by Berthezene *et al.*[26] The patient was a phenotypic female with female external genitalia, primary amenorrhea, and a chromatin-negative, 46,XY karyotype. The plasma T concentration was extremely low and did not increase in response to hCG administration. Plasma LH was high, but FSH was normal. Testicular biopsy showed hyalinization of tubules, normal Sertoli cells, rare germ cells, and no Leydig cells. After orchiectomy, the FSH rose. This case is the first example of one that can be presumed to reflect an isolated lack of Leydig cells. Since both differentiation and function of these cells depend on a response to gonadotropin—hCG during embryogenesis and LH during life—the disorder could be the result of an absence of the relevant receptor, rather than agenesis of the cell. A second important aspect of the disease is the presence of a normal plasma FSH concentration, despite complete aspermatogenesis. This suggests that the feedback inhibition of FSH is mediated by a substance from the Sertoli cells that, while it may usually correlate with the general level of spermatogenesis, is not directly linked thereto. A puzzling aspect of the patient was the presence of vas deferens and seminal vesicle, normally thought to require androgen. The authors speculate that a small amount of T was secreted during fetal life, and an accompanying editorial[27] draws an analogy to the vanishing testis syndrome,[28] but the issue remains problematic.

9.2.2. Testicular Function in Childhood

The plasma testosterone is high in infants of both sexes at birth; it then falls in both but rises again during the first month in the male. Follow-up studies of plasma steroids in infancy were reported by Winter et al.,[29] who measured T, estradiol (E_2), and 17-hydroxy progesterone (17-OHP). After a neonatal fall from high levels at birth, T and 17-OHP rose again, remained elevated for 4 months, and then gradually declined to prepubertal levels. In infant girls, levels of E_2 were very variable, but some were elevated during the first 6 months. Thereafter, they were at the low levels characteristic of midchildhood. Gonadotropin levels, measured in another study, were high at birth, fell during the first week, rose in the second week, and declined gradually by 4 or 6 months.[30] Although it is not yet possible to be sure of specific patterns and their universality, gonadotropin and gonadal steroid levels are higher in the first 6 months of life than at any time later until the prepubertal increases begin. The function of these early high levels is not yet known, but they may be significant in sexual dimorphism and later maturation.

9.3. Puberty

Excellent reviews of the endocrinology of puberty have been published by a number of authors.[30,31] As reviewed last year, the general view is that puberty results from a change in the brain's sensitivity to feedback inhibition by gonadal steroids. The first hormonal event in the initiation of puberty would thus be expected to be rising gonadotropin levels, but several studies have shown that gonadal or adrenal secretions or both rise before the measureable increases in gonadotropin, which themselves antedate clinical puberty by about 2 years. The paper by Odell and Swerdloff[32] showed that in the sexually maturing rat, the earliest event was the appearance of gonadal tissue receptors for LH, and that these appeared to be stimulated by low levels of FSH. With a gradual rise in testicular production of T, progressive maturation of the CNS could follow, with rising gonadotropin levels, further testicular response, and other developments. It is not possible to determine whether the gonadal maturation is due to cumulative effects of low FSH levels, biologically significant but imperceptible rises in FSH, or intrinsic maturation of the gonad. In a number of animals, the prepubertal testis responds very little to hCG unless pretreated with FSH. Similarly, in man, the child's testis responds much less to hCG than the adolescent's or adult's. Since FSH is known to rise before LH, and since LH responsiveness is correlated with age, testicular size, and basal levels of FSH and LH, Odell and Swerdloff suggest that a similar sequence occurs in man. Thus, gonadal maturation, perhaps induced by the low prepubertal levels of FSH, would include the development of LH receptors and thus the capacity to produce pubertal amounts of testosterone.

Ducharme's group has emphasized the role of adrenal steroids in pubertal maturation prior to frank gonadotropin elevation.[33,34] This work shows that androstenedione (A) and dehydroepiandrosterone (sulfate) (DHEA) rise in the first decade of life in a pattern that parallels but anticipates puberty; i.e., levels rise earlier in females than males, and in both sexes anticipate gonadotropin elevation by about 1.5–2 years. This cannot be attributed to adrenocorticotropic hormone (ACTH), since there is no comparable rise in cortisol or aldosterone secretion. Thus, there may be intrinsic maturation in the adrenal cells; one can imagine that its basis is the appearance and subsequent increase of ACTH receptors in cells that secrete androgen rather than cortisol.

Rayner[35] and Root and Reiter[36] reviewed clinical aspects of puberty and the evaluation and management of disorders causing pubertal delay. The use of LHRH to detect the early progress of puberty has been extended. Although LHRH responsiveness increases in parallel with the rising basal levels of FSH and LH, the response to LHRH reflects the progress of pubertal development better than basal levels of FSH and LH do.[37,38] From the practical standpoint, it should be noted that sophisticated longitudinal studies showed that testicular enlargement occurs before serum FSH has risen enough for an isolated value to be significant.[39] One can therefore use physical examination to assess the pubertal status.

An interesting study of LHRH infusion has served to highlight differences between the feedback control of gonadotropin and thyrotropin (TSH) secretion.[40] In most studies, continuous infusion of LHRH causes an initial sharp rise, followed by a progressive increase and then a sustained elevation of LH concentration in plasma. In contrast, during continuous infusion of thyrotropin-releasing hormone (TRH), serum TSH concentration rises initially and then falls. The latter is interpreted as being due to a negative-feedback effect on the pituitary by the small but significant increase in thyroid hormone secretion that occurs during the infusion. In contrast, even though plasma T concentration rises during continuous LHRH infusion, plasma LH concentration remains elevated. This suggests that the feedback effect of T is exerted on the hypothalamus, rather than the pituitary.

Few of the papers about puberty revealed anything novel, but a note by Santen et al.[41] showed an ingenious exploitation of the aldosterone antagonist, spironolactone. This drug is known to inhibit both the synthesis and the action of T. The drug was given, in rather large doses, to 7 boys with idiopathic delayed puberty. It produced a rise in LH in all 7, the change being significant in 5. The authors feel this to be the first evidence of a drug that can increase gonadotropin secretion by inhibiting negative feedback, exerted by T, but unfortunately plasma T concentrations were not measured.

Aynsley-Green et al.[42] reviewed the syndrome of anorchia, in which genetic males with normal fetal sex differentiation fail to undergo puberty. In 21 boys, growth was apparently normal, except for absence of a pubertal spurt. Plasma T was low, plasma LH and FSH were elevated, and the LH response to LHRH was also increased. Administration of T produced normal growth and bone maturation. Some urinary T was measurable in most patients, but presumably reflected hepatic conversion of adrenal androgen, since the level did not respond to HCG. The authors argue that if a patient with this disease shows no T response to administered hCG (as was true of most of their patients), surgical exploration is not necessary; whereas if there is a partial response to hCG, a search for intraabdominal testes is appropriate. The precise nosological status of these patients is unclear. Several recent papers have distinguished agonadism (46,XY patients with a female phenotype, but no uterus) from anorchia (same karyotype, but with embryonic virilization normally negotiated.[43-45] The difference between the two is presumed to be the timing of testicular regression. Since the underlying mechanisms are not known, since the disorder in some patients appears to be sporadic and in others familial, and since the patients fall along a continuous spectrum of adequacy with respect to male differentiation, it is not yet possible to categorize patients with confidence.

Longitudinal studies of two of the distressing accompaniments of puberty showed what many had anticipated, but had not been extensively documented. Lee[46] found that E_2 levels tended to be higher in boys with gynecomastia, and that this difference appeared before plasma T concentrations rose. The same author, in what may have been some of the same children, found that on average, boys who developed acne had higher plasma T values in the year before the acne appeared than did patients who failed to develop acne.[47] Those with severe acne did not always have high levels, however, and there was no threshold above which acne developed in all.

9.4. Adult Physiology

9.4.1. The Hypothalamus and Pituitary

Several comprehensive reviews of hypothalamic and pituitary function have been published recently. Schally *et al.*[48] summarized over 250 papers concerning LHRH, emphasizing research on analogues and the general usefulness of these compounds in diagnosis and therapy. Franchimont *et al.*[49] concluded that primary gonadal failure is the only disorder in which LHRH testing is pathognomonic. In hypogonadotropic states, LHRH elicits a variety of responses reflecting diverse functional states, rather than distinct diseases: "The same functional state may be found in different diseases and, in contrast, one disease can evolve through different functional states with time."[50] London *et al.*,[51] using LHRH diagnostically in hypogonad patients, found an exaggerated response only in patients with elevated basal FSH, and concluded that the test should not be needed in that circumstance; rather, its use should be confined to patients with low or normal FSH. Several workers have found specific binding sites for LHRH on anterior pituitary cells.[52,53] Indeed, there may be at least two sites, and, as suggested by Spona,[52] modulation of these receptors by gonadal steroids would provide an elegant means of controlling two pituitary gonadotropins with one releasing hormone.

If the stimulatory role of LHRH has become progressively clarified, the feedback regulation of gonadotropin secretion is still poorly understood. In a fine review of the problem as illustrated in the rat, Naftolin and Ryan[54] emphasize that the alternate pathways for androgen metabolism open the possibility for a complex set of controls:

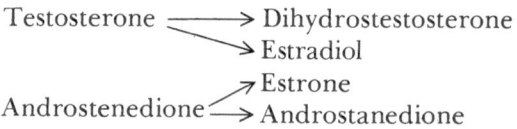

Secreted androgens could inhibit gonadotropin secretion directly, by reduction to other androgens, or by their conversion to estrogens. Further, given the potency of E_2, a minuscule amount produced intracellularly could easily account for the effect of androgens. In discussing the relative importance of gonadal steroids and inhibin as regulators of gonadotropin secretion, Baker et al.[55] pointed out that there is no need to consider one *or* the other as the sole mediator of feedback control—both inhibin and gonadal steroids may be involved, allowing greater flexibility and subtlety. In this connection, Dhont et al.[56] compared the effects of estrogen (E_2) and an antiestrogen (clomiphene) on basal and LHRH-stimulated gonadotropin levels in males. Clomiphene raised and E_2 lowered basal levels; both reduced the gonadotropin response to LHRH. Lasley et al.[57] also found diminished gonadotropin release after estrogen pretreatment. Both these papers therefore show a decided difference between the male and female, for in the female, estrogen pretreatment potentiates LHRH effect.[58,59] (Lasley's paper also showed that estrogen treatment lowered plasma T without lowering plasma LH; i.e., it appeared to exert a direct inhibition of T biosynthesis in the testis.) On the other hand, if clomiphene acts only by competing for estrogen-binding sites in the hypothalamus, the increase in basal gonadotropin levels in patients given clomiphene may mean that estrogen ordinarily has a positive feedback on gonadotropin responsiveness of the pituitary. In any case, the data suggest an important difference between male and female in regard to the effect of estrogen on pituitary responsiveness to LHRH. Kulin and Reiter[60] reported a slightly different finding: sustained administration of estrogen to adult males initially lowers both FSH and LH, but the LH later rises. In prepubertal or midpubertal boys, only the suppression was seen.

Several facts of practical value have emerged in regard to gonadotropins. The pulsatile and episodic secretion of LH, confirmed by Nankin and Troen,[61] and the variability of FSH at different times of day, have made some authors question the value of individual measurements. Penny and co-workers examined this question in several settings, and found that despite the pulsatile phenomenon, isolated values generally represented the overall level very well. When the measurement is important in a clinical decision, however, it should be repeated, and if necessary confirmed with multiple samples, as many groups are now doing. Timed urine collections may occasionally be valuable in circumventing difficulties posed in the interpretation of single plasma values.[62] Further, since there is heterogeneity of circulating LH, the availability of a sensitive bioassay of gonadotropins will likely provide a valuable index to correlate with immunoassay in interpreting puzzling clinical pictures.[63]

In some ways, this has been an important year for FSH—both in sharper delineation of its function and in the general acceptance of the existence and role of inhibin in regulating its secretion. Welsh and Wiebe[64] showed a direct effect of FSH on steroidogenesis in Sertoli cells; this effect is on the conversion of late-stage androgens, such as A to T, rather than on androgen precursors, such as progesterone or pregnenolone. Dorrington and Armstrong[65] showed that FHS stimulated aromatization of testosterone to E_2 in Sertoli cells. Davies and Lawrence[66] showed that FSH increased protein synthesis in germinal epithelium and Sertoli cells; the effect of FSH on the synthesis by Sertoli cells of androgen-binding protein (ABP) has been confirmed by many. Means et al.[67] reviewed the evidence concerning the mechanism of action of FSH in stimulating the production of ABP. FSH stimulates an adenylate cyclase and the formation of a specific RNA, but the generation of ABP is blocked by cycloheximide; i.e., it requires transcription. This group also showed that androgen induced ABP synthesis.[68]

Baker et al.[55] provide a comprehensive review of the testicular regulation of FSH secretion. The details are beyond the scope of this chapter, but those interested should read this excellent, balanced review of the long-postulated "inhibin." It seems no longer arguable that the seminiferous tubules produce a protein, molecular weight around 15,000–30,000, that inhibits the release of FSH from the anterior pituitary. This substance has been found in cultured Sertoli cells,[69] in bull seminal fluid,[70] and most recently in follicular fluid as well.[71] Many questions remain, including its cell of origin and mechanism of action, its interrelationship with sex steroids, and its correlation with defects in spermatogenesis.

9.4.2. The Testis

9.4.2.1. Steroidogenesis

Several papers have focused on the origin and interrelationships of androgens. Fiorelli et al.[72] compared the levels of A, T, and DHT in spermatic and peripheral venous blood in 24 men undergoing elective herniorrhaphy. The concentration of DHT was higher in spermatic than in peripheral vein blood, and in both sites it correlated with T, but not with A. It was concluded that T is the precursor of DHT in the testis as well as in androgen target tissues elsewhere in the body.

In normal males given either ACTH or dexamethasone, Vermeulen and Verdonck[73] found that (1) DHT, 17-OHP, and DHEA levels were lower in males after the age of 50 than earlier; (2) ACTH induced a small decrease in T, but an increase in A, DHEA, 17-OHP, and progesterone (P); and (3) hCG raised T, DHT, 17-OHP, and A levels, but not P or

DHEA levels. They concluded that in males, T, DHT, and 17-OHP are almost entirely of testicular origin, that A comes from both adrenal and testis, and that DHEA is mainly, and P exclusively, from the adrenal. Metcalf and Cowles[74] reconfirmed earlier work showing that for laboratories unable to measure plasma T concentration, three other steroid patterns can be used to monitor the response to hCG: androsterone plus etiocholanolone, 17-ketosteroids, or estrogen excretion rates.

Samuels et al.[75] reported elegant studies of the localization within the interstitial cells of the several biosynthetic steps between pregnenolone and estrogen. Since there are unique disorders of each of the five specific enzymes involved in the biosynthesis of T, this paper can be consulted for details of the sequence and its normal pattern (see also *The Year in Endocrinology 1975–1976*, Chapter 5). Specifically, pregnenolone was converted to P on the outer surfaces of the microsomes; P was metabolized to A within the microsomal membrane; and the A then diffused out and in the process underwent 17β-reduction to T. Vihko and Ruokonen[76] also worked on the pathways of T biosynthesis in the human testis, and concluded that the δ^5 pathway predominates. They found large amounts of sulphated steroids, and suggested that since synthesis of T uses these as precursors, one means of regulating T synthesis could be via testicular steroid sulphatase activity. This would be a novel mechanism.

Finally, there has been some illumination of the site of estrogen formation in the testis. Kelch et al.[77] had shown that E_2 is synthesized in the normal human testis, and in increased amounts in certain disorders. In a follow-up to this work, Payne et al.[78] compared the formation of estrogen from androgen in whole testicular tissue and in seminiferous tubules; finding the estrogen concentration greater in the intact tissues than in the tubules, they concluded that aromatization of C-19 steroids to estrogens occurs in the interstitial cells. E_2 was the principal steroid formed, regardless whether T or A was the precursor.

Since T and E_2 circulate bound to one plasma protein, the T–E_2-binding globulin, and since each influences the level of this protein, there is a potential for misunderstanding in measuring the whole blood sex steroid levels rather than the small amount of free biologically active steroid. Just as with thyroid hormone and the thyroid-hormone-binding proteins, measurement of the free T or E_2 has been technically difficult. Several approaches have been published, one being the T-free index, calculated in like manner to the free thyroxine.[79] The percentage of free T was measured by equilibrium dialysis. This was multiplied by the total T to give the T-free index. Values in normal males were 24.6–93.6 and in normal females, 0.8–3.8 ng/100 ml. The index was abnormal in 4 hirsute women who had normal plasma total T values; 20 other hirsute women had elevated total T values and would not have required the new test for their detection. It is early to evaluate this approach, but it seems likely to illuminate problems of hirsutism and androgen excess more than problems of androgen deficiency in the male.

Values for the plasma T concentration have been reported in a number of syndromes about which questions were previously raised. Free T concentrations were not elevated in 5 of 6 patients with the 47,XYY karotype[80]; plasma T values did not correlate with body composition or strength in a group of young adult male and female athletes[81]; and both LH and T concentrations rose during strenuous anaerobic exercise.[82] Finally, a follow-up study by Boyar *et al.*[83] showed that the sleep-related rise in LH that is characteristic of puberty (1) is reversed to the day when the waking–sleep pattern is reversed and (2) is not seen in the adult.

9.4.2.2. Spermatogenesis

Several reviews of spermatogenesis have been published,[84,85] but little major progress is evident. In patients with 5α-reductase deficiency, who convert little T to DHT, the testis shows active spermatogenesis.[19] This implies that T rather than DHT is the androgen required for spermatogenesis, yet most studies continue to show DHT produced in the seminiferous tubules, and in particular show it there at a time that spermatogenesis becomes active. Such were the findings in a paper by Rivarola *et al.*,[86] in both the rat and the human. Further work on the role of FSH has confirmed that it is not necessary throughout spermatogenesis, but that it plays a key role at several points. A major aspect of this is its action on the Sertoli cell, where it stimulates the formation of the ABP. A number of studies on the Sertoli cell-enriched testis—prepared by irradiating the tubules—have emphasized this role.[87,88] Means *et al.*[67,89] also did a series of studies that implicate the Sertoli cell as the target for FSH. In this thoughtful review, however, they warn against the facile assumption that the attachment of FSH to the plasma membrane and its stimulation of cAMP are directly linked to the synthesis of ABP. In this system, as in several others in which the ubiquitous second messenger is produced, the picture appears to be more complicated than had been assumed. Although FSH may act via cAMP to enhance ABP synthesis, androgen also stimulates the synthesis of ABP,[68,90] and thus androgen and FSH may have a synergistic effect. FSH also acts on the Leydig cells to stimulate the formation of LH receptors.[32] Thus, both gonadotropins are involved in both compartments of the testis, although not necessarily directly.

A valuable perspective on the ultrastructural changes that occur during spermatogenesis was provided by Gondos,[91] who reviewed his own and others' observations in a large series of normal testes. He suggested that electron microscopy could be used with advantage to understand disordered spermatogenesis, but unfortunately neither his own nor cited results illuminate the most troublesome cases—those in which the defect is intrinsic to the testis and not secondary to hormone lack.

9.4.2.3. Effect of Age on Testicular Function

The accumulation of information on the testicular function in older males is now quite impressive. Although there is no uniformity in the findings by different groups, the weight of evidence favors the following picture. Some time beyond the age of 40, and variably from one man to another, there is a gradual and incomplete decline in gonadal function. The evidence that this occurs includes:

1. Diminution in total and free T concentration in plasma
2. Diminution in DHT (varying in different reports)
3. Elevation in plasma FSH and LH (not necessarily both in each patient
4. A rise in total E_2, but a variable lowering of free E_2
5. An enhanced FSH response to LHRH[92]
6. A rise in sex-steroid-binding globulin concentration in plasma
7. Some diminution in testicular size (variable and hard to measure)
8. Decrease in sexual activity and "virility"

No study has demonstrated all the features listed, and no patient shows every change; thus far, all studies are of groups of patients of varying age, rather than longitudinal studies of individuals. Perhaps the most comprehensive report is that of Baker et al.,[93] covering 466 subjects from age 2 to 101 years. This paper differs in some particulars from others in the literature, but the general pattern is as outlined.

Analyses of particular aspects of aging are also available. Giusti et al.[94] measured A, T, and DHT in spermatic venous plasma in patients undergoing elective herniorrhaphy. T and DHT both decreased with age, but A was unchanged, leading the authors to speculate that since A is a direct precursor of T in the δ^4 pathway, there may be a change in that enzymatic step with senescence. Consistent with this have been numerous observations of diminished T and E_2 responses to administered hCG.[95] Most authors have attributed the age-related decline to changes in the testis, perhaps related to germinal cell depletion or vascular insufficiency. Hallberg et al.,[96] despite finding elevated LH with diminished T, argue that in addition to the testicular defect, there may also be a central defect, because the LH values were not as high as one would find in younger males with comparable lowering of the plasma T concentration.

Greenblatt et al.[97] compared normal young males with older males who had symptoms attributed to the male climacteric. The "climacteric" males had lower plasma T concentrations than the younger males did, but the study is flawed by a lack of age-matched controls; one cannot tell that the symptomatic patients are endocrinologically different from others of their own age without symptoms. The study does suggest, however, a rationale for hormone therapy in both male and female patients with declining gonadal function. Regrettably, there are no controlled observations to define whether the response is specific or the results of a placebo effect. But this paper is a reminder that we have little knowledge of the correlations between declining testicular function and the psychosexual changes of normal aging. What sexual drive and activity are "normal" for the 70-year-old male? Since therapy is not without its hazard (e.g., activation of prostatic carcinoma), one would like to know when a given clinical complaint is abnormal, when a given laboratory finding is abnormal, and what relationship between the two indicates that hormone replacement would be helpful and worth the risk.

Age-related changes may also occur in the peripheral metabolism of T. Several groups have shown an increased conversion of T to estrogen,[93] and Zumoff et al.[98] showed a decrease in the androsterone/etiocholanolone ratio after infusion of labeled T. Thus, the ratio of effective androgen to effective estrogen depends on many factors, including androgen secretory rates, plasma protein binding, peripheral metabolism, and androgen-to-estrogen conversion.

Feldman et al.[99] called attention to the presence of vaso-motor symptoms similar to those of the menopause in three young males with abrupt loss of testicular function. In each patient, testosterone therapy in doses adequate to suppress elevated gonadotropins corrected the symptoms. Although this study was not placebo-controlled, the implications for the traumatically castrate male are obvious.

9.5. Adult Pathophysiology

9.5.1. Gonadotropin Deficiencies

A conference on genetic disorders of sexual development has been published,[100] and the interested reader should consult this reference when confronted with a particular problem. Rabin[101] described the genetic heterogeneity in the hypogonadotropic disorders. Since LHRH tests have not yet been done in a large number, since the patients are usually infertile, and since males are affected far more commonly than females, it has been difficult to work out the genetics of these disorders. An interesting paper by Boyar et al.[102] purported to demonstrate two types of hypogonadotropic hypogonadism: one, a severe form, with small testes, low LH and T, and no difference in LHRH response between day and night; the second, a less severe form with almost adult-sized testes, definite tubular maturation, and a sleep-related increase in LH output similar to the CNS "program" of early puberty. Background for this interpretation is provided in a paper by Dickerman et al.,[103] which purports to separate hypothalamic–hypogonadotropic hypogonadism (tertiary) from pituitary–hypogonadotropic hypogonadism (secondary) from a combined lesion by comparing the acute response to LHRH before and after 5 days of LHRH administration. I thought the claim was not convincing, and others have not been able to reliably distinguish hypothalamic from pituitary deficiency by this approach. Certainly, however, a failure to respond to a single dose of LHRH should be followed by testing after a week of LHRH administration before concluding that the defect is an inability to make LH.

A fascinating paper by Park et al.[104] described a patient with an apparently new form of male pseudohermaphroditism. To masculinize in utero, the genetic male normally requires T secreted by the fetal Leydig cells in response to chorionic gonadotropin. Prior to this report, patients with hypogonadotropinism (e.g., Kallman's syndrome) have often been reported to have microphallus or undescended testes. But this patient had ambiguous external genitalia, bilateral immature testes, epididymis, but no uterus or Fallopian tubes. The plasma T was low but responded normally to hCG; administered T had an impressive virilizing effect. From the elevated plasma LH, the authors infer that the disease reflects an embryonic and pubertal androgen deficiency secondary to an altered LH molecule that is immunologically recognized but biologically inactive. They recognize, however, that this interpretation of the pseudohermaphroditism is not compatible with prior observations that fetal gonadotropin is not necessary for Leydig cell function. The case is therefore an enigma.

On the other side of the coin is a patient, reported by Snyder and Sterling,[105] who had a pituitary tumor, elevated levels of FSH and LH, and elevated T, DHT, and free T. Semen was not examined. It is interesting that the patient initially complained of impotence and decreased libido despite the very high T levels. Both FSH and LH responded to LHRH and, though less markedly, to TRH. After two subtotal hypophysectomies, all levels fell to normal and sexual function improved. The patient was considered to be the first example of a pituitary tumor hypersecreting both FSH and LH.

9.5.2. The Testis

9.5.2.1. Steroidogenesis

9.5.2.1a. Defects in Synthesis. The synthesis of T from pregnenolone requires five distinct enzymes; defects in each enzymatic step, producing male pseudohermaphroditism, have been described and were reviewed last year (see *The Year in Endocrinology 1975–1976,* Chapter 5). Tourniaire *et al.*[106] described a new patient with 17α-hydroxylase deficiency in both testis and adrenal. The patient was a phenotypic female with primary amenorrhea, a 46,XY karyotype, no breast development, and low plasma androgens and estrogens unresponsive to hCG or ACTH. Hypertension was attributed to high levels of corticosterone and 11-deoxycorticosterone. Schaison and Sitruk[107] report a third case of testicular 17-ketosteroid reductase deficiency *without* gynecomastia. The patient had elevated A and estrone, normal E_2, and low T concentrations in both peripheral blood and spermatic vein. FSH and LH were elevated. The absence of gynecomastia was attributed to failure to convert T and estrone to E_2. The authors speculate that there may also be a secondary decrease in 5α-reductase activity with a consequent peripheral androgen insensitivity; they point to the importance of measuring plasma A concentration in patients with incomplete pseudohermaphroditism. The pathogenesis of the elevated plasma A concentration that is the hallmark of the disorder was explored by Pittaway *et al.,*[108] who found an increased activity of the 3β-hydroxysteroid dehydrogenase step, and some interesting differences from normal in cofactor dependency.

9.5.2.1b. Defects in Transport, Binding, or Metabolism of Testosterone. The syndromes of androgen resistance continue to be exciting models both for understanding male pseudohermaphroditism and for deriving general principles of endocrine action. Testicular feminization (TF) is the polar syndrome. The patients are 46,XY males with testes, no male or female internal genitalia, a female external appearance, and spontaneous breast development at puberty. T production is normal or high for a male, but the hormone is ineffective because of the absence of its cytosol receptor from target tissues. The genetic aspects of TF were reviewed in several papers. A comprehensive lecture by McKusick[109] develops the relationship of TF to other hereditary diseases the mechanisms of which have been defined, and also reviews the methods for demonstrating X-linkage. Using cultured fibroblasts, Griffin et al.[110] studied DHT binding in 14 normals and 12 patients with various types of male pseudohermaphroditism. They found two types of androgen binding: high-affinity and low-affinity. High-affinity binding was normal in 5α-reductase deficiency and in 17-ketosteroid reductase deficiency, but low in patients with classic TF. Both high- and low-affinity binding were decreased in patients with incomplete TF and familial incomplete male pseudohermaphroditism, Type I. They infer that either partial androgen resistance is an allelic form of TF or at least two gene products are required for normal binding of DHT. A resounding echo of this interpretation was reported by Amrhein et al.,[111] who studied DHT binding to cultured skin fibroblasts. In 10 patients with phenotypically homogeneous TF, there were two patterns of response: 6 patients had diminished binding of DHT, but 4 patients had normal binding. The authors point to the similarity of the work of Tomkins and co-workers,[112,113] who had posited three types of hormone resistance: (1) impaired binding of hormone to receptor, (2) impaired attachment of hormone: receptor to chromatin, and (3) an abnormality beyond that step. Whatever the mechanism, the paper demonstrates that the syndrome of TF is genetically heterogeneous, and apparently involves more than one biochemical mechanism. Kaufman et al.[114] also showed, as had Griffin et al.[110] (see above), that genital skin is more useful than nongenital skin in revealing the binding abnormalities in TF. In an interesting paper that includes a patient who appeared to have both 47,XYY karyotype and TF, Kaufman et al.[115] urged that patients with male pseudohermaphroditism and a predominantly female phenotype be studied for the binding of DHT to their fibroblasts to predict whether they will virilize at puberty. This suggestion erroneously equates binding with androgen responsiveness; the papers cited above show that binding can occur without androgen effect.

An interesting case of TF was studied by Nusynowitz and Strader.[116] The pertinent point of their paper was the demonstration that prior to gonadectomy FSH was normal and LH slightly elevated. The latter was raised by clomiphene therapy, whereas postorchiectomy both FSH and LH were markedly elevated and were suppressed by E_2. Combined with the failure of a synthetic androgen to lower LH levels, this was taken to mean that in TF the steroid responsible for inhibition of LH is estrogen and not androgen.

The syndrome of TF has been used many times to study the factors that regulate gonadotropin secretion. Zarate et al.[117] gave clomiphene, LHRH, E_2, and E_2 followed by P to 7 patients with TF before and after gonadectomy. They found preoperatively that:

1. FSH was almost normal, but showed the brisk response to LHRH seen in patients with testicular deficiency.
2. LH was elevated, but both FSH and LH rose still further after surgery.
3. Clomiphene had no effect on either FSH or LH.
4. Estrogen readily suppressed both FSH and LH.

Using a similar protocol, Addison et al.[118] found that LHRH did not stimulate FSH release in two patients with TF. Now that genetic heterogeneity of the disease has been identified (see above), some of these differences among reports may be explained by genetic differences in the patients being studied.

TF is one of many diseases in which closely similar animal models provide useful opportunity for comparative studies. The Tfm rat was exploited in a fine paper by Naess et al.,[119] who showed that the defect in androgen binding in many tissues, including brain, was due to a defect in the number of DHT receptors, not to an abnormal receptor. In other animal models, Bardin et al.[120] and Verhoeven and Wilson[121] each produced valuable insights. The latter paper is of interest because it reexamines a finding that had previously proven confusing—namely, that the submandibular gland of the Tfm mouse has a cytosol protein that binds DHT, whereas this binding is absent in most other tissues in all TF models. The Dallas group speculates in this paper that since this was a small binding protein, whereas the active complex involves a larger molecule, perhaps the defect is one in the aggregation of small units into a functional binding protein. Alternatively, in some variants of the disease, target cells may bind DHT but not react to it; i.e., there may be genetic heterogeneity in the animal models, as there is in man.

Flatau et al.[122] reported gonadotropin dynamics in two brothers with Reifenstein's syndrome studied over an 18-month period. One brother had normal FSH and LH values and a normal response to LHRH early in puberty; when tested later, both brothers showed elevated basal FSH and LH values and a hyperresponse to LHRH, despite elevated plasma T levels. Thus, the androgen insensitivity postulated by Wilson is confirmed.

The disorders of sexual differentiation in man have been disappointing with respect to their yield of information about psychosexual differentiation. In general, most syndromes have been consistent with the view that gender identify in man is a reflection of early rearing experiences, and the latter are determined largely by the appearance of the neonate's external genitalia. But in a spirited exchange of letters in *Science*, Money[123] challenges, and Imperato-McGinley defends, the statement that the patients with testosterone 5α-reductase deficiency, initially raised as girls, switch atraumatically to a male role after their impressive pubertal virilization occurs. This syndrome remains the major challenge to the view that gender identity is indelibly imprinted in infancy, for these patients appear to show that imprinting of the brain by T during development and a definite male puberty can lead to adoption of a male role despite early female rearing. More knowledge is needed of the adjustment of these individuals, including the results of Rorschach and other projective tests that might reveal their self-image.

9.5.2.2. Tubular Defects

9.5.2.2a. Klinefelter's Syndrome. Several studies of the pathophysiology of Klinefelter's syndrome have been published. Smals *et al.*[124] found elevated gonadotropins that responded to a bolus of LHRH; in addition, an 8-hr infusion of LHRH elicited a rise in T as well, indicating that despite the resting hypergonadotropinism, the Leydig cells in Klinefelter's syndrome have a functional reserve. Kley *et al.*[125] studied E_2 as a monitor of testicular response to hCG or LHRH; although E_2 responses paralleled those of T, basal E_2 was less satisfactory than basal T in reflecting the presence of Klinefelter's syndrome and other hypogonadal disorders. Illig *et al.*[126] confirmed an earlier report that showed elevated gonadotropins in patients with Turner's syndrome before puberty but normal values in patients with Klinefelter's syndrome at the corresponding time. Raboch *et al.*[127] reported an absence of age-related changes of plasma T in Klinefelter's syndrome. Given the current evidence of decline in testicular function with age, and the older suspicion that Klinefelter's syndrome would, as an abiotrophy, show a significant decline of plasma T with age, it is unfortunate that this paper did not study individuals over 46, in whom significant decline might be expected. This paper did confirm, however, the lesser phenotypic defect in 46,XY/47,XXY mosaic patients.

Mention should be made of a paper from Johns Hopkins Hospital,[128] in which the principal discussant of the syndrome is Harry Klinefelter. He describes the original cases and the development of the concepts with Fuller Albright; in a companion portion, Cole highlights the association of this disease with cancer of the breast, including speculation on the possible role of the elevated estrogen/androgen ratio in these patients.

9.5.2.2b. Other Tubular Defects. In an excellent paper on the control of FSH secretion by products of the testis, Baker *et al.*[55] present one of the best-documented studies of gonadotropin and T levels in a variety of testicular diseases. The background of their findings is a study of 113 normal subjects from 19 to 45 years old. Having established normal values for testicular size as well as plasma steroid and peptide hormone concentrations, the authors present the values for a group of patients with progressively greater involvement of the testis. Patients with obstructive azoospermia were taken to be endocrinologically normal,

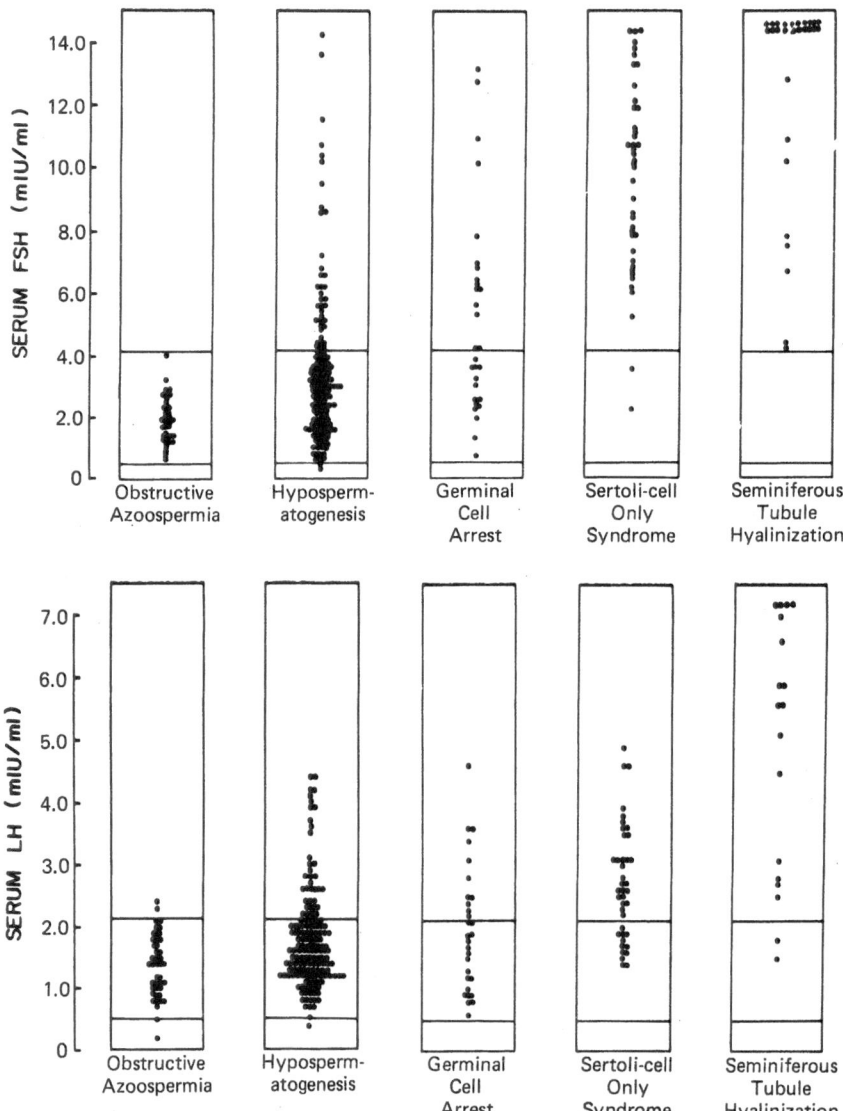

Fig. 1. Individual values for serum FSH, LH, and plasma T in patients with different testicular biopsy classifications. The horizontal lines represent the 95% range for the normal population. Only the lower limit of the T range is shown. Reprinted from Baker *et al.*, 1976, in: *Recent Progress in Hormone Research*, Vol. 32, pp. 435–436, Academic Press, New York.

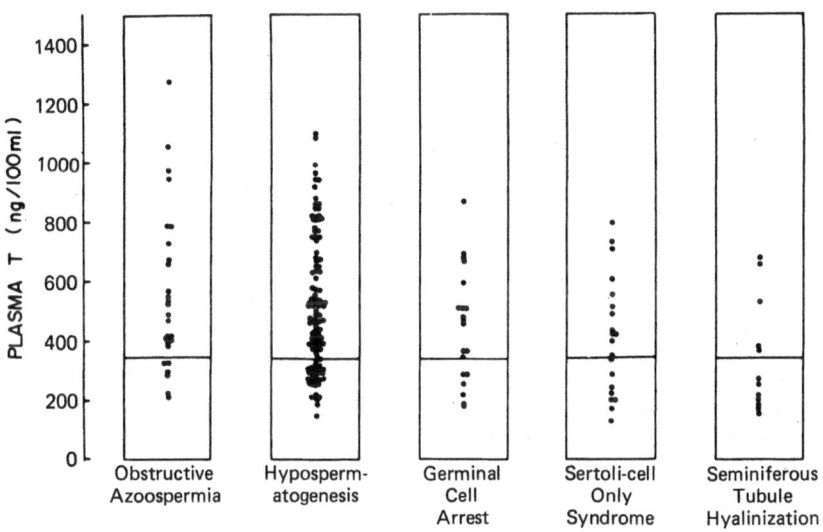

Fig. 1 (*continued*).

and indeed showed normal plasma LH and FSH concentrations, with perhaps a few low concentrations of T. In order of impairment, the other syndromes were idiopathic hypospermatogenesis, germinal cell arrest, Sertoli-cell-only syndrome, and seminiferous tubule hyalinization (see Fig. 1). The lessons to be learned include:

1. FSH was elevated in a significant number of patients with hypospermatogenesis (see last year's discussion of this point).
2. Elevation of LH was also seen in a significant number of patients with hypospermatogenesis, suggesting that Leydig cell impairment is a component of this disease.
3. LH was increased in a greater number of patients with germinal cell arrest and even more strikingly in patients with Sertoli-cell-only syndrome.
4. Plasma T levels were often abnormal in idiopathic hypospermatogenesis and were even more often so in the other three disorders.
5. FSH levels, but not LH levels, correlated inversely ($r = -0.5$) with spermatogonial numbers. Individual patients, however, showed marked discrepancies, confirming the fact that regulation of FSH secretion involves factors other than the absolute number of spermatogonia.
6. Dynamic studies with LHRH and hCG confirmed striking hyperresponsiveness of gonadotropin and diminished responsiveness of T in patients with supposedly pure defects of the germinal epithelium.

This comprehensive review reveals that Leydig cell impairment is also present in these disorders, which, other than Klinefelter's syndrome, were thought to involve only the tubules. The low plasma T and elevated plasma LH concentrations are definite, if not dramatic.

After a thoughtful historical review of the concept of inhibin, the authors review their own and others' experimental evidence. They conclude that the tubular Sertoli cells elaborate a protein that has a negative-feedback function in regulation of FSH (cf. Section 9.4.1). They believe that estrogen and perhaps other steroids may also play a role, and that the regulation of FSH is probably a complex result of all these factors.

There are several important clinical implications of this work. In addition to the true gonadal defects, a few patients with putative primary gonadal disorders were found to have low normal LH values and some response to LHRH. Patients with these findings who also have normal FSH may be appropriately treated with LHRH on a sustained basis, at least long enough to see whether fertility can be induced. Second, some patients may have a diminished but improvable response of the plasma T to hCG. Again, the combination of normal plasma FSH, LH. and T concentrations with subnormal fertility would seem to invite a trial of chorionic gonadotropin. Finally, the work confirms the older view that if the plasma FSH is elevated, the prognosis is extremely poor, and counseling and support, rather than desperate endocrine efforts, are appropriate.

A nice paper on Sertoli-cell-only syndrome confirmed the finding of elevated plasma LH and slightly diminished plasma T concentrations in this disorder,[129] supporting the interpretation that this disease involves an interstitial cell defect as well as a tubular abnormality.

9.5.2.2c. Infertility. Somehow things seemed a bit better this year in the most frustrating and ill-understood area of human testicular pathology—infertility. About 3–5% of adult males are subfertile or infertile. Craig[130] provided a valuable, well-supported review of the pathology of male infertility, and Tresidder[131] a comprehensive statement from the urologist's perspective. The previous section summarized several good papers on the endocrine pathophysiology of primary testicular disorders and suggested several additional avenues of therapy. Some comment should also be made about varicocele, chromosomal defects, nondescent of the testis, and miscellaneous other conditions.

Several new papers on varicocele have emphasized its importance. Schiff et al.[132] showed that endocrine functions are not abnormal in the unoperated patient and do not change after operation. Fernando et al.[133] described careful studies of 17 patients and, while confirming the variable defects in semen analysis that others have showed, plus the benefits of surgery, were unable to identify specific defects that would predict the success of surgery. An excellent report of results in 295 patients confirmed the value of surgery in patients with poor semen production.[134] The results were as follows:

	Improved semen (%)	Pregnancy (%)
Total	58	41
Counts under 10 million	46	35
Counts over 10 million	70	48

Men with moderate and large varicoceles fared better.

The influence of chromosomal abnormality on spermatogenesis has received further study. Whole-body defects such as Klinefelter's syndrome damage the testis severely and virtually interdict spermatogenesis. Mosaic sex-chromosome disorders are harder to detect, but may be very significant in the testis.[135] Meiotic abnormalities have been sought in consecutive patients in a number of series; they cannot be suspected from somatic chromosome studies. Hendry et al.[136] found meiotic abnormalities in 20% of patients; these do not necessarily render the patient infertile, and pregnancy can be undertaken with the likelihood that only normal sperm will be competitive. They advise amniocentesis, however, in pregnant wives of patients with known meiotic defects. Several groups have reported an unfavorable influence of balanced translocations elsewhere in the complement.[137-139] One of the more common chromosomal abnormalities in man is a translocation such as D/D—a centric fusion of a 13 and a 14 chromosome. This variant is found with undue frequency among patients with unexplained subfertility, and it seems likely that it contributes to abnormal spermatogenesis.

The role of cryptorchidism in male infertility has been debated for many years, but there are few good follow-up studies. The disadvantages of cryptorchidism include subfertility, risk of trauma, and risk of malignancy. There has been disagreement on the time at which histological abnormality appears in the prepubertal boy and no conscensus on the benefit from surgery. Unilateral cryptorchidism has been thought by some not to have any implications for fertility; yet many papers have shown abnormality in the contralateral testis, and subfertility has often been seen postorchiopexy. Several good papers have illuminated the problem. Werder et al.[140] reported a follow-up study of 48 patients, and Lipshultz critically reviewed the whole problem[141] while also reporting follow-up studies of their operated patients.[142] Both groups agree that unilateral nondescent is associated with a significant defect in spermatogenesis and fertility, and that this is not regularly corrected by surgery, regardless when the surgery is done. Lipshultz stresses that the truly undescended testis—not the retractile one, which can be diagnosed by a response to hCG—does not descend after the first year of life. He emphasizes that intraabdominal residence adds a further insult to the congenital defect; that histological abnormality can be detected within the first 5 years; and that surgery should therefore be done by age 3. Except for the last point, which is well-argued but unproved, the paper seems to me one of the best on the subject in a long while.

Except in the few patients with acquired or congenital hypogonado-tropinism, endocrine aspects of the diagnosis and therapy of infertility remain as puzzling as ever. One report[143] of three patients with hyperthy-roidism and impaired fertility, with improvement on therapy of the thyroid disorder, was therefore most welcome. Otherwise, there are the usual papers reporting benefit in sperm count, volume, or motility after various endocrine manipulations, but without adequate documentation to allow full understanding.

9.5.2.2d. Control of Fertility. Several studies of endocrine function following vasectomy were reported.[144-148] Although a few showed some statistically significant changes in hormone levels postoperatively, these differences were in general either temporary, or within the normal range and of no clear biological significance. Bremner and deKretser[149] reviewed the possible male contraceptives, but it is safe to say that no consistently effective and acceptable means of controlling male fertility has yet been provided.

9.6. Influence of Other Diseases on Testicular Function

Alcoholic liver disease, accompanied by loss of virility and appearance of estrogenic manifestations, continues to receive much attention. The results from different groups do not agree closely, and no mechanism yet explains all the clinical phenomena. Baker *et al.*,[150] in studies of 117 men with hepatic cirrhosis, found decreased values of the plasma T and free T concentrations, and decreased T clearance and production rates. Levels of the sex-steroid-binding protein were increased. Mean serum LH and FSH concentrations were increased, but the ranges were actually broader than normal, with a few individual values below the normal, many within, and a significant group above the normal range. E_2 levels tended to be higher than normal, but E_2 production rate was not high, even though the conversion of T to E_2 was increased. The authors conclude that in most patients, cirrhosis induces a primary testicular defect, with compensatory elevation of gonadotropin secretion. They could not account for all the clinical features, but they reject the older view that attributed the feminization to diminished estrogen clearance.

Gordon et al.[151] and Van Thiel and Lester[152,153] propose that the liver disease is only part of the picture, and that a direct effect of alcohol on the testis or the hypothalamic–pituitary axis or both is important as well. They find that alcoholism is accompanied by elevations of serum prolactin and estradiol, with diminished plasma gonadotropin and T concentrations. The discrepancy between these findings with respect to gonadotropin and those of Baker et al.[150] remains unexplained.

9.7. The H-Y Antigen

Within the past several years, an exciting convergence of information in immunology and genetics has affected theories of testicular differentiation. It had been known for 20 years that female mice would reject skin grafts from males of the same strain.[154] This was attributed to the presence in the male of a histocompatibility antigen called the H-Y antigen. In 1971, Goldberg et al.[155] developed a cytotoxicity assay in which serum from female mice repeatedly transplanted with isogenic male skin grafts would kill sperm from the same strains when incubated with complement. Such serum, presumed to contain anti-H-Y antibody, has been used as a probe for the purported H-Y antigen. Although the methodology leaves much to be desired, there is evidence that H-Y antigen is expressed in the eight-celled embryo[156] and in the Tfm mouse,[157] i.e., in the presence of complete androgen resistance. Expression of the H-Y antigen is therefore independent of testosterone action. H-Y antigen has since been found in (1) the sex-reversed (Sxr/+) mouse,[158] an XX mouse with a male phenotype; (2) the 46,XX male[159]; and (3) 46,XX true hermaphrodites,[160] i.e., one murine and two human disorders in which testicular differentiation occurs without a visible Y chromosome. It is also found in the gonad of the XX freemartin,[161] where it is thought to function as a soluble antigen that diffuses from Y-bearing cells and "entices" XX cells to differentiate along male lines. The antigen is known to be extensively conserved through long stretches of evolution, since it is found in mammals, reptiles, amphibians, and birds.[162] Ohno and Wachtel have thus argued that there is a locus on the Y chromosome, probably on the short arm near the centromere, that codes for a weak transplantation antigen that is simultaneously the signal for testicular differentiation of the indifferent embryonic gonad.[163,164] As indicated above, the method for demonstrating the H-Y antigen is technically demanding and so far depends almost exclusively on one fortuitously raised antibody. If the findings are confirmed and generalized, however, they suggest that a single genetic locus, conserved across millions of years of evolution, governs two far-reaching biological differentiations:

"I" vs. "all others" (i.e., transplantation identity)
"Us" vs. "them" (i.e., male vs. female)

While not endocrinology in the ordinary sense, the unfolding of knowledge in this area should be one of the extraordinary developments in our understanding of the testis.

ACKNOWLEDGMENT

Mrs. Janet Morgan has again provided invaluable assistance in the preparation of this chapter.

References

1. Josso, N., Forest, M. G., and Picard, J.-Y., 1975, Müllerian-inhibiting activity of calf fetal testes: Relationship to testosterone and protein synthesis, *Biol. Reprod.* **13:**163–167.
2. Picard, J.-Y., and Josso, N., 1976, Anti-Müllerian hormone: Estimation of molecular weight by gel filtration, *Biomedicine* **25:**147–150.
3. Picon, R., 1976, Testicular inhibition of fetal Mullerian ducts *in vitro;* Effect of dibutyryl cyclic AMP, *Mol. Cell. Endocrinol.* **4:**35–42.
4. Clements, J. A., Reyes, F. I., Winter, J. S. D., and Faiman, C., 1976, Studies on human sexual development. III. Fetal pituitary and serum, and amniotic fluid concentrations of LH, CG, and FSH, *J. Clin. Endocrinol. Metab.* **42:**9–19.
5. Reyes, F. I., Boroditsky, R. S., Winter, J. S. D., and Faiman, C., 1974, Studies on human sexual development. II. Fetal and maternal serum gonadotropin and sex steroid concentrations, *J. Clin. Endocrinol. Metab.* **38:**612–617.
6. Schindler, A. E., 1975, Steroid metabolism of fetal tissues. II. Conversion of androstenedione to estrone, *Am. J. Obstet. Gynecol.* **123:**265–268.
7. Schindler, A. E., 1976, Steroid metabolism in foetal tissues—IV. Conversion of testosterone to 5α-dihydrotestosterone in human foetal brain, *J. Steroid Biochem.* **7:**97–100.
8. Groom, G. V., and Boyns, A. R., 1973, Effect of hypothalamic releasing factors and steroids on release of gonadotrophins by organ cultures of human foetal pituitaries, *J. Endocrinol.* **59:**511–522.
9. Tamura, T., Minaguchi, H., and Sakamoto, S., 1973, Responsiveness of human fetal pituitary to hypothalamic hormones *in vitro, Endocrinol. Jpn.* **20:**545–553.
10. Gennser, G., Liedholm, P., and Thorell, J., 1976, Pituitary hormone levels in plasma of the human fetus after administration of LRH, *J. Clin. Endocrinol. Metab.* **43:**470–473.
11. Stallings, M. W., Rose, A. H., Auman, G. L., and Cunningham, R. D., 1976, Persistent Mullerian structures in a male neonate, *Pediatrics* **57:**568–569.

THE TESTIS

281

12. Caterine, J. M., Valestin, R. F., and Song, J., 1975, Male with a uterus and fallopian tubes: A rare disorder of sexual development, *J. Iowa Med. Soc.* **65:**385–387.
13. Sloan, W. R., and Walsh, P. C., 1976, Familial persistent Müllerian duct syndrome, *J. Urol.* **115:**459–461.
14. Aimakhu, V. E., Park, I. J., and Jones, H. W., Jr., 1976, Male hermaphroditism with bilateral testes, well-formed Müllerian structures, and 45,X chromosome complement, *Obstet. Gynecol.* **48**(1 Suppl.):25s–28s.
15. Allen, T. D., 1976, Disorders of sexual differentiation, *Urology* **7**(4 Suppl.):1–32.
16. Odell, W. D., and Swerdloff, R. S., 1976, Male hypogonadism, *West. J. Med.* **124:**446–475.
17. Park, I. J., Aimakhu, V. E., and Jones, H. W., Jr., 1975, An etiologic and pathogenetic classification of male hermaphroditism, *Am. J. Obstet. Gynecol.* **123:**505–518.
18. Imperato-McGinley, J., and Peterson, R. E., 1976, Male pseudohermaphroditism: The complexities of male phenotypic development, *Am. J. Med.* **61:**251–272.
19. Peterson, R. E., Imperato-McGinley, J., Gautier, T., and Sturla, E., 1977, Male pseudohermaphroditism due to steroid 5α-reductase deficiency, *Am. J. Med.* **62:**170–191.
20. Pinsky, L., 1974, Human male sexual maldevelopment: Teratogenetic classification of monogenic forms, *Teratology* **10:**193–203.
21. Canty, T. G., 1976, Evaluation and management of the neonate with ambiguous genitalia, *J. Ky. Med. Assoc.* **74:**75–82.
22. Dewhurst, C. J., 1975, The aetiology and management of intersexuality, *Clin. Endocrinol.* **4:**625–642.
23. Donahoe, P. K., and Hendren, W. H., 1976, Evaluation of the newborn with ambiguous genitalia, *Pediatr. Clin. North Am.* **23:**361–370.
24. Hendren, W. H., and Crawford, J. D., 1972, The child with ambiguous genitalia, *Curr. Prob. Surg.* (Nov., 1972) 1–64.
25. Laurance, B. M., Darby, C. W., and Vanderschueren-Lodeweyckx, M., 1976, Two XX males diagnosed in childhood: Endocrine, renal and laboratory findings, *Arch. Dis. Child.* **51:**144–148.
26. Berthezène, F., Forest, M. G., Grimaud, J. A., Claustrat, B., and Mornex, R., 1976, Leydig cell agenesis: A cause of male pseudohermaphroditism, *N. Engl. J. Med.* **295:**969–972.
27. Ohno, S., 1976, Editorial: Sexual differentiation and testosterone production, *N. Engl. J. Med.* **295:**1011–1012.
28. Bardin, C. W., Bullock, L. P., Sherins, R. J., Mowszowicz, I., and Blackburn, W. R., 1973, Part II. Androgen metabolism and mechanism of action in male pseudohermaphroditism: A study of testicular feminization, *Recent Prog. Horm. Res.* **29:**65–109.
29. Winter, J. S. D., Hughes, I. A., Reyes, F. I., and Faiman, C., 1976, Pituitary–gonadal relations in infancy. 2. Patterns of serum gonadal steroid concentrations in man from birth to two years of age, *J. Clin. Endocrinol. Metab.* **42:**679–686.
30. Forest, M. G., De Peretti, E., and Bertrand, J., 1976, Hypothalamic–pituitary–gonadal relationships in man from birth to puberty, *Clin. Endocrinol.* **5:**551–569.
31. Swerdloff, R. S., and Odell, W. D., 1975, Hormonal mechanisms in the onset of puberty, *Postgrad. Med. J.* **51:**200–208.

32. Odell, W. D., and Swerdloff, R. S., 1976, Etiologies of sexual maturation: A model system based on the sexually maturing rat, *Recent Prog. Horm. Res.* **32:**245–288.
33. Ducharme, J.-R., Forest, M. G., De Peretti, E., Sempé, M., Collu, R., and Bertrand, J., 1976, Plasma adrenal and gonadal sex steroids in human pubertal development, *J. Clin. Endocrinol. Metab.* **42:**468–476.
34. Collu, R., and Ducharme, J. R., 1975, Role of adrenal steroids in the regulation of gonadotropin secretion at puberty, *J. Steroid Biochem.* **6:**869–872.
35. Rayner, P. H. W., 1976, Puberty: Precocious and delayed, *Br. Med. J.* **1:**1385–1387.
36. Root, A. W., and Reiter, E. O., 1976, Evaluation and management of the child with delayed pubertal development, *Fertil. Steril.* **27:**745–755.
37. Winter, J. S. D., 1976, Editorial: Analysis of clinical studies with LH-RH in children and adolescents, *Am. J. Dis. Child.* **130:**590–592.
38. Dickerman, Z., Prager-Lewin, R., and Laron, Z., 1976, Response of plasma LH and FSH to synthetic LH-RH in children at various pubertal stages, *Am. J. Dis. Child.* **130:**634–638.
39. Faiman, C., and Winter, J. D. S., 1974, Gonadotropins and sex hormone patterns in puberty: Clinical data, in: *Control of the Onset of Puberty* (M. M. Grumbach, G. D. Grave, and F. E. Mayer, eds.), pp. 32–61, John Wiley and Sons, New York.
40. DeLange, W. E., Sluiter, W. J., Van Zanten, A. K., and Doorenbos, H., 1974, The effect of injection and infusion of LH-RH on serum LH and FSH in normal males and in boys with delayed puberty, *Neth. J. Med.* **17:**196–201.
41. Santen, R. J., Kulin, H. E., Loriaux, D. L., and Friend, J., 1976, Spironolactone stimulation of gonadotropin secretion in boys with delayed adolescence, *J. Clin. Endocrinol. Metab.* **43:**1386–1390.
42. Aynsley-Green, A., Zachmann, M., Illig, R., Rampini, S., and Prader, A., 1976, Congenital bilateral anorchia in childhood: A clinical, endocrine and therapeutic evaluation of twenty-one cases, *Clin. Endocrinol.* **5:**381–391.
43. Edman, C. D., Winters, A. J., Porter, J. C., Wilson, J., and MacDonald, P. C., 1977, Embryonic testicular regression: A clinical spectrum of XY agonadal individuals, *Obstet. Gynecol.* **49:**208–217.
44. Penney, L. L., and Betz, G., 1977, Agonadism: Case report and review, *Am. J. Obstet. Gynecol.* **127:**299–301.
45. Wu, R. H., Boyar, R. M., Knight, R., Hellman, L., and Finkelstein, J. W., 1976, Endocrine studies in a phenotypic girl with XY gonadal agenesis, *J. Clin. Endocrinol. Metab.* **43:**506–511.
46. Lee, P. A., 1975, The relationship of concentrations of serum hormones to pubertal gynecomastia, *J. Pediatr.* **86:**212–215.
47. Lee, P. A., 1976, Acne and serum androgens during puberty, *Arch. Dermatol.* **112:**482–484.
48. Schally, A. V., Kastin, A. J., and Coy, D. H., 1976, LH-releasing hormone and its analogues: Recent basic and clinical investigations, *Int. J. Fertil.* **21:**1–30.
49. Franchimont, P., Demoulin, A., and Bourguignon, J. P., 1975, Clinical use of LH-RH test as a diagnostic tool, *Horm. Res.* **6:**177–191.
50. Franchimont, P., Demoulin, A., and Bourguignon, J. P., 1975, Clinical use of LH-RH test as a diagnostic tool, *Horm. Res.* **6:**177–191.
51. London, D. R., Butt, W. R., Rudd, B. T., Holder, G., Robinson, W. R.,

Duignan, N., and Logan-Edwards, R., 1975, Gonadotrophin secretion in androgen disorders, *Proc. R. Soc. Med.* **68:**75–76.

52. Spona, J., 1975, Sex steroids influence LH-RH-receptor interaction, *Endocrinol. Exp.* **9:**167–176.

53. Marshall, J. C., Shakespear, R. A., and Odell, W. D., 1976, LHRH-pituitary plasma membrane binding: The presence of specific binding sites in other tissues, *Clin. Endocrinol.* **5:**671–677.

54. Naftolin, F., and Ryan, K. J., 1975. The metabolism of androgens in central neuroendocrine tissues, *J. Steroid Biochem.* **6:**993–997.

55. Baker, H. W. G., Bremner, W. J., Burger, H. G., de Kretser, D. M., Dulmanis, A., Eddie, L. W., Hudson, B., Keogh, E. J., Lee, V. W. K., and Rennie, G. C., 1976, Testicular control of follicle-stimulating hormone secretion, *Recent Prog. Horm. Res.* **32:**429–476.

56. Dhont, M. De Gezelle, H., and Vandekerckhove, D., 1976, Modulation of pituitary responsiveness to exogenous LHRH by an oestrogenic and an anti-oestrogenic compound in the normal male, *Clin. Endocrinol.* **5:**175–180.

57. Lasley, B. L., Wang, C. F., and Yen, S. S. C., 1976, Assessments of the functional capacity of the gonadotrophs in men: Effects of estrogen and clomiphene, *J. Clin. Endocrinol. Metab.* **43:**182–189.

58. Young, J. R., and Jaffe, R. B., 1976, Strength–duration characteristics of estrogen effects on gonadotropin response to gonadotropin-releasing hormone in women. II. Effects of varying concentrations of estradiol, *J. Clin. Endocrinol. Metab.* **42:**432–442.

59. Yen, S. S. C., Vandenberg, G., and Siler, T. M., 1974, Modulation of pituitary responsiveness to LRF by estrogen, *J. Clin. Endocrinol. Metab.* **39:**170–177.

60. Kulin, H. E., and Reiter, E. O., 1976, Gonadotropin and testosterone measurements after estrogen administration to adult men, prepubertal and pubertal boys, and men with hypogonadotropism: Evidence for maturation of positive feedback in the male, *Pediatr. Res.* **10:**46–51.

61. Nankin, H. R., and Troen, P., 1974, Oscillatory changes in LH secretion in men, in: *Biorhythms and Human Reproduction* (M. Ferin, F. Halberg, R. M., Richart, and R. L. Vande Wiele, eds.), pp. 457–468, John Wiley and Sons, New York.

62. Penny, R., Goldstein, I. P., and Frasier, S. D., 1976, Overnight follicle stimulating hormone (FSH) and luteinizing hormone (LH) excretion in normal males, *J. Clin. Endocrinol. Metab.* **43:**1394–1397.

63. Dufau, M. L., Pock, R., Neubauer, A., and Catt, K. J., 1976, *In vitro* bioassay of LH in human serum: The rat interstitial cell testosterone (RICT) assay, *J. Clin. Endocrinol. Metab.* **42:**958–969.

64. Welsh, M. J., and Wiebe, J. P., 1976, Sertoli cells from immature rats: *In vitro* stimulation of steroid metabolism by FSH, *Biochem. Biophys. Res. Commun.* **69:**936–941.

65. Dorrington, J. H., and Armstrong, D. T., 1975, Follicle-stimulating hormone stimulates estradiol-17β synthesis in cultured Sertoli cells, *Proc. Natl. Acad. Sci. U.S.A.* **72:**2677–2681.

66. Davies, A. G., and Lawrence, N. R., 1976, Proceedings: Stimulation of nuclear protein synthesis in testicular germinal and Sertoli cells by follicle-stimulating hormone, *J. Physiol.* **257:**18P–19P.

67. Means, A. R., Fakunding, J. L., and Tindall, D. J., 1976, Follicle stimulating

hormone regulation of protein kinase activity and protein synthesis in testis, *Biol. Reprod.* **14:**54–63.

68. Tindall, D. J., and Means, A. R., 1976, Concerning the hormonal regulation of androgen binding protein in rat testis, *Endocrinology* **99:**809–818.

69. Steinberger, A., and Steinberger, E., 1976, Secretion of an FSH-inhibiting factor by cultured Sertoli cells, *Endocrinology* **99:**918–921.

70. Franchimont, P., Chari, S., Hagelstein, M. T., and Duraiswami, S., 1975, Existence of a follicle-stimulating hormone inhibiting factor (inhibin) in bull seminal plasma, *Nature (London)* **257:**402–404.

71. De Jong, F. H., and Sharpe, R. M., 1976, Evidence for inhibin-like activity in bovine follicular fluid, *Nature (London)* **263:**71–72.

72. Fiorelli, G., Borrelli, D., Forti, G., Gonnelli, P., Pazzagli, M., and Serio, M., 1976, Simultaneous determination of androstenedione, testosterone and 5α-dihydrostestosterone in human spermatic and peripheral venous plasma, *J. Steroid Biochem.* **7:**113–116.

73. Vermeulen, A., and Verdonck, L., 1976, Radioimmunoassay of 17β-hydroxy-5α-androstan-3-one, 4-androstene-3,17-dione, dehydroepiandrosterone, 17-hydroxyprogesterone and progesterone and its application to human male plasma, *J. Steroid Biochem.* **7:**1–10.

74. Metcalf, M. G., and Cowles, R. J., 1976, Response of plasma testosterone, urinary 17-oxosteroids, oestrogens, and androsterone plus aetiocholanolone to human chorionic gonadotrophin in dexamethasone-suppressed men, *Clin. Endocrinol.* **5:**235–243.

75. Samuels, L. T., Bussmann, L., Matsumoto, K., and Huseby, R. A., 1975, Organization of androgen biosynthesis in the testis, *J. Steroid Biochem.* **6:**291–296.

76. Vihko, R., and Ruokonen, A., 1975, Steroid sulphates in human adult testicular steroid synthesis, *J. Steroid Biochem.* **6:**353–356.

77. Kelch, R. P., Jenner, M. R., Weinstein, R., Kaplan, S. L., and Grumbach, M. M., 1972, Estradiol and testosterone secretion by human, simian and canine testes, in males with hypogonadism and in male pseudohermaphrodites with the feminizing testes syndrome, *J. Clin. Invest.* **51:**824–830.

78. Payne, A. H., Kelch, R. P., Musich, S. S., and Halpern, M. E., 1976, Intratesticular site of aromatization in the human, *J. Clin. Endocrinol. Metab.* **42:**1081–1087.

79. Clark, A. F., Marcellus, S., deLory, B., and Bird, C. E., 1975, Plasma testosterone free index: A better indicator of plasma androgen activity?, *Fertil. Steril.* **26:**1001–1005.

80. Pelzmann, K. S., and Brodie, H. K. H., 1976, Circulating plasma testosterone in the XYY male, *Life Sci.* **18:**1207–1212.

81. Fahey, T. D., Rolph, R., Moungmee, P., Nagel, J., and Mortara, S., 1976, Serum testosterone, body composition, and strength of young adults, *Med. Sci. Sports* **8:**31–34.

82. Kuoppasalmi, K., Näveri, H., Rehunen, S., Harkonen, M., and Adlercreutz, H., 1976, Effect of strenuous anaerobic running exercise on plasma growth hormone, cortisol, luteinizing hormone, testosterone, androstenedione, estrone, and estradiol, *J. Steroid Biochem.* **7:**823–829.

83. Boyar, R. M., Rosenfeld, R. S., Finkelstein, J. W., Kapen, S., Roffwarg, H. P., Weitzman, E. D., and Hellman, L., 1975, Ontogeny of luteinizing hormone and testosterone secretion, *J. Steroid Biochem.* **6:**803–808.

84. Lostroh, A. J., 1976, Hormonal control of spermatogenesis, in: *Regulatory*

Mechanisms of Male Reproductive Physiology (C. H. Spilman, T. J. Lobl, and K. T. Kirton, eds.), pp. 13–27, Excerpta Medica, Amsterdam.

85. Frick, J., 1974, Effect of androgens and progestins on spermatogenesis, in: *Male Fertility and Sterility: Proceedings of the Serono Symposium,* Vol. 5 (R. E. Mancini and L. Martini, eds.), pp. 441–457, Academic Press, London.

86. Rivarola, M. A., Podestá, E. J., Chemes, H. E., and Calandra, R. S., 1975, Androgen metabolism and concentration in the seminiferous tubules at different stages of development, *J. Steroid Biochem.* **6**:365–369.

87. Fakunding, J. L., Tindall, D. J., Dedman, J. R., Mena, C. R., and Means, A. R., 1976, Biochemical actions of follicle-stimulating hormone in the Sertoli cell of the rat testis, *Endocrinology* **98**:392–402.

88. Fritz, I. B., Rommerts, F. G., Louis, B. G., and Dorrington, J. H., 1976, Regulation by FSH and dibutyryl cyclic AMP of the formation of androgen-binding protein in Sertoli cell-enriched cultures, *J. Reprod. Fertil.* **46**:17–24.

89. Means, A. R., Fakunding, J. L., Huckins, C., Tindall, D. J., and Vitale, R., 1976, Follicle-stimulating hormone, the Sertoli cell, and spermatogenesis, *Recent Prog. Horm. Res.* **32**:477–528.

90. Weddington, S. C., Hansson, V., Purvis, K., Varaas, T., Verjans, H. L., Eik-Nes, K. B., Ryan, W. H., French, F. S., and Ritzen, E. M., 1976, Biphasic effect of testosterone propionate on Sertoli cell secretory function, *Mol. Cell. Endocrinol.* **5**:137–145.

91. Gondos, B., 1975, Testicular changes associated with the initiation of spermatogenesis, *Ann. Clin. Lab. Sci.* **5**:4–13.

92. Lindholm, J., Korsgaard, O., Rasmussen, P., and Micic, S., 1976, Luteinizing hormone and follicle stimulating hormone and the response to luteinizing hormone releasing hormone in relation to sex and age, *Eur. J. Clin. Invest.* **6**:249–254.

93. Baker, H. W. G., Burger, H. G., de Kretser, D. M., Hudson, B., O'Connor, S., Wang, C., Mirovics, A., Court, J., Dunlop, M., and Rennie, G. C., 1976, Changes in the pituitary–testicular system with age, *Clin. Endocrinol.* **5**:349–372.

94. Giusti, G., Gonnelli, P., Borrelli, D., Fiorelli, G., Forti, G., Pazzagli, M., and Serio, M., 1975, Age-related secretion of androstenedione, testosterone and dihydrotestosterone by the human testis, *Exp. Gerontol.* **10**:241–245.

95. Longcope, C., 1973, The effect of human chorionic gonadotropin on plasma steroid levels in young and old men, *Steroids* **21**:583–592.

96. Hallberg, M. C., Wieland, R. G., Zorn, E. M., Furst, B. H., and Wieland, J. M., 1976, Impaired Leydig cell reserve and altered serum androgen binding in the aging male, *Fertil. Steril.* **27**:812–814.

97. Greenblatt, R. B., Oettinger, M., and Bohler, C. S.-S., 1976, Estrogen–androgen levels in aging men and women: Therapeutic considerations, *J. Am. Geriatr. Soc.* **24**:173–178.

98. Zumoff, B., Bradlow, H. L., Finkelstein, J., Boyar, R. M., and Hellman, L., 1976, The influence of age and sex on the metabolism of testosterone, *J. Clin. Endocrinol. Metab.* **42**:703–706.

99. Feldman, J. M., Postlethwaite, R. W., and Glenn, J. F., 1976, Hot flashes and sweats in men with testicular insufficiency, *Arch. Intern. Med.* **136**:606–608.

100. Bergsma, D. (ed.), 1975, *Genetic Forms of Hypogonadism, Birth Defects: Orig. Artic. Ser.* **11**(4), Stratton, New York.

101. Rabin, D., 1975, The syndromes of isolated gonadotropin deficiency, *Birth Defects: Orig. Artic. Ser.* **11**(4):73–80.

102. Boyar, R. M., Wu, R. H. K., Kapen, S., Hellman, L., Weitzman, E. D., and Finkelstein, J. W., 1976, Clinical and laboratory heterogeneity in idiopathic hypogonadotropic hypogonadism, *J. Clin. Endocrinol. Metab.* **43:**1268–1275.
103. Dickerman, Z., Prager-Lewin, R., and Laron, Z., 1976, The effect of repeated injections of synthetic luteinizing hormone-releasing hormone on the response of plasma luteinizing hormone and follicle-stimulating hormone in young hypogonadotropic–hypogonadal patients, *Fertil. Steril.* **27:**162–166.
104. Park, I. J., Burnett, L. S., Jones, H. W., Jr., Migeon, C. J., and Blizzard, R. M., 1976, A case of male pseudohermaphroditism associated with elevated LH, normal FSH and low testosterone possibly due to the secretion of an abnormal LH molecule, *Acta Endocrinol.* **83:**173–181.
105. Snyder, P. J., and Sterling, F. H., 1976, Hypersecretion of LH and FSH by a pituitary adenoma, *J. Clin. Endocrinol. Metab.* **42:**544–550.
106. Tourniaire, J., Audi-Parera, L., Loras, B., Blum, J., Castelnovo, P., and Forest, M. G., 1976, Male pseudohermaphroditism with hypertension due to a 17α-hydroxylation deficiency, *Clin. Endocrinol.* **5:**53–61.
107. Schaison, G., and Sitruk, L. R., 1976, Male pseudohermaphroditism due to testicular 17-ketosteroid reductase deficiency, *Horm. Metab. Res.* **8:**307–310.
108. Pittaway, D. E., Andersen, R. N., and Givens, J. R., 1976, Deficient 17β-hydroxysteroid oxidoreductase activity in testes from a male pseudohermaphrodite, *J. Clin. Endocrinol. Metab.* **43:**457–461.
109. McKusick, V. A., 1976, The Jeremiah Metzger lecture of the American Clinical and Climatological Association 1975: New genetic insight into old diseases, *Trans. Am. Clin. Climatol. Assoc.* **87:**193–213.
110. Griffin, J. E., Punyashthiti, K., and Wilson, J. D., 1976, Dihydrotestosterone binding by cultured human fibroblasts: Comparison of cells from control subjects and from patients with hereditary male pseudohermaphroditism due to androgen resistance, *J. Clin. Invest.* **57:**1342–1351.
111. Amrhein, J. A., Meyer, W. J., III, Jones, H. W., Jr., and Migeon, C. J., 1976, Androgen insensitivity in man: Evidence for genetic heterogeneity, *Proc. Natl. Acad. Sci. U.S.A.* **73:**891–894.
112. Sibley, C. H., and Tomkins, G. M., 1974, Mechanisms of steroid resistance, *Cell* **2:**221–227.
113. Gehring, U., and Tomkins, G. M., 1974, A new mechanism for steroid unresponsiveness: Loss of nuclear binding activity of a steroid hormone receptor, *Cell* **3:**301–306.
114. Kaufman, M., Straisfeld, C., and Pinsky, L., 1976, Male pseudohermaphroditism presumably due to target organ unresponsiveness to androgens: Deficient 5α-dihydrotestosterone binding in cultured skin fibroblasts, *J. Clin. Invest.* **58:**345–350.
115. Kaufman, M., Straisfeld, C., and Pinsky, L., 1976, Specific 5α-dihydrostestosterone binding in labial skin fibroblasts cultured from patients with male pseudohermaphroditism, *Clin. Genet.* **9:**567–574.
116. Nusynowitz, M. L., and Strader, W. J., III, 1975, Regulation of gonadotropin response in testicular feminization syndrome, *Am. J. Med. Sci.* **270:**491–496.
117. Zárate, A., Soria, J., and Canales, E. S., 1975, LH and FSH releasing mechanism in the testicular feminization syndrome, *J. Steroid Biochem.* **6:**1043–1046.
118. Addison, W. A., Hammond, C. B., Tyrey, L., and Schomberg, D. W., 1976,

Gonadotropin release in patients with androgen insensitivity: Testicular feminization syndrome, *Obstet. Gynecol.* **47**:331–336.

119. Naess, O., Haug, E., Attramadal, A., Aakvaag, A., Hansson, V., and French, F., 1976, Androgen receptors in the anterior pituitary and central nervous system of the androgen "insensitive" (Tfm) rat: Correlation between receptor binding and effects of androgens on gonadotropin secretion, *Endocrinology* **99**:1295–1303.

120. Bardin, C. W., Bullock, L. P., Jänne, O., and Jacob, S. T., 1975, Genetic regulation of the androgen receptor—a study of testicular feminization in the mouse, *J. Steroid Biochem.* **6**:515–520.

121. Verhoeven, G., and Wilson, J. D., 1976, Cytosol androgen binding in submandibular gland and kidney of the normal mouse and the mouse with testicular feminization, *Endocrinology* **99**:79–92.

122. Flatau, E., Josefsberg, Z., Prager-Lewin, R., Markman-Halabe, E., Kaufman, H., and Lardon, Z., 1975, Response to LH-RH and HCG in two brothers with the Reifenstein syndrome, *Helv. Paediatr. Acta* **30**:377–383.

123. Money, J., 1976, Letter: Gender identity and hermaphroditism, *Science* **191**:872.

124. Smals, A. G. H., Kloppenborg, P. W. C., Lequin, R. M., and Benraad, T. J., 1976. The effect of gonadotrophin releasing hormone on pituitary–gonadal function in Klinefelter's syndrome, *Acta Endocrinol.* **83**:829–838.

125. Kley, H. K., Nieschlag, E., Wiegelmann, W., and Krüskemper, H. L., 1976, Oestrone, oestradiol and testosterone in normal and hypogonadal men following LH-RH or HCG stimulation, *Acta Endocrinol.* **81**:616–622.

126. Illig, R., Tolksdorf, M., Mürset, G., and Prader, A., 1975, LH and FSH response to synthetic LH-RH in children and adolescents with Turner's and Klinefelter's syndrome, *Helv. Paediatr. Acta* **30**:221–231.

127. Raboch, J., Neuwirth, J., and Stárka, L., 1975, Plasmatic testosterone values in 105 Klinefelters, *Andrologia* **7**:77–83.

128. Griesemer, D. A., 1976, Clinical conference at the Johns Hopkins Hospital: Klinefelter syndrome and breast cancer, *Johns Hopkins Med. J.* **138**:102–108.

129. Ishida, H., Isurugi, K., Aso, Y., Takayasu, H., and Tamaoki, B., 1976, Endocrine studies in Sertoli-cell-only syndrome, *J. Urol.* **116**:56–58.

130. Craig, J. M., 1975, The pathology of infertility, *Pathol. Annu.* **10**:299–328.

131. Tresidder, G. C., 1975, Male fertility, *Proc. R. Soc. Med.* **68**:291–298.

132. Schiff, I., Wilson, E., Newton, R., Shane, J., Kates, R., Ryan, K. J., and Naftolin, F., 1976, Serum luteinizing hormone, follicle-stimulating hormone and testosterone responses to gonadotropin-releasing factor in males with varicoceles, *Fertil. Steril.* **27**:1059–1061.

133. Fernando, N., Leonard, J. M., and Paulsen, C. A., 1976, The role of varicocele in male fertility, *Andrologia* **8**:1–9.

134. Brown, J. S., 1976, Varicocelectomy in the subfertile male: A ten-year experience with 295 cases, *Fertil. Steril.* **27**:1046–1053.

135. Jones, T. M., Amarose, A. P., and Lebowitz, M., 1976, Testicular chromosomal mosaicism and infertility, *J. Clin. Endocrinol. Metab.* **42**:888–893.

136. Hendry, W. F., Polani, P. E., Pugh, R. C. B., Sommerville, I. F., and Wallace, D. M., 1976, 200 infertile males: Correlation of chromosome, histological, endocrine and clinical studies, *Br. J. Urol.* **47**:899–908.

137. Plymate, S. R., Bremner, W. J., and Paulsen, C. A., 1976, The association of D-group chromosomal translocations and defective spermatogenesis, *Fertil. Steril.* **27**:139–144.

138. Millet, D., Plachot, M., Lety, M. A., De Grouchy, J., and Netter, A., 1975, Chromosomal anomalies in male secretory infertility, *J. Genet. Hum.* **23**(Suppl.):121–122.

139. Zuffardi, O., Maraschio, P., and Pasquali, F., 1975, Chromosome abnormalities and male sterility, *J. Genet. Hum.* **23**(Suppl.):136.

140. Werder, E. A., Illig, R., Torresani, T., Zachmann, M., Baumann, P., Ott, F., and Prader, A., 1976, Gonadal function in young adults after surgical treatment of cryptorchidism, *Br. Med. J.* **2**:1357–1359.

141. Lipshultz, L. I., 1976, Cryptorchidism in the subfertile male, *Fertil. Steril.* **27**:609–620.

142. Lipshultz, L. I., Caminos-Torres, R., Greenspan, C. S., and Snyder, P. J., 1976, Testicular function after orchiopexy for unilaterially undescended testis, *N. Engl. J. Med.* **295**:15–18.

143. Clyde, H. R., Walsh, P. C., and English, R. W., 1976, Elevated plasma testosterone and gonadotropin levels in infertile males with hyperthyroidism, *Fertil. Steril.* **27**:662–666.

144. Whitby, M., Gordon, R. D., Seeney, N., and Thomas, M. J., 1976, Vasectomy: A long-term study of its effects on testicular endocrine function in man, *Andrologia* **8**:55–59.

145. Skegg, D. C. G., Mathews, J. D., Guillebaud, J., Vessey, M. P., Biswas, S., Ferguson, K. M., Kitchin, Y., Mansfield, M. D., and Sommerville, I. F., 1976, Hormonal assessment before and after vasectomy, *Br. Med. J.* **1**:621–622.

146. Smith, K. D., Tcholakian, R. K., Chowdhury, M., and Steinberger, E., 1976, An investigation of plasma hormone levels before and after vasectomy, *Fertil. Steril.* **27**:145–151.

147. Purvis, K., Saksena, S. K., Cekan, Z., Diczfalusy, E., and Giner, J., 1976, Endocrine effects of vasectomy, *Clin. Endocrinol.* **5**:263–272.

148. Kobrinsky, N. L., Winter, J. S. D., Reyes, F. I., and Faiman, C., 1976, Endocrine effects of vasectomy in man, *Fertil. Steril.* **27**:152–156.

149. Bremner, W. J., and de Kretser, D. M., 1976, The prospects for new, reversible male contraceptives, *N. Engl. J. Med.* **295**:1111–1117.

150. Baker, H. W. G., Burger, H. G., de Kretser, D. M., Dulmanis, A., Hudson, B., O'Connor, S., Paulsen, C. A., Purcell, N., Rennie, G. C., Seah, C. S., Taft, H. P., and Wang, C., 1976, A study of the endocrine manifestations of hepatic cirrhosis, *Q. J. Med.* **45**:145–178.

151. Gordon, G. G., Altman, K., Southern, A. L., Rubin, E., and Lieber, C. S., 1976, Effect of alcohol (ethanol) administration on sex-hormone metabolism in normal men, *N. Engl. J. Med.* **295**:793–797.

152. Van Thiel, D. H., and Lester, R., 1976, Alcoholism: Its effect on hypothalamic pituitary gonadal function, *Gastroenterology* **71**:318–327.

153. Van Thiel, D. H., and Lester, R., 1976, Sex and alcohol: A second peek, *N. Engl. J. Med.* **295**:835–836.

154. Gasser, D. L., and Silvers, W. K., 1972, Genetics and immunology of sex-linked antigens, *Adv. Immunol.* **15**:215–247.

155. Goldberg, E. H., Boyse, E. A., Bennett, D., Scheid, M., and Carswell, E. A., 1971, Serological demonstration of H-Y (male) antigen on mouse sperm, *Nature (London)* **232**:478–480.

156. Krco, C. J., and Goldberg, E. H., 1976, H-Y (male) antigen: Detection on eight-cell mouse embryos, *Science* **193**:1134–1135.

157. Bennett, D., Boyse, E. A., Lyon, M. F., Mathieson, B. J., Scheid, M., and Yanagisawa, K., 1975, Expression of H-Y (male) antigen in phenotypically female Tfm/Y mice, *Nature (London)* **257**:236–238.

158. Bennett, D., Mathieson, B. J., Scheid, M., Yanagisawa, K., Boyse, E. A., Wachtel, S., and Cattanach, B. M., 1977, Serological evidence for H-Y antigen in Sxr,XX sex-reversed phenotypic males, *Nature (London)* **265:**255–257.
159. Wachtel, S. S., Koo, G. C., Breg, W. R., Thaler, H. T., Dillard, G. M., Rosenthal, I. M., Dosik, H., Gerald, P. S., Saenger, P., New, M., Lieber, E., and Miller, O. J., 1976, Serologic detection of a Y-linked gene in XX males and XX true hermaphrodites, *N. Engl. J. Med.* **295:**750–754.
160. Saenger, P., Levine, L. S., Wachtel, S. S., Korth-Schutz, S., Doberne, Y., Koo, G. C., Lavengood, R. W., Jr., German, J. L., III, and New, M. I., 1976, Presence of H-Y antigen and testis in 46XX true hermaphroditism, evidence for Y-chromosomal function, *J. Clin. Endocrinol. Metab.* **43:**1234–1239.
161. Ohno, S., Christian, L. C., Wachtel, S. S., and Koo, G. C., 1976, Hormone-like role of H-Y antigen in bovine freemartin gonad, *Nature (London)* **261:**597–599.
162. Wachtel, S. S., Koo, G. C., and Boyse, E. A., 1975, Evolutionary conservation of H-Y ("male") antigen, *Nature (London)* **254:**270–272.
163. Ohno, S., 1976, Major regulatory genes for mammalian sexual development: Review, *Cell* **7:**315–321.
164. Wachtel, S. S., Ohno, S., Koo, G. C., and Boyse, E. A., 1975, Possible role for H-Y antigen in the primary determination of sex, *Nature (London)* **257:**235–236.

The Sympathoadrenal System

Lewis Landsberg

10.1 Introduction: Regulation of the Sympathoadrenal System

In considering the role of catecholamines in the regulation of physiological processes, it is important to remember that the sympathetic nerve
endings and the adrenal medulla are extensions of the CNS. The sympathetic nerves function as neurochemical transducers, converting electrical
impulses in the nervous system to a chemical messenger that is decoded
locally in the innervated tissue by specialized receptors that mediate the
physiological response characteristic of the innervated tissue. The chemical messenger of the sympathetic nerves is, of course, norepinephrine
(NE), the prototypic neurotransmitter. The adrenal medulla is entirely
analogous; it converts neural impulses into a circulating messenger or
hormone, epinephrine (E), the message of which is decoded in tissues

LEWIS LANDSBERG • Associate Professor of Medicine at Beth Israel Hospital,
Harvard Medical School, and Associate Chief, Department of Medicine, Beth Israel Hospital,
Boston, Massachusetts

throughout the body. The diverse physiological manifestations that result depend on the characteristics of the particular tissue that is stimulated by E. As an extension of the nervous system, the physiological effects of the sympathoadrenal system are induced rapidly and dissipated quickly, in distinction to the slower, more prolonged effects of other hormones. In common with that of the other major divisions of the nervous system, sympathoadrenal outflow represents the integrated response of central neurons to a vast array of afferent neural inputs as well as the intrinsic activity of many central nervous structures. The central nervous connections involved in the regulation of sympathoadrenal outflow are complex and incompletely understood.[1] It is of interest to note, however, that many of these central pathways involve catecholamine-containing neurons,[2] including the descending tracts from the brainstem centers that innervate the preganglionic cholinergic neurons of the intermediolateral cell column of the spinal cord. Recent evidence, in fact, suggests that these descending adrenergic tracts excite preganglionic sympathetic neurons by an alpha-receptor mechanism.[3]

Knowledge of the function of the sympathoadrenal system has been significantly advanced by careful analysis of recordings made directly from the cut ends of autonomic nerves of experimental animals.[4] These studies permit comparison of activity in sympathetic nerves innervating different organs under a variety of physiological and pathophysiological conditions. The important conclusion to be drawn from these studies is that sympathetic outflow to different organs is regulated independently. Thus, changes in sympathetic inpulse traffic in response to changes in blood pressure differ in sympathetic nerves supplying heart, kidney, spleen, and stomach of experimental animals.[4,5] Changes in blood pressure affect renal sympathetic nerve activity much more than gastric sympathetic nerve activity, while hypoxia affects impulse traffic similarly in the nerves of both organs.[5] The adrenal and renal nerves respond similarly to changes in blood pressure, while only the activity of the adrenal nerve increases in response to hypoglycemia.[6,7] Thus, sympathetic outflow to different tissues is apparently controlled by different pools of central autonomic motor neurons[1]; contrary to previous thoughts, the sympathetic nervous system is therefore capable of discriminant and selective responses, not merely gross discharge. The precise regulation of diverse visceral functions by the sympathoadrenal system clearly requires just such an arrangement.

The capability for selective responses on the part of the sympathoadrenal system is supported by the more limited information available from studies of plasma catecholamines in man. Postural increases in plasma NE are much more marked than concomitant changes in E, indicating that orthostatic stress stimulates the sympathetic nerves more than the adrenal medulla.[8] Hypoglycemia, on the other hand, stimulates predominantly E secretion,[9,10] indicating primary stimulation of the adrenal medulla rather than of the sympathetic nerves under these circumstances. Plasma catecholamine levels, of course, provide no information on sympathetic nervous activity in different sympathetically innervated tissues, unless specific cannulation of a particular vascular bed (such as the coronary sinus) is undertaken.

Another approach to the assessment of sympathetic activity in individual organs of experimental animals is the measurement of NE turnover.[11-13] Since steady-state levels of NE reflect the density of the sympathetic innervation, rather than the functional status of the sympathetic nerves, tissue NE levels are not usually helpful in assessing sympathetic activity. NE turnover, however, appears to reflect sympathetic activity, and has been useful in identifying adrenergic factors in the pathophysiology of various states relative to disease in man.[13,14] The advantages of this technique are that it can be applied to unanesthetized animals with a minimum of interventions that might affect sympathetic activity.

Of all the afferent pathways that must be involved in the regulation of sympathoadrenal activity, only the classic baroreceptor reflexes have been well characterized. The inhibition of sympathoadrenal activity that follows baroreceptor activation consequent to a rise in blood pressure is mediated by the nucleus of the tractus solitarius.[15] Central adrenergic pathways with an alpha-receptor synapse are involved in the inhibition of sympathetic outflow that characterizes the baroreceptor vasodepressor response.[16] Vagal afferents are also involved in the reflex regulation of the circulation via the sympathetic nervous system.[17,18] The participation of the sympathoadrenal system in the regulation of visceral function clearly requires a vast array of afferent pathways that have not as yet been identified or well characterized. Of particular interest in this regard is the recent demonstration that an artificially induced increase in local tissue (hindlimb) metabolism in dogs increased cardiac output and blood pressure by a neurogenic mechanism,[19] an effect presumably mediated by the sympathetic nervous system. The afferent limb in this case appears to be responsive to a change in tissue metabolism, but the precise metabolic alteration or tissue receptor thereof has not been characterized.

The barest outlines of the basic organization of the sympathoadrenal system are indicated in Fig. 1. Brainstem centers give rise to descending noradrenergic tracts that innervate the preganglionic neurons in the intermediolateral column of the spinal cord; the preganglionic neurons directly innervate the adrenal medulla or synapse with postganglionic neurons in the sympathetic ganglia; the postganglionic nerve endings supply the vasculature and viscera throughout the body. The basic organization of the sympathoadrenal system favors amplification of central adrenergic outflow, since each preganglionic fiber synapses with several postganglionic neurons, and circulating E generally reinforces the effects

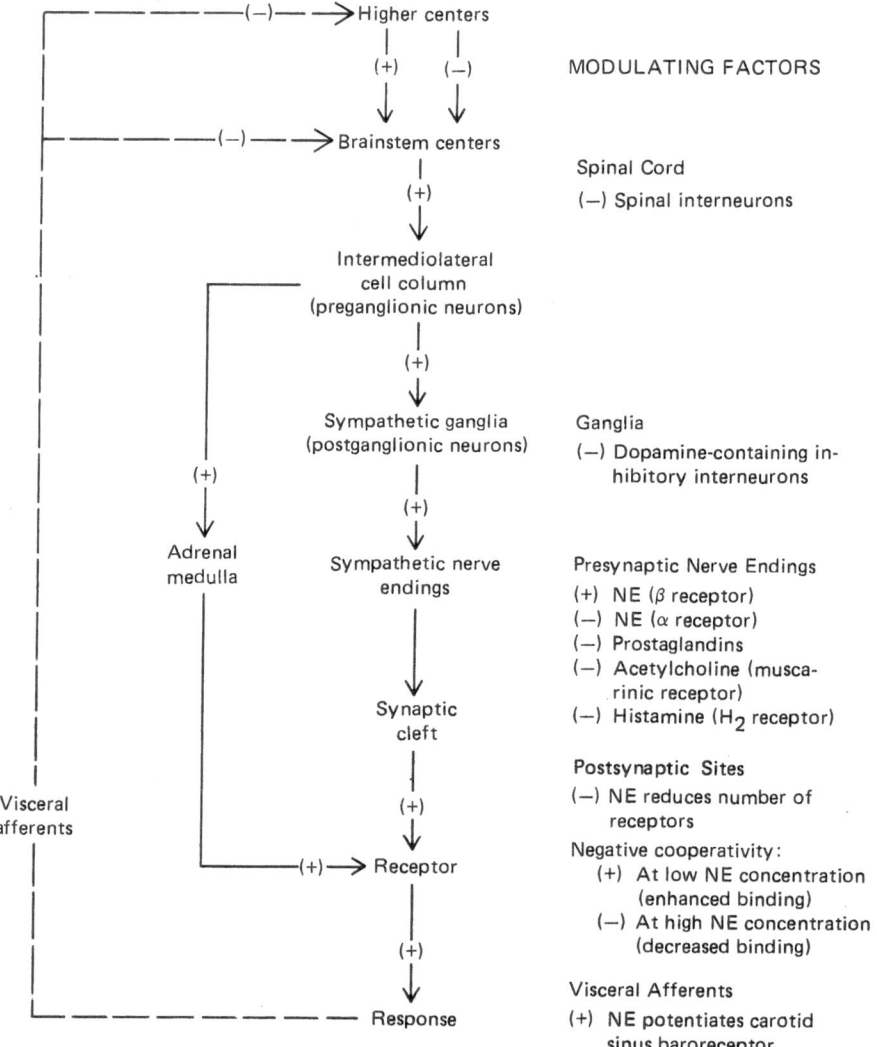

Fig. 1. Simplified scheme of the regulation of central sympathetic outflow. Except for the baroreceptors, the visceral afferents are poorly characterized but are probably extensive and capable of stimulating or suppressing sympathetic output. The negative feedback system shown here is an extreme oversimplification. Modulating factors are shown with their site of effect on the side of the figure. (+), stimulation; (−), inhibition.

of locally released NE. There is, in addition, a series of modulators that adjust the expression of central sympathetic outflow. These regulatory factors (Fig. 1), which have been described only recently, serve to emphasize the tremendous complexity involved in the regulation of the sympathoadrenal system. It is noteworthy that the predominant effect of these modulating factors is either to dampen sympathetic outflow and guard against excessive discharge or to decrease the responsiveness of tissues to released NE. As noted in Fig. 1, the potential for down-regulation of sympathetic outflow exists at every level.

With respect to the spinal cord itself, recent neurophysiological evidence suggests the possibility of an inhibitory interneuron between the brainstem and the preganglionic neurons.[20] In the sympathetic ganglia, a population of "small intensely fluorescent cells" (SIF) resembling chromaffin cells has been identified[21]; these appear to be interneurons stationed between some of the preganglionic and postganglionic cells.[22] Dopamine is concentrated in storage vesicles within these cells and appears to be the neurotransmitter. Interestingly, the postganglionic nerve cells possess a dopamine-sensitive adenylate cyclase[23] that activates a protein kinase that eventually results in hyperpolarization of the postganglionic cells.[24] It appears, therefore, that these interneurons exert an inhibitory influence on the postganglionic neurons. Dopamine is also stored in the Type I cell of the carotid body, where it appears to exert a direct inhibitory effect on chemoreceptor afferent output.[25]

Additional inhibitory influences come into play at the presynaptic axonal membrane of the sympathetic nerve ending.[26] NE in the synaptic cleft feeds back on the nerve ending to inhibit further neurotransmitter release by an alpha-receptor mechanism in the presynaptic nerve ending.[2,27] Alpha-receptor blocking agents enhance neurotransmitter release by blocking this inhibition.[28] Interestingly, a beta-receptor mechanism for augmenting NE release is present on the presynaptic membrane.[29,30] Since beta receptors tend to be more sensitive than alpha receptors to low levels of agonists, it is possible that at low stimulation frequency (or at the beginning of NE discharge, when the concentration of NE in the synaptic cleft is low), the beta mechanism augments secretion. At higher stimulation frequencies (or late in the course of discharge, when the NE concentration is higher), the alpha-receptor mechanism inhibits release. Prostaglandins of the E series may be released from the nerve endings of the effector tissue during nerve stimulation and may then feed back on the presynaptic nerves to reduce the amount of NE released by a mechanism independent of the alpha receptor.[31-33] This decrease in NE release is antagonized by the inhibition of prostaglandin synthesis and stimulated by the provision of substrates for prostaglandin E (PGE) synthesis.[34] Cholinergic receptors of the muscarinic type also mediate an inhibitory effect on

NE release.[26,35] An inhibitory effect on NE release from sympathetic nerve endings in heart can be demonstrated by vagal stimulation,[36] but might also result from ACh release from sympathetic nerve endings. Histamine may also depress NE release from the presynaptic nerve endings, an effect mediated by the H_2 receptor.[37] lhe physiological significance and relative importance of these various presynaptic inhibitory influences is not clear at present.

Postsynaptic modulation may occur at the level of the adrenergic receptor. Recent evidence suggests that in some isolated systems, exposure of effector cell membranes to high concentrations of catecholamines leads to a decrease in catecholamine binding, with kinetics that suggest a decrease in the number of receptor sites.[38] In other experiments, negative cooperativity was apparently demonstrated[39] between catecholamines and membrane receptors, so that the affinity of receptors for agonists changes reciprocally with changes in the ambient agonist concentration. At low concentrations of agonists, binding is enhanced, whereas at high concentrations, binding is inhibited. The general significance of these findings for catecholamine–receptor interactions in a wide variety of tissues is not established.

The ultimate form of postsynaptic regulation is, of course, activation of the afferent limb of reflex arcs that inhibit central sympathetic outflow. Even the afferent limb, however, is subject to inhibitory modulation. Sympathetic stimulation has been shown to sensitize the baroreceptors of the carotid sinus,[40] and thus to potentiate the vasodepressor reflexes that inhibit sympathetic outflow.

The relative significance of these many factors (Fig. 1) that are reported to regulate the expression of central sympathoadrenal activity remains to be established. There appears to be ample machinery, however, for fine-tuning of the entire system at many levels. Having briefly considered the regulation of the sympathoadrenal system, we will now direct attention to the role of the sympathoadrenal system in the regulation of other hormones and to the possible role of catecholamines in the pathogenesis of essential hypertension.

10.2. The Sympathoadrenal System and the Integration of Endocrine Responses

10.2.1 Background

Neural regulation of endocrine responses is well established in the case of the anterior and posterior pituitary. The hypothalamus directly controls the storage and release of hormones from the posterior pituitary;

the hypothalamus indirectly controls the secretion of anterior pituitary hormones via releasing factors that directly regulate anterior pituitary secretion or modify the feedback relationship between the trophic hormones of the pituitary and the peripheral hormones under anterior pituitary control. It seems likely, in addition, that catecholamine stimulation of other endocrine cells represents another type of central regulation of the endocrine system. Numerous effects of catecholamines on the secretion of peptide hormones have been demonstrated over the past decade. The role of catecholamines in endocrine integration is however obscure; the various hormones influenced by catecholamines respond to well-described feedback loops that are, for the most part, independent of direct neural control. It seems likely that catecholamines, via the sympathoadrenal system, have an important role in regulating the functions of various endocrine organs in accord with the needs of the organism as perceived by the CNS. When the matter is viewed in this light, it is possible to make sense out of a bewildering mass of information related to the effects of catecholamines and sympathetic nerve stimulation on a variety of endocrine systems. Some of these catecholamine effects are shown in Table I along with the usual feedback loops that regulate the release of the particular hormones.

10.2.2. Renin

Renin is secreted by the juxtaglomerular cells of the kidney in response to changes in perfusion pressure at the afferent arteriole and sodium concentration in the distal tubule.[41,42] Catecholamines and renal nerve stimulation are also known to increase renin secretion[43,44] independently of changes in both renal hemodynamics and the filtered load of sodium.

10.2.2.1. Effects of Catecholamines on Renin Release

10.2.2.1a. Sympathetic Innervation of the Juxtaglomerular Apparatus. The juxtaglomerular apparatus is heavily innervated with sympathetic nerve endings, as demonstrated by electron-microscopic and histochemical fluorescent techniques.[45-47] The extent of sympathetic innervation varies among different species, reflecting, perhaps, the presence or absence of upright posture in the particular species under study. The macula densa is apparently not innervated. Anatomical evidence of sympathetic innervation is thus consistent with a role for the sympathetic nervous system in the regulation of renin release.

10.2.2.1b. Nerve Stimulation. Stimulation of the renal nerves in a

Table I. Some Effects of Catecholamines on Endocrine Secretion

Hormone	Stimulation(↑) or inhibition(↓)	Receptor	Usual feedback loop	Possible role in fight-or-flight response
Glucagon	↑	β	Plasma substrate levels	Rapid mobilization of glucose, free fatty acids
Insulin	↓	α	Plasma substrate levels	Rapid mobilization of glucose, free fatty acids
Thyroxine	↑	β	TSH	Potentiates effects of catecholamines
PTH	↑	β	Plasma ionized calcium	Increases [CA^{2+}] for blood clotting and muscle contraction
Calcitonin	↑	β	Plasma ionized calcium	Defends against hypercalcemia
Renin	↑	β	Distal tubular [Na^+]: renal baroreceptor	Increases blood pressure by generation of angiotensin II Increases sodium conservation and potassium excretion via aldosterone
Erythropoietin	↑	β	Arterial pO_2	Increases oxygen-carrying capacity
Gastrin	↑	β	Gastric luminal pH	Decreases acidosis by intraluminal buffering capacity and "alkaline tide"

variety of experimental animals causes the release of renin via the activation of the beta receptor.[48,49] Both electrical stimulation of centers in the brain[50,51] and activation of reflex arcs that increase sympathetic activity have been shown to increase renin release; the increase in renin under these circumstances can be prevented by beta-receptor blockade.[52,53] Thus, direct and reflex stimulation of renal sympathetic activity increases renin secretion.

Experiments with infusions of adrenergic agonists and blocking agents also support beta-mediated stimulation of renin secretion in experimental animals and man.[54–57]

10.2.2.1c. Renin Release from Isolated Preparations. Studies from isolated cells and kidney tissue slices show clearly that catecholamines have a direct effect on renin release independently of catecholamine-induced changes in blood pressure, cardiac output, renal perfusion pressure, and intrarenal distribution of blood flow. In these preparations, isoproterenol consistently increases renin secretion, an increase that is abolished by β-blockade.[58–60] This response appears to be mediated by activation of adenylate cyclase and the intracellular accumulation of cAMP.[61] A possible alpha-mediated inhibition of renin secretion by catecholamines has been suggested,[58,60] but is unproved.

Thus, catecholamines clearly can stimulate renin secretion directly, independently of hemodynamic changes; *in vivo,* it is likely that sympathoadrenal stimulation induces hemodynamic changes (particularly afferent arteriolar vasoconstriction) that summate with the direct effects of catecholamines to enhance renin output. The direct effect of catecholamines can be demonstrated, however, even in the absence of these hemodynamic changes.

10.2.2.2. Physiological Role of Catecholamines in Stimulating Renin Release

Catecholamines appear to be important in stimulating renin output in response to abrupt physiological or pathophysiological changes.

10.2.2.2a. Upright Posture. The acute or chronic administration of propranolol abolishes the well-recognized stimulation of renin that occurs with the assumption of upright posture.[62–64] Patients with postural hypotension secondary to autonomic neuropathy have deficient renin responses consistent with inadequate sympathetic response to orthostatic stress.[65–68] Recipients of renal transplants have been shown to increase their plasma renin concentration with postural change,[69] even though the transplanted kidney is denervated. However, the effects of circulating catecholamines and regrowth of sympathetic nerves into the transplant have apparently not been excluded in the reported cases.

10.2.2.2b. Acute Volume Depletion. An acute reduction in renal perfusion pressure secondary to hemorrhage, peripheral vasodilation, or intravenous furosemide all cause an abrupt increase in renin secretion that is diminished by adrenergic blocking agents.[62,70–73] The evidence thus suggests that the elevation of plasma renin in response to reduction in renal perfusion pressure is mediated at least in part via the sympathetic nervous system; the more acute the drop in pressure, the greater the sympathetic contribution appears to be.

10.2.2.2c. Other Physiological and Pathophysiological States. Adrenal medullary secretion of E appears to be responsible for the increase in renin that occurs in hypoglycemia.[74,75] The increase in plasma renin induced by exercise is prevented by chronic β-blockade.[76] Stressful psychological stimuli are also associated with increased renin levels that are diminished by β-blockade.[77,78]

On the other hand, fasting is known to be associated with an inappropriately low renin response in the face of the marked natriuresis that occurs early in the fast.[79] This diminished renin response may reflect the withdrawal of sympathetic activity, since fasting was recently shown to decrease markedly sympathetic activity in rats.[80]

10.2.2.2d. Chronic Sodium Depletion. The rise in renin secretion that accompanies chronic salt depletion, on the other hand, does not appear to require a functionally intact sympathetic nervous system. β-Blockade does not abolish the renin response to chronic salt depletion.[64,81,82] There is some evidence, however, that the acute administration of propranolol can significantly reduce elevated plasma renin in subjects with chronic sodium depletion.[81,83] The increase in plasma renin with sodium depletion despite sympathetic blockade may reflect the absence of sympathetic control of the macula densa. Renal sympathetic activity, although not essential for the renin response to chronic salt depletion, probably augments the increase in renin secretion that occurs in this state.

In summary, the sympathetic nervous system appears to be most important in stimulating renin release in those physiological circumstances that require an acute response. Upright posture, acute volume depletion, and a variety of stressful pathophysiological situations are associated with increased renin secretion; in these circumstances, the increase appears to be mediated via catecholamines. In long-term sodium or volume depletion, on the other hand, nonsympathetic factors are adequate to support enhanced renin output.

10.2.3. Insulin and Glucagon

The secretion of insulin and glucagon from the beta cells and alpha cells, respectively, of the pancreatic islets is governed by an interplay of many factors. The level of various substrates in the blood, the concentrations of a variety of other hormones (secretagogues), and catecholamines all influence the release of insulin and glucagon.[84-86] The evidence that catecholamines suppress insulin release and stimulate the release of glucagon is well established. The importance of catecholamines in regulating insulin and glucagon secretion in a variety of physiological and pathophysiological states is not so well clarified, however. The parasympathetic nervous system stimulates the secretion of both insulin and glucagon directly, and may have an important physiological role under certain conditions.

10.2.3.1. Effects of Catecholamines on Insulin and Glucagon Secretion

10.2.3.1a. Sympathetic Innervation of the Pancreatic Islets. Sympathetic and parasympathetic nerve endings have been demonstrated in close association with the secretory cells of the pancreatic islets in most vertebrate species.[86]

10.2.3.1b. Nerve Stimulation. When cholinergic effects are blocked by atropine, stimulation of splanchnic nerves in a variety of mammalian species decreases the insulin response to infused glucose.[87-90] The importance of the parasympathetic nervous system is indicated by the fact that splanchnic stimulation in the absence of cholinergic blockade increases insulin levels.[89] Sympathetic nerve stimulation increases glucagon secretion.[91] Electrical stimulation of the ventromedial hypothalamus likewise suppresses insulin and increases glucagon secretion[92,93]; the suppression of insulin secretion under these circumstances is abolished by alpha-receptor antagonists.[92] Thus, stimulation of peripheral autonomic nerves and central hypothalamic centers affects insulin and glucagon secretion via the stimulation of adrenergic receptors.

10.2.3.1c. Infusions of Adrenergic Agonists and Antagonists. E infusions are regularly associated with hyperglycemia and a failure of plasma insulin to rise appropriately in response to the elevated level of plasma

glucose.[94-96] The suppressive effect of E on insulin release is antagonized by α-adrenergic blockade. Infusions of E and other beta-receptor
agonists increase glucagon secretion,[97] an effect that is blocked by propranolol and other beta-receptor antagonists.[98,99] Patients with pheochromocytoma have a blunted insulin response to a glucose challenge,[100,101] an effect that is overcome by alpha-receptor blockade and
surgical removal of the tumor. Adequate data on glucagon levels in
patients with pheochromocytoma are not available.

10.2.3.1d. Isolated Preparations. A variety of *in vitro* studies employing incubated tissues or perfusion of isolated pancreas demonstrate that
catecholamines modify the hormonal response to prevailing glucose
concentrations. E and NE decrease insulin and increase glucagon release
at a given glucose level in the supporting medium.[102-107] Pure beta
agonists, such as isoproterenol or E in combination with alpha-receptor
blockade, increase insulin release, an increase that is prevented by β-
blockade. Thus, beta-receptor stimulation increases insulin release, but
under usual physiological circumstances, alpha-receptor-mediated inhibition of insulin release is the predominant effect. Whether or not alpha-
receptor stimulation suppresses glucagon secretion is unclear. Theophylline and cAMP stimulate both insulin and glucagon secretion in
these *in vitro* systems.[107,108] This indicates that beta-receptor stimulation
of insulin and glucagon may be mediated by increased intracellular
cAMP and raises the possibility that alpha-receptor stimulation leads to
decreased cAMP and inhibition of hormone release.

10.2.3.2. Physiological Role of Catecholamines in the Regulation of Insulin and Glucagon Secretion

10.2.3.2a. Fasting and Feeding. Catecholamines probably have no
role in the suppressed insulin and elevated glucagon levels associated
with fasting. Although fasting has traditionally been thought to be
associated with increased sympathetic activity, recent studies in the rat
showed that a brief fast is associated with diminished sympathetic activity.[80] Direct measurement of pancreatic NE turnover in fasted rats
demonstrates a reduction in sympathetic activity to the pancreas and no
rise in urinary E excretion.[109] In fasting man, insulin and glucagon levels
are unaffected by propranolol or phentolamine infusion[110] or by prior
sympathetic decentralization resulting from spinal cord transection.[111]
Thus, the changes in insulin and glucagon secretion that occur during
fasting appear to be completely independent of sympathetic control.

There is considerable evidence that the acute response to feeding
involves enhanced sympathetic activity, as well as the better-recognized

increase in parasympathetic activity.[86,112] During feeding, parasympathetic stimulation of insulin release appears to override sympathetic inhibition of insulin, while both parasympathetic and sympathetic activation may contribute to the augmentation of glucagon release during this "cephalic" phase of hormone secretion. The subsequent responses of insulin, following the acute stimulation related to feeding, depend to a greater extent on postabsorptive substrate levels than on neurogenic factors.

10.2.3.2b. Hypoglycemia. In hypoglycemia, glucagon secretion is stimulated and insulin secretion inhibited, but the relative importance of catecholamines and decreased glucose delivery to the islets in mediating these responses is unclear. Studies with 2-deoxy-D-glucose in rats implicated the adrenal medullary secretion of E as an important factor in the inhibition of insulin release,[113] and, in dogs, suppressed insulin release in response to hypoglycemia was attributed to direct neural inhibition of the endocrine pancreas.[114] The importance of catecholamines as compared with deficient islet supply of glucose is uncertain. In man, adrenergic blockade,[110] adrenalectomy,[115] and sympathetic decentralization from prior cervical cord transection[116] all have no effect on the magnitude of the glucagon response to hypoglycemia. The direct effect of low glucose delivery would appear to be more important than neural factors in augmenting islet glucagon output during hypoglycemia.

10.2.3.2c. Other Pathophysiological States. Catecholamines appear to be importantly involved in the suppression of insulin and stimulation of glucagon secretion that occurs in a variety of pathophysiological states. Thus, catecholamines have been implicated in the altered insulin and glucagon secretion associated with trauma,[111] hypoxia,[118] hypothermia,[119–122] severe burn,[123–125] hemorrhagic shock,[126–129] sepsis,[130] myocardial infarction,[131–134] and laboratory stress in animals.[135,136] The altered glucose metabolism in these states probably reflects both the direct effects of catecholamines on the mobilization of stored fuels and the indirect effects resulting from suppressed insulin and stimulated glucagon release. The relative importance of the adrenal medulla and the sympathetic nervous system in initiating these changes is unknown, although it is likely that both are involved. In exercise, the hyperglucagonemia that occurs is probably related to catecholamines.[137–139]

Thus, catecholamines probably play no role in the suppressed insulin and elevated glucagon secretion associated with fasting, but appear to have a major role in the altered insulin and glucagon secretion that occurs with major disruptions in the integrity of the internal environment.

10.2.4. Other Hormones

10.2.4.1. Thyroid Hormones

The regulation of thyroid hormone biosynthesis and release depends on pituitary TSH. Despite the overriding importance of pituitary TSH, iodine is known to exert an important influence on the biosynthesis and release of thyroid hormones. In recent years, evidence has accumulated to suggest that catecholamines may play a role in the regulation of these processes as well. The thyroid gland has long been known to be innervated with sympathetic nerve fibers from the superior cervical ganglion. Although such innervation was originally thought to be exclusively perivascular, the application of newer morphological techniques, including fluorescent histochemical staining and electron microscopy, has provided convincing evidence that the thyroid follicular epithelium itself is innervated.[140–142] Experiments with isolated thyroid cells and tissue slices have demonstrated that catecholamines increase iodine accumulation and organification and iodothyronine synthesis.[143,144] The relationship of these changes to catecholamine-stimulated generation of intracellular cAMP is unclear.[145] Stimulation of the superior cervical ganglion in animals causes an increase in the formation of colloid droplets, an indication of endocytosis of thyroglobulin correlated with increased release of thyroid hormone; nerve stimulation also causes an increase in blood radioiodine levels after prelabeling of intrathyroidal iodine stores with ^{131}I.[146] The opposite effects can be demonstrated transiently after chemical or surgical sympathectomy.[141] Infusions of catecholamines in hypophysectomized or thyroxine-treated mice, in which TSH is completely suppressed, were shown to increase thyroid hormone secretion.[147,148] These effects appear to be subserved by the beta receptor.[149] The administration of sympatholytic agents to intact rats was also shown to decrease the secretory rate of thyroid hormone.[150] The data thus strongly suggest that catecholamines have the potential to influence thyroid hormone secretion. Although it seems reasonable to speculate that sympathetic stimulation might transiently increase thyroid hormone output, there is no definite evidence that relates catecholamines to a sustained change in thyroid hormone secretion.

10.2.4.2. Gastrin

Gastrin is secreted by the "G" cells of the gastric antrum and proximal duodenum. Ingested foodstuffs, gastric distention, intraluminal pH, parasympathetic effects, and catecholamines may all influence the release of this hormone. Morphological studies clearly demonstrate adrenergic

nerve fibers in the mucosal and submucosal layers of stomach and duodenum in many mammalian species.[151,152] In addition to rich perivascular
innervation of the submucosa, specific adrenergic fluorescence has been
demonstrated at the basal surface of the glandular epithelium. Stimulation of the splanchnic nerves in anesthetized animals results in important
changes in blood flow, but definite effects on gastrin have not been
established. Infusions of E and isoproterenol, on the other hand, do
increase gastrin levels acutely; the stimulatory effect of catecholamine
infusions is abolished by β-blockade.[153-156] Thus, catecholamines appear
to stimulate gastrin release by a beta-receptor mechanism.

The physiological role of catecholamines in the stimulation of gastrin
is unknown. β-Blockade has no effect on the increase in gastrin secretion
produced by food intake.[157] Similarly, an additive effect of food ingestion
and isoproterenol on gastrin secretion has been demonstrated; propranolol prevented the increase in response to isoproterenol but did not affect
the increase related to ingestion of the meal.[156] In various pathophysiological states the elevation of gastrin that occurs appears to reflect the effects
of catecholamines. In hypoglycemia, for example, the rise in plasma
gastrin levels was shown to correlate with the level of plasma epinephrine,[158] and is reduced by pretreatment with propranolol.[159,160] In patients
with severe burns, gastrin levels are significantly increased, and the
increase is greater in those patients with the more serious injuries.
Changes in gastrin secretion tend to parallel those of glucagon, but are not
as marked. In two studies systemic acidosis was associated with stimulation
of gastrin secretion.[125,161] Pretreatment with propranolol prevents the rise
in gastrin in response to respiratory acidosis.[161] These findings raise the
interesting possibility that catecholamine-mediated gastrin secretion
increases gastric acid output as a compensatory mechanism in systemic
acidosis, although direct evidence for this hypothesis is lacking. Some
patients with peptic duodenal ulcers are known to hypersecrete gastrin in
response to beta-receptor stimulation by isoproterenol[156] and by hypoglycemia,[162] as well as in response to a protein meal.[156] The significance of this
increased responsiveness of the gastrin system to catecholamines in
patients with ulcer is unknown, but is intriguing and deserves further
investigation. Stress ulceration of the stomach may also be related to
sympathetic factors; the development of restraint ulcers in rats is associated with increased gastric sympathetic tone as measured by NE turnover;
this is blocked by alpha-receptor blocking agents.[13]

10.2.4.3. Calcitonin

Calcitonin is synthesized and stored in the parafollicular or "C" cells
of the thyroid gland. The serum calcium level is the major factor regulat-

ing its rate of secretion.[163-165] A number of other hormones such as glucagon, enteroglucagon, gastrin, pancreozymin, prolactin, prostaglandins, and thyroxine, as well as the catecholamines, have been shown to increase calcitonin secretion, although the actual role of these various agents in regulating calcitonin release is unknown at present. There is no direct evidence of adrenergic innervation of the parafollicular cells. Studies performed to date, however, have not been extensive enough to rule out a sympathetic supply to the "C" cells. *In situ* perfusion of canine thyroids with isoproterenol or dibutyryl cAMP and theophylline increases circulating calcitonin levels.[166] Perfusion with E is without effect, except when combined with α-adrenergic blockade, in which case E significantly increases calcitonin output. Studies in other mammalian species confirm β-adrenergic stimulation and alpha-receptor-mediated inhibition of calcitonin release.[167.-169] *In vitro* experiments also demonstrate the importance of cAMP in the release of calcitonin from isolated porcine thyroid slices.[170,171] The evidence thus raises the possibility that catecholamines may stimulate calcitonin secretion.

The physiological significance of catecholamine-stimulated calcitonin release is uncertain. As noted above, feeding appears to increase sympathetic activity; in feeding sheep, calcitonin levels rise transiently within 15 min after presentation of food, well before significant calcium absorption could take place. In these experiments, perfusion of the animals's thyroid with a β-adrenergic blocker prevents the increase in calcitonin secretion.[172] Similar increases in calcitonin secretion with feeding have been noted in other mammalian species in circumstances in which calcium could not be the stimulant.[173,174] It thus seems possible that calcitonin, under the influence of catecholamines, helps defend against alimentary hypercalcemia, but studies adequate to test this hypothesis have not yet been done.

10.2.4.4 Parathyroid Hormone

The secretion of PTH by the chief cells of the parathyroid glands is regulated primarily by the serum calcium concentration. A reasonable amount of evidence has accumulated recently indicating that catecholamines as well can influence PTH secretion. Morphological studies have shown that human parathyroids are richly innervated with adrenergic nerve endings that terminate directly on chief cells.[175,176] Catecholamines stimulate PTH release *in vitro* by a β-adrenergic mechanism.[177] Intracellular levels of cAMP appear to be the mediator of PTH secretion.[178] The receptor sites on the parathyroid cells appear to be different for catecholamines and calcium, since PTH release from both stimuli is additive.[179] Infusion studies in humans have demonstrated that beta-receptor agonists increase plasma PTH levels without concomitant alteration in the serum calcium concentration[180]; simultaneous infusion of calcium with E does not induce the PTH rise seen with E alone.[181] Insulin-induced hypoglycemia in man was also shown to elevate PTH levels without associated change in serum calcium concentration.[182] It is possible that concomitant changes in calcitonin in these studies prevent an elevation of calcium in response to the elevated PTH. There is thus considerable evidence that catecholamines can influence PTH secretion, although the physiological role of catecholamines in this context is not clear.

Some patients with pheochromocytoma have mild hypercalcemia that disappears following resection of the tumor.[183-185] It is not likely, however, that catecholamines are responsible for the hyperparathyroidism that occurs in patients with Sipple's syndrome (MEA II; see *The Year in Endocrinology 1975–76*, Chapter 8, Section 8.2.2). Elevated levels of PTH have not been demonstrated in patients with hypercalcemia and pheochromocytoma, and there is some thought that catecholamines may directly affect calcium release from bone.[185] The incidence of hyperparathyroidism appears to be increased only in those patients with pheochromocytoma who have Sipple's syndrome.[186]

10.2.4.5. Erythropoietin

Erythropoietin is a glycoprotein secreted by the kidney; the cell of origin is as yet unidentified.[187] The secretion of this hormone is thought to be regulated by arterial PO_2 via the adenylate cyclase system. NE infusions were shown to increase plasma erythropoietin levels in dogs,[188] and two reports of elevated erythropoietin levels in patients with pheochromocytoma have appeared.[189,190]

Of interest is that the acute erythropoietin response to hypoxia can be reduced by sympathetic denervation of the kidney[191,192] or by β-adrenergic blockade.[193] These studies indicate that the sympathetic innervation of the kidney may have an important role in regulating the release of erythropoietin, but further studies are necessary before firm conclusions can be drawn. The development of a reliable radio-immunoassay for erythropoietin and the demonstration of the cell of origin of erythropoietin in the kidney are also necessary for a full understanding of the role of catecholamines in erythropoietin secretion.

10.2.5. Hypothesis: Role of Catecholamines in the Integration of Endocrine Secretion

A summary of the effects of catecholamines on the eight hormones reviewed here appears in Table I. All, with the exception of the thyroid hormones, are peptide hormones not directly controlled by the pituitary. The regulation of the secretion of these eight hormones appears to depend on the adenylate cyclase–cAMP system. Both catecholamines and the usual feedback mechanism influence secretion by affecting intracellular cAMP. The receptor sites for stimulation of adenylate cyclase by catecholamines and by the usual feedback loop are, however, different. Utilization of the adenylate cyclase–cAMP system by both catecholamines and the usual feedback loop via different receptors is an economical arrangement for allowing dual stimulation of a final common pathway.

In addition, the particular secretory cells for some of these hormones are members of the APUD cell series (see *The Year in Endocrinology 1975–76*, Chapter 8, Section 8.2.4.1). Since APUD cells, as well as the sympathoadrenal system, are thought to derive from embryonic neural crest, the association between these secretory cells and the sympathoadrenal system may begin at a very early stage of development. These similarities raise the possibility that the secretion of other peptide hormones synthesized by APUD cells, such as secretin and enteroglucagon, may also be influenced by catecholamines and that the renin and erythropoietin secretory cells may belong to the APUD cell series.

The physiological role of catecholamines in influencing the secretion of the various hormones considered here is not known. Each of these hormones is regulated in important ways by factors other than catecholamines. There is, however, an important difference between catecholamine-induced stimulation of these various hormones and stimulation by the usual feedback loop. The sympathoadrenal system is geared for quick response, and catecholamines induce rapid changes in effector cells. As a result, the activation of the sympathoadrenal system can quickly mobilize stored hormones and result in a prompt change in hormone secretion. In contrast, changes operating through the usual feedback loop are likely to develop more slowly. Catecholamine-induced alterations in hormone secretion are probably more rapid and operate in the short run as compared with the more usual feedback loops, which operate in the long run and respond to slower, more sustained changes in the environment. Furthermore, catecholamine-induced changes in hormone secretion can anticipate required changes in the hormonal milieu; the usual feedback loops can respond only to changes that have already taken place. The sympathoadrenal system thus allows the CNS to initiate an integrated endocrine response in accord with the perceived needs of the organism as a whole.

In extreme circumstances, the endocrine changes induced by catecholamines may be considered the appropriate hormonal set for the "fight-or-flight" response. The effects of catecholamines on the various hormones tend to reinforce the direct effects of catecholamines on metabolism and on the circulation. Thus, in strenuous exercise and in a variety of pathophysiological states associated with a threat to the constancy of the internal environment, activation of the sympathoadrenal system provides for an endocrine response that may be useful in combating the associated problems of (1) hypotension from fluid loss, hemorrhage, or shunting of blood through muscle vascular beds; (2) acidosis; (3) electrolyte change; and (4) increased demands for metabolic substrates, particularly glucose and free fatty acids. The response to hypotension includes not only the direct effects of catecholamines, which raise the blood pressure and redistribute blood flow to the heart and the brain, but also the increase in renin secretion, which reinforces the effects of catecholamines on blood pressure through increased generation of angiotensin II and encourages sodium conservation and potassium excretion via the stimulation of aldosterone. The increased demands for metabolic energy are met in part through direct stimulation by catecholamines of glycogenolysis, gluconeogenesis, and lipolysis; concomitant suppression of insulin and stimulation of glucagon secretion provides the hormonal milieu to allow full expression of the effects of catecholamines. The catabolic–hormonal balance that results provides an adequate supply of glucose and free fatty acids at the expense of stored body fuels. Stimulation of thyroid hormone release by catecholamines may potentiate the metabolic effects of catecholamines. Stimulation of PTH secretion by catecholamines ensures an adequate supply of ionized calcium for muscle contraction and blood clotting. The simultaneous stimulation of calcitonin protects against the development of pronounced hypercalcemia. Catecholamine-induced increase in gastrin may, if gastric acid secretion ensues, serve to protect against an acute acid load by transiently sequestering hydrogen ions within the GI tract, utilizing intraluminal buffering capacity, and by the generation of an "alkaline tide." Catecholamine-induced release of erythropoietin would provide an anticipatory stimulation of red cell production and increase in oxygen-carrying capacity. After the acute event has passed and sympathetic activity is restored to basal levels, the usual control of hormonal secretion may then be reestablished.

Feeding is another area in which catecholamines may provide an endocrine milieu that protects against undue changes in the internal environment. During feeding, the organism must be prepared to defend its internal environment against perturbations caused by ingested foodstuffs and minerals and by the large volume of intestinal secretions and the hyperosmolarity of the intestinal contents. The responses outlined above would clearly be of benefit in this regard.

Although direct evidence for the participation of catecholamines in many of the responses described above is lacking, the hypothesis that these catecholamine-induced changes in endocrine secretion provide the metabolic set for "fight-or-flight" is not unreasonable. Viewed as a whole, these changes in endocrine secretion may represent an expression of the integrated response of the CNS to a present or impending alteration in the internal milieu.

10.3. Catecholamines and Essential Hypertension

10.3.1. Background

The role of catecholamines in the pathogenesis of essential hypertension has been debated for decades. The critical question of whether excessive sympathetic stimulation occurs in patients with primary essential hypertension is still unanswered. The available evidence indicates[194-196] that in hypertensive patients, the sympathetic nervous system remains responsive to changes in blood pressure; therefore, central sympathetic outflow has at least a permissive role in the maintenance of the hypertensive state. Whether the central sympathetic outflow is abnormally increased as a primary event in essential hypertension constitutes the subject of the continued debate.

Some investigators have long held that catecholamines and the sympathetic nervous system are involved in the pathogenesis of essential hypertension.[197] That the sympathetic nervous system regulates the cardiac output and the distribution of blood flow supports this viewpoint (Fig. 2). The potent pressor effects of catecholamines and their ubiquitous distribution in the cardiovascular system, coupled with the fact that antiadrenergic agents lower the blood pressure more in hypertensive than in normotensive subjects, also favor involvement of the sympathetic system in the hypertensive state. Nonetheless, the traditional viewpoint has been to deny an important role for catecholamines in the pathogenesis of essential hypertension,[198,199] largely because direct and unequivocal evidence of increased sympathetic activity in hypertensive subjects has been lacking. Recent studies, have, however, called the traditional views into question, and although the issue is by no means settled, evidence from several sources, coupled with a greater understanding of the central mechanisms involved in blood pressure regulation, indicates that the sympathetic nervous system may well have a role in the pathogenesis of essential hypertension in some patients. The technological problems that relate to the difficulty in assessing sympathetic activity in man (see *The Year in Endocrinology 1975–76*, Chapter 8, Section 8.3) continue to compound the problem.

There are several ways in which the sympathoadrenal system can

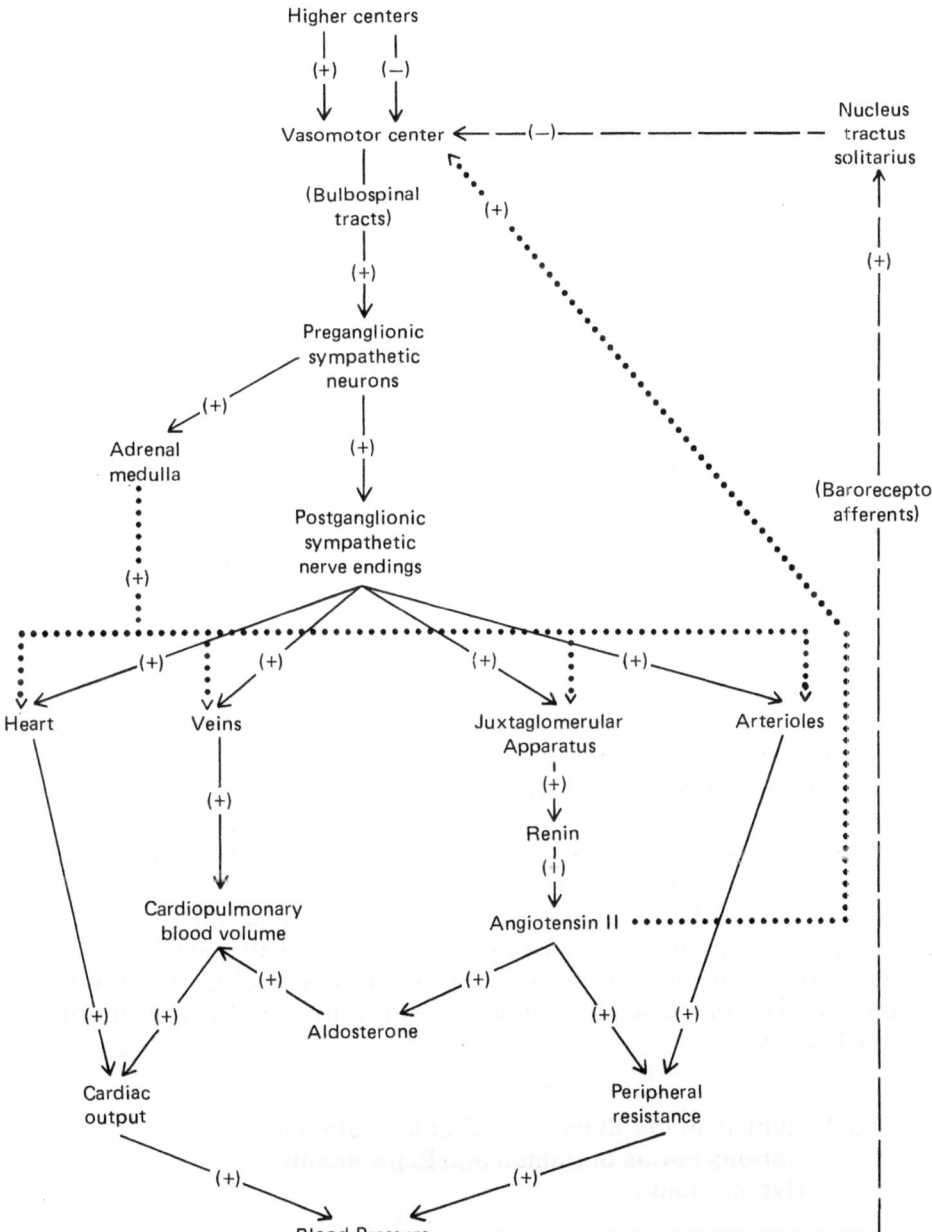

Fig. 2. Simplified scheme of the regulation of blood pressure by the sympathoadrenal system. See text for details. Figure shows the possible consequences of increased central sympathetic stimulation. (+), stimulation; (−); inhibition.

influence blood pressure (Fig. 2). Catecholamines increase arteriolar resistance directly by alpha-mediated vasoconstriction and indirectly via the beta-receptor stimulation of renin output and the generation of angiotensin II. Catecholamines also increase cardiac output directly by an effect on cardiac contractility and heart rate and indirectly by increasing the venous return, the latter by inducing venoconstriction and reducing the capacitance vessels while stimulating the retention of sodium via the renin–angiotension–aldosterone system. Central sympathetic outflow, which ultimately determines the catecholamine-mediated events shown in Fig. 2, is responsive to both central and peripheral influences. Baroreceptor afferents in the aortic arch and carotid sinus respond acutely to changes in blood pressure with reciprocal stimulation or depression of the sympathetic outflow and a corresponding rise or fall in blood pressure toward normal. Baroreceptor afferents terminate in the nucleus of the tractus solitarius (NTS); an inhibitory pathway from the NTS decreases the outflow of the vasomotor center. Other central stimulatory and inhibitory tracts impinge on the vasomotor center as well. As least one of the inhibitory systems is responsive to adrenergic stimuli, so that centrally active α-adrenergic agonists are capable of lowering the blood pressure. There appears to be, in addition, a central noradrenergic pathway capable of inhibiting the outflow of the vasomotor center, so that increased turnover of a brainstem noradrenergic pathway is associated with decreased blood pressure. Noradrenergic fibers from the vasomotor center descend in the bulbospinal tracts and stimulate the cholinergic preganglionic sympathetic neurons in the intermediolateral column of the spinal cord. These, in turn, stimulate the postganglionic sympathetic nerve endings that innervate the heart and vasculature.

Evidence relating to a role of the sympathoadrenal system in essential hypertension involves: (1) direct indices of sympathoadrenal activity in experimental and human hypertension; (2) physiological and biochemical changes in experimental and human hypertension that might reflect increased adrenergic activity; and (3) beneficial effects of treatment with certain agents or techniques that decrease the activity of the sympathoadrenal system.

10.3.2. Activity of the Sympathoadrenal System in Various Forms of Human and Experimental Hypertension

10.3.2.1. Animal Models of Hypertension

An intact sympathoadrenal system is required for the development of high blood pressure in a wide variety of animal models of hypertension.[200]

In some, an increase in sympathoadrenal outflow appears to be the inciting or initiating event. Although no form of experimental hypertension is directly analogous to human hypertension, the involvement of central and peripheral adrenergic pathways in many experimental models that may have relevance for human disease is of considerable interest.

10.3.2.1a. Spontaneously Hypertensive Rat. The spontaneously hypertensive rat (SHR) is a selectively inbred strain of Wistar rat developed at Kyoto University in Japan. It is considered by many to be the best animal model of human essential hypertension available at present. One hundred percent of these animals develop hypertension without obvious renal or endocrine lesions as a cause. The increase in blood pressure is due to an increase in peripheral vascular resistance, and is preceded by a prehypertensive phase of predictable length (about 60 days). Although the mechanisms involved in the development of hypertension in the SHR are not completely elucidated, a substantial amount of evidence points to an important role of the sympathetic nervous system in the initiation and perhaps the maintenance of the hypertensive state. Direct recordings from the cut ends of sympathetic nerves in the SHR demonstrate increased activity,[201,202] an increase that correlates with the degree of hypertension.[202] The turnover of cardiac NE is also increased in the SHR during the development of hypertension, but not after it is sustained.[201,203] Similarly, serum dopamine-β-hydroxylase (DBH) levels are increased in the SHR only during the development of hypertension.[204] The activity of phenylethanolamine-N-methyl transferase (PNMT) in discrete brainstem nuclei of the SHR that contain E was also shown to be increased.[205] The SHR rat shows a greater fall in blood pressure after treatment with sympatholytic agents than comparably hypertensive rats with renovascular hypertension.[206] In contrast, the renin–angiotensin system in the SHR is suppressed.[207] Hypothalamic stimulation results in a greater increase in blood pressure in the SHR as compared with normotensive controls.[208] Intraventricular injection of 6-hydroxydopamine reduces the blood pressure in the SHR, whereas peripheral sympathectomy with 6-hydroxydopamine has a limited effect.[16] The SHR also displays a resetting of the baroreceptors.[209] Although there is some question about the sensitivity of the blood vessels in the SHR,[210] recent evidence indicates that increased responsiveness may be present.[211,212] All considered, the evidence for the participation of adrenergic factors in the development of hypertension in the SHR is quite impressive.

10.3.2.1b. Buffer Nerve Denervation and Lesions of the Nucleus of the Tractus Solitarius. The role of the arterial baroreceptors in the autoregulation of the blood pressure is well established.[213] In animals, denervation of the peripheral baroreceptors produces a centrally mediated increase in blood pressure.[214] Interestingly, there is a human counterpart to this animal model.[215] The elevated blood pressure in this model appears to result from disinhibition of the sympathetic vasomotor centers in the brainstem. Brainstem lesions in the rat that destroy the NTS lead to a much more severe and fulminant hypertension[216] due to central deafferentiation of the baroreceptor reflexes. This hypertension is blocked by alpha-receptor-blocking agents, ganglionic blockade, and reserpine, and by a combination of peripheral 6-hydroxydopamine and adrenalectomy; peripheral 6-hydroxydopamine alone is without effect, indicating a significant role for the adrenal medulla. Intracisternal 6-hydroxydopamine, however, does prevent the development of hypertension.[217] These results indicate that central sympathetic outflow mediates the blood pressure changes that occur following NTS ablation. NTS lesions in the cat produce a less severe, nonfatal, labile hypertension.[15] Lesions of the anterior hypothalamus in the rat produce a fulminant form of hypertension due entirely to catecholamine release from the adrenal medulla.[218]

10.3.2.1c. The DOCA–Salt Hypertensive Rat. Rats made hypertensive by the administration of desoxycorticosterone acetate (DOCA) and salt display increased NE turnover[219] in the heart and other organs.[220,221] Ganglionic blockade reduces both the blood pressure and the increase in NE turnover. Plasma levels of NE are also increased in this model.[222,223] Peripheral sympathetic ablation with 6-hydroxydopamine only partially decreases the blood pressure, but the combination of adrenalectomy and 6-hydroxydopamine restores the blood pressure to normal.[224] On the other hand, central administration of 6-hydroxydopamine (cerebral ventricle) prevents both the increase in blood pressure and the rise in plasma NE,[223,225] since central 6-hydroxydopamine effectively decentralizes both the sympathetic nerves and the adrenal medulla. Thus, DOCA–salt hypertension in the rat clearly depends on central sympathetic activity.

10.3.2.1d. Renal and Renovascular Hypertension. Although there is a substantial amount of evidence that implicates the adrenergic system in the expression of renal and renovascular hypertension in experimental animals,[200,226,227] a recent report questioned the importance of the sympathoadrenal system in one-kidney, low-renin, renovascular hypertension in the rat.[228] This discrepancy may reflect differences in the renin–angiotensin system in different renovascular models. Since the stimulation of adrenergic centers in the brainstem by angiotensin II may be involved in the development of increased blood pressure in some of these animal models,[229–231] the participation of the sympathetic nervous system may depend on whether renin is high or low in the particular model of renal hypertension under study.

Thus, even in nonneurogenic forms of hypertension, there is evidence to implicate the sympathoadrenal system.

10.3.2.2. Indices of Sympathoadrenal Activity in Patients with Essential Hypertension

10.3.2.2a. Urinary Norepinephrine. Studies of urinary catecholamine excretion in hypertensive patients have variously shown increased, unchanged, or decreased quantities of catecholamines and metabolites as compared with values in normal subjects.[232–235] The reason for the conflicting results is not entirely clear, although the vagaries of the urinary methods, including failure to consider renal function, posture, exercise, and the like, may be involved. A more important reason for the discrepancies may be that hypertensives are a nonhomogeneous group; failure to identify and separate significant subgroups would be expected to obscure any real changes in particular subgroups. Recent evidence does suggest that patients with labile hypertension have increased urinary catecholamine excretion when compared with those with stable hypertension,[234,236] along with greater than normal increases in urinary catecholamines in response to stressful situations.[234]

10.3.2.2b. Norepinephrine Turnover Rates. DeQuattro and Sjoerdsma[194] infused [³H]-L-DOPA into normotensive and hypertensive subjects and found no difference in the specific activity of urinary NE. The use of labeled L-DOPA, however, is subject to theoretical limitations when used in the measurement of NE turnover, since the formation of substrate levels of dopamine creates an invalid tracer experiment from a kinetic standpoint. Moreover, the dopamine formed from L-DOPA may release NE from the nerve endings.[237,238] The authors conclude, nonetheless, that NE turnover was not altered in patients with essential hypertension. Gitlow *et al.*,[239] on the other hand, found that a bolus of [³H]-D,L-NE was more rapidly excreted by patients with essential hypertension than by normotensive controls. They invoked decreased uptake or storage of the tracer NE, but the results appear to be consistent with increased NE turnover.

10.3.2.2c. Urinary HVA and Dopamine. Dopamine is a precursor of NE, and homovanillic acid (HVA) is the major metabolite of dopamine. Increased excretion of dopamine and HVA in patients with hypertension was recently reported.[236] The increase in urinary HVA was quite striking (approximately a 5-fold increase) in patients with labile hypertension, and dopamine excretion was significantly increased as well. The meaning of this is not clear, but it is conceivable that it reflects increased activity in the sympathetic system. Since the rate of intraneuronal hydroxylation of tyrosine, and hence and the formation of dopa and dopamine, is known to be accelerated by increased sympathetic activity, it is conceivable that entrance of dopamine into the storage particles where β-hydroxylation to NE occurs might become the rate-limiting step in NE biosynthesis[240] under circumstances of increased sympathetic activity. The excess dopamine outside the storage particle would be deaminated and eventually O-methylated to yield HVA. This interpretation is supported by the recent report[241] of increased HVA excretion in quadriplegic patients with neurogenic hypertension secondary to urinary bladder distention. This type of hypertension is known to be associated with increased sympathetic outflow, and in this study, dopamine-β-hydroxylase (DBH) and other catecholamine metabolities were increased as well. The value of urinary HVA and dopamine in the assessment of sympathetic activity needs further study.

10.3.2.2d. Plasma Catecholamines in Hypertension. Whether plasma catecholamine levels in hypertension are elevated is still uncertain. Three groups of investigators have reported increased total catecholamine levels in plasma.[194,222,242,243] The increases were small (30–50%) and were due to elevation of NE rather than E. In two studies, the increase in NE levels on standing was of the same magnitude in hypertensive and normotensive subjects.[194,244] Another group showed [195,196] a consistent relationship between resting diastolic blood pressure and plasma NE concentration, a correlation that holds when the blood pressure is lowered with a ganglionic blocking agent or clondine (an agent that decreases central sympathetic outlfow). Plasma renin activity, in comparison, did not correlate with resting blood pressure or NE levels in the latter study.[196] Comparison with normotensive subjects was not made, so it is not clear that the NE levels in the hypertensive subjects in these studies were elevated. The correlation of plasma NE level with blood pressure, and the orthostatic rise in NE levels in the hypertensive patients, indicate that in hypertensives, as well as in normal subjects, sympathetic activity is important in regulating circulatory adjustments and controlling the blood pressure; therefore, the sympathetic nervous system must have at least a permissive role in maintaining the increased blood pressure in hypertension.

At least three studies have failed to confirm an increase in plasma NE concentration in hypertensive patients. Christensen and Christensen,[245] using the Engelman technique, found no difference between catecholamine levels of normal subjects and hypertensive patients. Another group using fluorescent assay also failed to confirm an increase in plasma catecholamines in hypertension.[246] In a recent report, Lake *et al.*,[244] using a high-quality NE assay, were not able to show a difference in plasma NE in hypertensives as compared with control subjects when the plasma NE levels were corrected for the age of the patients; other investigators, however, have not found age to be a significant factor in the elevated plasma NE levels found in hypertensives.[30] It is worth emphasizing in this regard that plasma NE levels may be a relatively insensitive indicator of sympathetic activity. In an interesting study of plasma catecholamine levels in the neurogenic hypertension of quadriplegic subjects, it was shown that paroxysms of hypertension were associated with a significant elevation of the plasma NE level; about a 3-fold increase in plasma NE was associated with an increase in mean arterial pressure from 75 to 114 mm Hg. To achieve a similar elevation in blood pressure by NE infusion, however, it was necessary to elevate the NE level over 20-fold.[247] This indicates that NE locally released from the sympathetic nerve endings can have potent effects on the cardiovascular system that are reflected only partially by changes in plasma catecholamine levels.

More data are clearly needed, and with the greater availability of high-quality assays for NE, more will be forthcoming. At present, there is at least a strong suggestion that plasma NE levels are elevated in some patients with essential hypertension. In any event, NE levels are not suppressed, and since plasma NE levels in hypertensive patients appear to retain their responsiveness to physiological and pharmacological manifestations, it seems likely that the level of sympathetic nervous activity is inappropriate for the elevated blood pressure.

10.3.2.2e. DBH Levels in Hypertension. There is disagreement as to whether DBH levels are significantly greater in hypertensive patients than in normotensive controls. It seems clear that there is considerable overlap between normotensive healthy subjects and patients with primary essential hypertension as regards plasma DBH activity. Some workers[248–250] have argued that both patients with labile hypertension and "normal" subjects with variable blood pressure have significantly higher DBH levels than do normals with stable blood pressure and higher DBH levels than do patients with essential hypertension that is sustained. This same group noted small but statistically significant increases in plasma DBH activity in women who became hypertensive on oral contraceptive agents as compared with women whose blood pressure did not change.[251] This finding awaits confirmation.

Other groups have not found significant differences in plasma DBH activity in hypertensive as compared with normal subjects.[252–254] DBH levels have been reported, however, to correlate with diastolic blood pressure[255] in patients with essential hypertension, and in labile hypertensives, the DBH level is said to correlate with diastolic blood pressure, cardiac output, and cardiopulmonary blood volume.[254] In patients with established hypertension, these hemodynamic measurements correlate poorly with DBH activity.[254]

The disagreement in the studies described above may reflect patient sellection, since significant subgroups within the hypertensive population probably exist: Labile hypertensives appear to have higher DBH levels (which correlate with the cardiovascular functional status) than patients with established hypertension, and patients with renal and other secondary forms of hypertension may well have lower DBH levels than normal. Delineation of appropriate subgroups and careful characterization of the hypertensive population is clearly important. Methodological differences continue to be a problem with the DBH assay, and may contribute to some of the discrepant results obtained by different investigators.

10.3.2.3. Features of Essential Hypertension Consistent with Increased Sympathetic Activity

In addition to the direct evidence of increased sympatheitc activity provided by studies of plasma and urinary NE levels and of plasma DBH activity, certain characteristics of patients with essential hypertension suggest increased adrenergic activity. Elevated plasma renin levels and increased cardiac output are found in some patients with labile, borderline, or mild essential hypertension. Although factors other than increased adrenergic activity may cause these same changes, the evidence in favor of sympathetic mediation of these changes is considerable.

10.3.2.3a. Plasma Renin Activity. The significance of peripheral renin levels in patients with essential hypertension has been a subject of considerable interest. Although most hypertensive patients have normal plasma renin activity, distinct subgroups with either low or high plasma renin levels have been described.[256] The high-renin subgroup classically consists of patients with malignant hypertension; in these patients, evidence of severe arteriolar disease in the form of retinopathy or nephropathy can usually be found, and the proximate cause of the increased renin appears to be renal ischemia secondary to the inflammatory and obstructive lesions of the renal arterioles.[257] Recently, however, a subgroup of patients with borderline or mild essential hypertension and high plasma renin activity was identified.[258,259] Patients in this group are clearly clinically distinct from patients with malignant hypertension and those with renal artery stenosis. In patients with mild high-renin hypertension, the increased renin may be a manifestation of increased sympathetic activity, rather than the cause of the hypertension.[258,259] In support of this concept that mild high-renin hypertension is a hyperadrenergic or neurogenic form of hypertension, the following evidence has been accumulated: (1) values of the urinary NE excretion[235] and plasma NE level[259] are increased in the high-renin population as compared with those in hypertensive patients with normal plasma renin activity; (2) increased sympathetic stimulation of the heart has been noted in patients with high as compared with normal renin levels,[258,259] as evidenced by an increase in heart rate, cardiac output, indices of contractility, and a greater response to β-adrenergic blockade[260]; and (3) the fall in peripheral vascular resistance and blood pressure that occurs during α-adrenergic blockade is greater in patients with high-renin hypertension than in those wih low-renin hypertension.[259] Conversely, patients with low-renin hypertension have decreased plasma NE levels[261] and decreased DBH activity,[250] consistent with suppression of the sympathetic nervous system. It appears that high plasma renin activity may be a marker for increased sympathetic activity in this group of patients, since it correlates with other evidence of increased adrenergic stimulation. The size of this subset of patients within the hypertensive population is not known with certainty. Esler *et al.*[259] estimate 15–30%, but this is higher than that reported by other investigators. As discussed below, however, increased adrenergic activity in borderline, labile, or mild hypertension may be a stage through which many patients with essential hypertension pass. In a later stage, increased sympathetic activity, having acted as an initiating event in the hypertension, may no longer be demonstrable.

10.3.2.3b. Cardiac Output. It has been well recognized for some time that many patients with labile, borderline, or mild hypertension have an increase in cardiac output.[262,263] The significance of this increase for the subsequent development of sustained hypertension with increased total peripheral resistance and normal cardiac output has been debated.[264] The theory of total body autoregulation, in which the increased cardiac output leads to secondary increase in total peripheral resistance that becomes fixed, has been criticized[263,264] on several grounds, including the fact that elevation of peripheral resistance can be demonstrated during the phase of increased cardiac output. Furthermore, in the SHR, which passes through a phase of increased cardiac output, blockade of the increase in cardiac output with beta-receptor antagonists does not prevent or delay the development of severe hypertension.[265] It does appear that increased cardiac output, like elevated plasma renin activity, is a concomitant of sympathetic stimulation, a manifestation of the hyperadrenergic state that causes the high blood pressure, but not the proximate cause of the high blood pressure itself.

Another way in which adrenergic factors could affect cardiac output, apart from direct sympathetic stimulation of the heart, is by increased venomotor tone with venoconstriction, increased venous return, and increased cardiopulmonary blood volume. Increased cardiopulmonary blood volume has in fact been noted in some studies of labile or borderline hypertensive patients[254,266] but not in others.[267] Decreased venous capacity has been demonstrated in animal models of hypertension,[268] but the decreased capacity may not be attributable solely to adrenergic factors.

10.3.2.3c. Renal Vascular Tone. Increased renal vascular tone has been described in about two-thirds of patients with essential hypertension.[269] Response to phentolamine indicates that this may be sympathetically mediated. Whether this has special significance in terms of the pathogenesis of essential hypertension or is a well-studied example of a generalized increase in adrenergic activity is not clear.

10.3.3. Response to Treatment

In recent years, a substantial literature has accumulated that indicates that many drugs useful in the treatment of hypertension have a central mechanism of action. This is consistent with a role for the sympathetic nervous system in the maintenance, if not the initiation, of the hypertensive process. Both clonidine and α-methyldopa[270-274] depress central sympathetic outflow by stimulating central α-adrenergic receptors. Although the mechanism of action of propranolol and other β-blocking agents in lowering the blood pressure is complex and controversial, the evidence that propranolol has central effects is compelling. Thus, propranolol is concentrated in human brain in levels that reduce the blood pressure in experimental animals.[275] Agents that penetrate the brain affect the blood pressure in the SHR more than do peripheral β-blockers.[276] Furthermore, it was recently shown that propranolol inhibits centrally mediated sympathetic activity. Direct recording of nerve impulses from the splanchnic nerves in conscious rabbits shows a significant reduction in sympathetic nerve activity and mean arterial pressure[277] after intravenous administration of propranolol. Hypertensive patients treated with propranolol have significantly smaller increases in NE excretion in response to mild industrial stress after treatment with propranolol than they do before.[278] It is clear that both propranolol and the α-adrenergic agonists clonidine and methyldopa have important, presumably different, central actions that relate to their hypotensive effects.

The relative importance of renin suppression in the hypotensive action of propranolol[279-284] is controversial and beyond the scope of this chapter. It is fair to say, however, that a significant body of literature indicates that the hypotensive effects of propranolol are not adequately explained by suppression of renin.[285-292]

Studies of the effect on blood pressure of biofeedback[293] and of relaxation or meditational techniques provide additional evidence in favor of a role of central sympathetic outflow in the initiation or maintenance of essential hypertension. Small but statistically significant decreases in mean arterial pressure have been produced by various relaxation techniques,[294-297] and in one study, a small decrease in plasma DBH activity was noted as well.[297] These results are consistent with stimulation of an inhibitory pathway (or inhibition of a stimulatory pathway), with reduction in vasomotor center outflow. Although the clinical usefulness of these techniques remains to be demonstrated, the fact that blood pressure can be reduced in hypertensive patients by a specific mental process is consistent with the participation of central sympathetic outflow in the maintenance or initiation of hypertension.

10.3.4. Summary: Does the Sympathetic Nervous System Have a Primary Role in the Development of Essential Hypertension?

The following conclusions appear justified on the basis of the evidence reviewed above: (1) The sympathetic nervous system remains responsive and is not suppressed in most hypertensive patients; centrally active drugs that decrease sympathetic activity lower the blood pressure more in hypertensive than in normotensive patients. The sympathetic nervous system therefore has at least a permissive role in the maintenance of increased blood pressure in almost all hypertensive patients. (2) A wide variety of experimental models of hypertension require an intact sympathoadrenal system for the development of elevated blood pressure and display evidence of enhanced sympathetic activity during or preceding the development of the hypertensive state. DOCA–salt, SHR, renovascular, buffer nerve, and NTS hypertension are the most prominent examples. (3) In patients with essential hypertension, direct evidence of increased sympathetic activity is equivocal. This may reflect, in part, the low sensitivity of the methods available clinically for the assessment of sympathetic activity. Of greater significance in many studies is the error introduced by grouping together all patients with hypertension, since significant subgroups clearly exist. Patients with borderline, labile, or hyperkinetic hypertension quite regularly have evidence of enhanced sympathetic stimulation. Just as the biochemical evidence for increased sympathetic activity is more compelling for patients with labile hypertension, physiological studies show that labile hypertensives are the patients with the physiological alterations (increased cardiopulmonary blood volume, increased heart rate, increased cardiac output) that suggest increased adrenergic activity.[254,266] The relationship between these hypertensive patients with physiological and biochemical evidence of adrenergic over-activity and other patients with sustained hypertension in whom it is more difficult to demonstrate increased sympathetic activity and who lack the physiological changes consistent with increased sympathetic activity is uncertain. Are the patients with borderline hypertension and evidence of increased sympathetic input to the heart and vasculature a discrete and distinct subgroup of the hypertensive population? Or do they represent, at one point in time, a stage in the development of essential hypertension through which many patients with sustained essential hypertension have passed? Only time and further studies will tell, but it is indeed possible that increased sympathoadrenal activity is present in the early stages of essential hypertension in many patients; the increased blood pressure itself or the enhanced sympathetic stimulation of the arteries[298,299] may eventually lead to thickening of the arteriolar wall and to a sustained increase in peripheral resistance not directly attributable to increased sympathetic activity. This sequence is supported by animal studies show-ing an early elevation of plasma DBH activity and an increase in cardiac NE turnover rate in the SHR, with normalization later in the course,[201,204] and by studies showing that sympathetic ablation is much more effective in preventing the development of certain forms of experimental hyper-tension than in eradicating it once established.[226] Further careful study of labile hypertensive patients over prolonged periods is essential to ade-quately characterize the role of the sympathetic nervous system in the pathogenesis of essential hypertension.

10.4. Update of Previously Reviewed Subjects

Background information on the subjects described in this section was provided in last year's edition.

10.4.1. Catecholamines and Hyperthyroidism

10.4.1.1. Propranolol in Preparation for Thyroid Surgery

Interest continues in the use of propranolol as the sole agent for the preoperative preparation of hyperthyroid patients being treated with subtotal thyroidectomy.[300–302] It is clear that many patients have been safely operated under emergent and elective conditions with propranolol as the sole preparative agent. Of particular note is the indication in a recent study that thyroid vascularity is significantly reduced by propranolol treatment.[302] (Could the effect on vascularity be due to an inhibition of adenylate cyclase by the local-anesthetic properties of propranolol?[303]) Preparation with propranolol has the advantages of greater speed and simplicity as compared with the conventional regimen of a thionamide plus inorganic iodide. The conventional regimen has withstood the test of time, however, and further evaluation of propranolol is needed before propranolol alone can be recommended for general use in elective thyroid surgery. The use of propranolol in emergent situations and as an adjunct to the conventional regimen is, on the other hand, well established. The recent report of thyroid storm developing in two patients receiving large doses of propranolol (in addition to propylthiouracil)[304] is particularly troublesome in this regard.

10.4.1.2. Thyroid Hormones and Sensitivity to Catecholamines

The question whether propranolol increases sensitivity to the vascular effects of catecholamines is still unanswered. Many studies currently in progress should help resolve the question. Studies on the effect of thyroid hormone on adrenergic receptors may be particularly interesting. Recent reports[305,306] have, in fact, demonstrated increased binding of labeled [³H]-alprenolol, a potent β-blocker, to cardiac membrane preparations from hyperthyroid rats. The increase in binding sites has been interpreted as indicating an increased number of beta receptors. An increase in the number of beta receptors in heart could certainly explain enhanced cardiovascular responses to catecholamines in hyperthyroidism. It remains to be demonstrated, however, that increased binding can be directly correlated with enhanced responses in hyperthyroid animals.

Furthermore, a change in sensitivity by itself would not adequately explain a sustained hyperadrenergic state in hyperthyroidism, since the sympathetic nervous system is not maximally suppressed in the hyperthyroid state. In addition to a change in sensitivity, a change in central sympathetic outflow with decreased suppressibility would appear to be required. Changes in central monamine metabolism in experimental hyperthyroidism continue to be described,[307] and some of these changes may relate to central sympathetic outflow. Another intriguing possibility is that thyroid-induced hypermetabolism indirectly stimulates central sympathetic outflow. Afferents from hypermetabolic muscle were demonstrated recently,[19] and such afferent impulse traffic is a probable source of sympathetic stimulation.[285]

10.4.2. Pheochromocytoma in MEA Syndromes

The occurrence of adrenal medullary hyperplasia as both a precursor of pheochromocytoma and an early feature of clinical involvement in Sipple's syndrome (MEA-II) was noted in two large kindreds.[308,309] The lesions are diffusely hyperplastic or display multifocal nodular proliferation of adrenal medullary tissue; ultimately, bilateral and multicentric pheochromocytomas result. The biochemical correlate is an increase in urinary E excretion, which, as noted previously (see *The Year in Endocrinology 1975–76*, Chapter 8, Section 8.2.2.3), makes measuring urinary E especially valuable for screening purposes.

That as many as 30% of the deaths in MEA-II may be attributed to pheochromocytoma has been emphasized.[309] Of interest in the Mayo Clinic series is that of 19 patients with adrenal medullary disease, 4 had local recurrence and metastases, and in an additional 3 cases, the tumor was locally invasive. This is a disturbingly high incidence of malignancy, which in sporadic cases of pheochromocytoma is said to be about 5%. It will be of interest to see whether this is the pattern in other large kindreds.

In a recent review of von Hipple–Lindau disease,[310] pheochromocytoma was noted in 10% of the 50 affected cases reviewed. Of these 5 cases of pheochromocytoma, 4 occurred in one family, raising the possibility that only certain families with von Hipple–Lindau trait have increased risk of developing pheochromocytoma. Of the 5 cases, 2 were bilateral. In a concomitant autopsy series reviewed at the same time (29 cases),[310] 25% of the cases had pheochromocytoma, the majority of which were not diagnosed clinically. Of the 7 cases of pheochromocytoma in the autopsy series, two were extraadrenal. No information is available as to whether the pheochromocytomas in this syndrome resembled the MEA-II pheochromocytomas with respect to the preponderant secretion of E.

Another recent study emphasized the importance of ganglioneuromatosis of the alimentary tract as a manifestation of the MEA-III syndrome (the mucosal neuroma syndrome).[311] The ganglioneuromata may be associated with motility problems causing constipation, diarrhea, and occasionally megacolon. Sometimes these symptoms may be the earliest manifestation of the disease.

The recent report of a crisis induced by saralasin in a patient with pheochromocytoma and neurofibromatosis[312] serves to emphasize the hazard that a variety of agents pose in patients who harbor an unsuspected pheochromocytoma. ACTH has been reported to cause crises in patients with pheochromocytoma as well. The complexity of the effect of catecholamines on renin levels in patients with pheochromocytoma is demonstrated by a recent report.[313] Renin levels tend to be elevated in patients with pheochromocytoma, particularly in those with elevated E secretion.

Although most of the literature on the MEA syndromes suggests that MEA I, II, and III and the phacomatoses are genetically and clinically distinct, a recent report indicates that tumors characteristic of one of these groups may, in an individual patient, occur in association with a neoplasm typical of another group.[314] We recently noted one patient with a pancreatic islet cell carcinoma whose brother died of medullary carcinoma of the thyroid and had unsuspected bilateral pheochromocytomas at autopsy. Careful study of the individuals and the families of such patients with "crossover" syndromes may provide interesting clues to the pathogenesis of the MEA syndrome as well as useful clinical information.

10.4.3. Plasma Catecholamines

10.4.3.1. Upright Posture, Volume Depletion, Isometric Hand Grip, and Cigarette Smoking

By means of sensitive isotope derivative techniques involving either catechol-O-methyl transferase[8] or phenolethanolamine-N-methyl transferase (PNMT),[315] it was shown that basal levels of NE average 0.2–0.3 ng/ml, and rise about 0.25 ng/ml after 5 min of standing and an additional 0.25 ng/ml after 5 min of isometric hand-grip exercise. Patients with extracellular fluid volume depletion have both elevated basal supine levels (about 0.5–1 ng/ml) and an exaggerated rise on standing.[316] Interestingly, α-adrenergic blockade is associated with a significant rise in plasma NE (as would be expected).[317] Cigarette smoking has also been shown to cause significant elevation of both plasma NE and E.[317]

10.4.3.2. Autonomic Neuropathies

Plasma NE measurements have provided some useful information about the pathogenesis of several disorders of the peripheral sympathetic nerves. Patients with familial dysautonomia have normal plasma NE levels when supine, but, concomitant with a fall in blood pressure and unchanging pulse rate, fail to increase plasma NE levels on assuming the upright posture.[318] Patients with idiopathic orthostatic hypotension also fail to raise the NE level in response to upright posture.[319] These patients may be separated into two groups, however, by the basal NE level: those with normal basal levels had evidence of CNS disease in addition to orthostatic hypotension, indicating that a central lesion is operative in the genesis of the orthostatic defect; those with low basal levels had no disorder of CNS function, implicating the peripheral sympathetic nervous system in the pathogenesis of the postural hypotension. Studies of other forms of neuropathy are currently in progress.[316]

References

1. Korner, P. I., 1976, Central control of blood pressure: Implications in the pathophysiology of hypertension, in: *Regulation of Blood Pressure by the Central Nervous System* (G. Onesti, M. Fernandes, and K. E. Kim, eds.), pp. 3–20, Grune & Stratton, New York.
2. Starke, K., Endo, T., and Taube, H. D., 1976, Central noradrenergic mechanisms of neurotransmission. in: *Regulation of Blood Pressure by the Central Nervous System* (G. Onesti, M. Fernandes, and K. E. Kim, eds.), pp. 21–34, Grune & Stratton, New York.
3. Taylor, D. G., and Brody, M. J., 1976, Spinal adrenergic mechanisms regulating sympathetic outflow to blood vessels, *Circ. Res.* (Suppl. II) **38**:II-10–II-20.
4. Ninomiya, I., Nisimaru, N., and Irisawa, H., 1971, Sympathetic nerve activity to the spleen, kidney, and heart in response to baroceptor input, *Am. J. Physiol.* **221**:1346–1351.
5. Nisimaru, N., 1971, Comparison of gastric and renal nerve activity, *Am. J. Physiol.* **220**:1303–1308.
6. Niijima, A., 1976, Baroreceptor effects on renal and adrenal nerve activity, *Am. J. Physiol.* **230**:1733–1736.
7. Niijima, A., 1975, The effect of 2-deoxy-D-glucose and D-glucose on the efferent discharge rate of sympathetic nerves, *J. Physiol. (London)* **251**:231–243.
8. Cryer, P. E., Santiago, J. V., and Shah, S., 1974, Measurement of norepinephrine and epinephrine in small volumes of human plasma by a single isotope derivative method: Response to the upright posture, *J. Clin. Endocrinol. Metab.* **39**:1025–1029.
9. Garber, A. J., Cryer, P. E., Santiago, J. V., Haymond, M. W., Pagliara, A. S., and Kipnis, D. M., 1976, The role of adrenergic mechanisms in the substrate and hormonal response to insulin-induced hypoglycemia in man, *J. Clin. Invest.* **58**:7–15.
10. Young, J. B., Landsberg, L., and Knopp, R. H., 1976, Effect of intravenous glucagon on urinary catecholamine excretion in normal man, *Metabolism* **25**:233–237.
11. Landsberg, L., and Axelrod, J., 1968, Influence of pituitary, thyroid, and adrenal hormones on norepinephrine turnover and metabolism in the rat heart, *Circ. Res.* **22**:559–571.
12. Taubin, H. L., Djahanguiri, B., and Landsberg, L., 1972, Noradrenaline concentration and turnover in different regions of the gastrointestinal tract of the rat: An approach to the evaluation of sympathetic activity in the gut, *Gut* **13**:790–795.
13. Djahanguiri, B., Taubin, H. L., and Landsberg, L., 1973, Increased sympathetic activity in the pathogenesis of restraint ulcer in rats, *J. Pharmacol. Exp. Ther.* **184**:163–168.
14. Young, J. B., and Landsberg, L., 1977, Suppression of the sympathetic nervous system during fasting, *Science* **196**:1473–1475.
15. Reis, D. J., Doba, N., and Nathan, M. A., 1976, Neurogenic arterial hypertension produced by brainstem lesions, in: *Regulation of Blood Pressure by the Central Nervous System* (G. Onesti, M. Fernandes, and K. E. Kim, eds.) , pp. 35–51, Grune & Stratton, New York.

16. Haeusler, G., 1976, Central adrenergic neurons in experimental hypertension, in: *Regulation of Blood Pressure by the Central Nervous System* (G. Onesti, M. Fernandes, and K. E. Kim, eds.), pp. 53–64, Grune & Stratton, New York.

17. Thorén, P. N., Donald, D. E., and Shepherd, J. T., 1976, Role of heart and lung receptors with nonmedullated vagal afferents in circulatory control, *Cir. Res. (Suppl. II)* **38**:II-2–II-9.

18. Vatner, S. F., and McRitchie, R. J., 1976, Reflex limb dilatation following norepinephrine and angiotensin II in conscious dogs, *Am. J. Physiol.* **230**:557–563.

19. Liang, C.-S., and Hood, W. B., Jr., 1976, Afferent neural pathway in the regulation of cardiopulmonary responses to tissue hypermetabolism, *Circ. Res.* **38**:209–214.

20. Gebber, G. L., and McCall, R. B., 1976, Identification and discharge patterns of spinal sympathetic interneurons, *Am. J. Physiol.* **231**:722–733.

21. Blaschko, H., 1973, Catecholamine biosynthesis, *Br. Med. Bull.* **29**:105–109.

22. Williams, T. H., and Palay, S. L., 1969, Ultrastructure of the small neurons in the superior cervical ganglion, *Brain Res.* **15**:17–34.

23. Kebabian, J. W., and Greengard, P., 1971, Dopamine-sensitive adenyl cyclase: Possible role in synaptic transmission, *Science* **174**:1346–1349.

24. Greengard, P., 1972, Adenosine 3′:5′-cyclic monophosphate as a mediator in the action of neurohumoral agents, *Biochem.* **128**:75P–77P.

25. Sampson, S. R., Aminoff, M. J., Jaffe, R. A., and Vidruk, E. H., 1976, Analysis of inhibitory effect of dopamine on carotid body chemoreceptors in cats, *Am. J. Physiol.* **230**:1494–1498.

26. Smith, A. D., 1973, Mechanisms involved in the release of noradrenaline from sympathetic nerves, *Br. Med. Bull.* **29**:123–129.

27. Enero, M. A., Langer, S. Z., Rothlin, R. P., and Stefano, F. J. E., 1972, Role of α-adrenoceptor in regulating noradrenaline overflow by nerve stimulation, *Br. J. Pharmacol.* **44**:672–688.

28. Häggendal, J., 1973, Regulation of catecholamine release, in: *Frontiers in Catecholamine Research* (E. Usdin and S. H. Snyder, eds.), pp. 531–535, Pergamon Press, New York.

29. Adler-Graschinsky, E., and Langer, S. Z., 1975, Possible role of the β-adrenoceptor in regulation of noradrenaline release by nerve stimulation through a positive feed-back mechanism, *Br. J. Pharmacol.* **53**:43–50.

30. de Champlain, J., 1977, The sympathetic system in hypertension, *Clin. Endocrinol. Metab.* **6**:Chapter 5.

31. Hedqvist, P., 1969, Modulating effect of prostaglandin E_2 on noradrenaline release from the isolated cat spleen, *Acta Physiol. Scand.* **75**:511–512.

32. Hedqvist, P., 1970, Control by prostaglandin E_2 of sympathetic neurotransmission in the spleen, *Life Sci.* **9**:269–278.

33. Horton, E. W., 1973, Prostaglandins at adrenergic nerve-endings, *Br. Med. Bull.* **29**:148–151.

34. Malik, K. U., Ryan, P., and McGiff, J. C., 1976, Modification by prostaglandins E_1 and E_2, indomethacin, and arachidonic acid of the vasoconstrictor responses of the isolated perfused rabbit and rat mesenteric arteries to adrenergic stimuli, *Circ. Res.* **39**:163–168.

35. Vanhoutte, P. M., and Verbeuren, T. J., 1976, Inhibition by acetylcholine of the norepinephrine release evoked by potassium in canine saphenous veins, *Circ. Res.* **39**:263–269.

36. Levy, M. N., and Blattberg, B., 1976, Effect of vagal stimulation on the overflow of norepinephrine into the coronary sinus during cardiac sympathetic nerve stimulation in the dog, *Circ. Res.* **38**:81–85.

37. McGrath, M. A., and Shepherd, J. T., 1976, Inhibition of adrenergic neurotransmission in canine vascular smooth muscle by histamine; mediation by H_2-receptors, *Circ. Res.* **39**:566–573.

38. Lefkowitz, R. J., 1976, The β-adrenergic receptor, *Life Sci.* **18**:461–472.

39. Limbird, L. E. De Meyts, P., and Lefkowitz, R. J., 1975, β-Adrenergic receptors: Evidence for negative cooperativity, *Biochem. Biophys. Res. Commun.* **64**:1160–1168.

40. Bolter, C. P., and Ledsome, J. R., 1976, Effect of cervical sympathetic nerve stimulation on canine carotid sinus reflex, *Am. J. Physiol.* **230**:1026–1030.

41. Vander, A. J., 1967, Control of renin release, *Physiol. Rev.* **47**:359–382.

42. Oparil, S., and Haber, E., 1974, The renin–angiotensin system, *N. Engl. J. Med.* **291**:389–401, 446–457.

43. Ganong, W. F., and Reid, I. A., 1976, Role of the sympathetic nervous system and central α- and β-adrenergic receptors in regulation of renin secretion, in: *Regulation of Blood Pressure by the Central Nervous System* (G. Onesti, M. Fernandes, and K. E., Kim, eds.), pp. 261–280, Grune & Stratton, New York.

44. Zanchetti, A., Stella, A., Leonetti, G., Morganti, A., and Terzoli, L., 1976, Control of renin release: A review of experimental evidence and clinical implications, *Am. J. Cardiol.* **37**:675–691.

45. Barajas, L., 1964, The innervation of the juxtaglomerular apparatus; an electron microscopic study of the innervation of the glomerular arterioles, *Lab. Invest.* **13**:916–929.

46. Nilsson, O., 1965, The adrenergic innervation of the kidney, *Lab. Invest.* **14**:1392–1395.

47. Wågermark, J., Ungerstedt, U., and Ljungqvist, A., 1968, Sympathetic innervation of the juxtaglomerular cells of the kidney, *Circ. Res.* **22**:149–153.

48. Loeffler, J. R., Stockigt, J. R., and Ganong, W. F., 1972, Effect of alpha- and beta-adrenergic blocking agents on the increase in renin secretion produced by stimulation of the renal nerves, *Neuroendocrinology* **10**:129–138.

49. Taher, M. S., McLain, L. G., McDonald, K. M., and Schrier, R. W., 1976, Effect of beta adrenergic blockade on renin response to renal nerve stimulation, *J. Clin. Invest.* **57**:459–465.

50. Ganong, W. F., 1973, Biogenic amines, sympathetic nerves, and renin secretion, *Fed. Proc. Fed. Am. Soc. Exp. Biol.* **32**:1782–1784.

51. Richardson, D., Stella, A., Leonetti, G., Bartorelli, A., and Zanchetti, A., 1974, Mechanisms of renal release of renin by electrical stimulation of the brainstem in the cat, *Circ. Res.* **34**:425–434.

52. Yun, J. C. H., Delea, C. S., Bartter F. C., and Kelly, G., 1976, Increase in renin release after sinoaortic denervation and cervical vagotomy, *Am. J. Physiol.* **230**:777–783.

53. Zehr, J. E., Hasbargen, J. A., and Kurz, K. D., 1976, Reflex suppression of renin secretion during distention of cardiopulmonary receptors in dogs, *Circ. Res.* **38**:232–239.

54. Leenen, F. H. H., Redmond, D. P., and McDonald, R. H., Jr., 1975, Alpha and beta adrenergic-induced renin release in man, *Clin. Pharmacol. Ther.* **18**:31–38.

55. Johnson, J. A., Davis, J. O., Gotshall, R. W., Lohmeier, T. E., Davis, J. L., Braverman, B., and Tempel, G. E., 1976, Evidence for an intrarenal beta receptor in control of renin release, *Am. J. Physiol.* **230**:410–418.
56. Johns, E. J., and Singer, B., 1974, Specificity of blockade of renal renin release by propranolol in the cat, *Clin. Sci. Mol. Med.* **47**:331–343.
57. Weber, M. A., Stokes, G. S., and Gain, J. M., 1974, Comparison of the effects on renin release of beta adrenergic antagonists with differing properties, *J. Clin. Invest.* **54**:1413–1419.
58. Desaulles, E., Forler, C., Velly, J., and Schwartz, J., 1975, Effect of catecholamines on renin release *in vitro, Biomedicine* **22**:433–439.
59. Weinberger, M. H., Aoi, W., and Henry, D. P., 1975, Direct effect of beta-adrenergic stimulation on renin release by the rat kidney slice *in vitro, Circ. Res.* **37**:318–324.
60. Capponi, A. M., and Vallotton, M. B., 1976, Renin release by rat kidney slices incubated *in vitro;* role of sodium and of α- and β-adrenergic receptors, and effect of vincristine, *Circ. Res.* **39**:200–203.
61. Nolly, H. L., Reid, I. A., and Ganong, W. F., 1974, Effect of theophylline and adrenergic blocking drugs on the renin response to norepinephrine *in vitro, Circ. Res.* **35**:575–579.
62. Leonetti, G., Mayer, G., Morganti, A., Terzoli, L., Zanchetti, A., Biachetti, G., Di Salle, E., Morselli, P. L., and Chidsey, C. A., 1975, Hypotensive and renin-suppressing activities of propranolol in hypertensive patients, *Clin. Sci. Mol. Med.* **48**:491–499.
63. Davies, R., and Slater, J. D. H., 1976, Is the adrenergic control of renin release dominant in man?, *Lancet* **2**:594–596.
64. Michelakis, A. M., and McAllister, R. G., 1972, The effect of chronic adrenergic receptor blockade on plasma renin activity in man, *J. Clin. Endocrinol. Metab.* **34**:386–394.
65. Christlieb, A. R., Munichoodappa, C., and Braaten, J. T., 1974, Decreased response of plasma renin activity to orthostasis in diabetic patients with orthostatic hypotension, *Diabetes* **23**:835–840.
66. Wilcox, C. S., Aminoff, M. J., Kurtz, A. B., and Slater, J. D. H., 1974, Comparison of the renin response to dopamine and noradrenaline in normal subjects and patients with autonomic insufficiency, *Clin. Sci. Mol. Med.* **46**:481–488.
67. Gordon, R. D., Kuchel, O., Liddle, G. W., and Island, D. P., 1967, Role of the sympathetic nervous system in regulating renin and aldosterone production in man, *J. Clin. Invest.* **46**:599–605.
68. Božović, L., Castenfors, J., and Orö, L., 1970, Plasma renin activity in patients with disturbed sympathetic vasomotor control (postural hypotension), *Acta Med. Scand.* **188**:385–388.
69. Lewis, E. J., Blaufox, M. D., and Hickler, R. B., 1966, Renin secretion by the denervated kidney, *Br. Med. J.* **2**:1430–1431.
70. Attman, P. O., Aurell, M., and Johnsson, G., 1975, Effects of metoprolol and propranolol on furosemide-stimulated renin release in healthy subjects, *Eur. J. Clin. Pharmacol.* **8**:201–204.
71. Pettinger, W. A., and Keeton, K., 1975, Altered renin release and propranolol potentiation of vasodilatory drug hypotension, *J. Clin. Invest.* **55**:236–243.
72. O'Malley, K., Velasco, M., Wells, J., and McNay, J. L., 1975, Control

plasma renin activity and changes in sympathetic tone as determinants of minoxidil-induced increase in plasma renin activity, *J. Clin. Invest.* **55:**230–235.

73. Bunag, R. D., Page, I. H., and McCubbin, J. W., 1966, Neural stimulation of release of renin, *Circ. Res.* **19:**851–858.
74. Lowder, S. C., Frazer, M. G., and Liddle, G. W., 1975, Effect of insulin-induced hypoglycemia upon plasma renin activity in man, *J. Clin. Endocrinol. Metab.* **41:**97–105.
75. Hansson, B.-G., and Hökfelt, B., 1976, Long term treatment of moderate hypertension with penbutolol (Hoe 893d). II. Effect on the response of plasma catecholamines and plasma renin activity to insulin-induced hypoglycemia, *Eur. J. Clin. Pharmacol.* **9:**245–251.
76. Hansson, B.-G., and Hökfelt, B., 1975, Long term treatment of moderate hypertension with penbutolol (Hoe 893d). I. Effects of blood pressure, pulse rate, catecholamines in blood and urine, plasma renin activity and urinary aldosterone under basal conditions and following exercise, *Eur. J. Clin. Pharmacol.* **9:**9–19.
77. Blair, M. L., Feigl, E. O., and Smith, O. A., 1976, Elevation of plasma renin activity during avoidance performance in baboons, *Am. J. Physiol.* **231:**772–776.
78. Clamage, D. M., Sanford, C. S., Vander, A. J., and Mouw, D. R., 1976, Effects of psychosocial stimuli on plasma renin activity in rats, *Am. J. Physiol.* **231:**1290–1294.
79. Boulter, P. R., Spark, R. F., and Arky, R. A., 1974, Dissociation of the renin-aldosterone system and refractoriness to the sodium-retaining action of mineralocorticoid during starvation in man, *J. Clin. Endocrinol. Metab.* **38:**248–254.
80. Young, J. B., and Landsberg, L., 1977, Suppression of the sympathetic nervous system during fasting, *Science* **196:**1473–1475.
81. Bravo, E. L., Tarazi, R. C., and Dustan, H. P., 1974, On the mechanism of suppressed plasma-renin activity during beta-adrenergic blockade with propranolol, *J. Lab. Clin. Med.* **83:**119–128.
82. Bravo, E. L., Tarazi, R. C., and Dustan, H. P., 1975, β-adrenergic blockade in diuretic-treated patients with essential hypertension, *N. Engl. J. Med.* **292:**66–70.
83. Sullivan, J. M., Adams, D. F., and Hollenberg, N. K., 1976, β-Adrenergic blockade in essential hypertension; reduced renin release despite renal vasoconstriction, *Circ. Res.* **39:**532–536.
84. Mayhew, D. A., Wright, P. H., and Ashmore, J., 1969, Regulation of insulin secretion, *Pharmacol. Rev.* **21:**183–212.
85. Porte, D., Jr., and Bagdade, J. D., 1970, Human insulin secretion: An integrated approach, *Annu. Rev. Med.* **21:**219–240.
86. Woods, S. C., and Porte, D., Jr., 1974, Neural control of the endocrine pancreas, *Physiol. Rev.* **54:**596–619.
87. Bloom, S. R., Edwards, A. V., and Vaughan, N. J. A., 1973, The role of the sympathetic innervation in the control of plasma glucagon concentration in the calf, *J. Physiol. (London)* **233:**457–466.
88. Bloom, S. R., and Edwards, A. V., 1975, The release of pancreatic glucagon and inhibition of insulin in response to stimulation of the sympathetic innervation, *J. Physiol. (London)* **253:**157–173.

89. Porte, D., Jr., Girardier, L., Seydoux, J., Kanazawa, Y., and Posternak, J., 1973, Neural regulation of insulin secretion in the dog, *J. Clin. Invest.* **52:**210–214.

90. Marliss, E. B., Girardier, L., Seydoux, J., Wollheim, C. B., Kanazawa, Y., Orci, L., Renold, A. E., and Porte, D., Jr., 1973, Glucagon release induced by pancreatic nerve stimulation in the dog, *J. Clin. Invest,* **52:**1246–1259.

91. Esterhuizen, A. C., and Howell, S. L., 1970, Ultrastructure of the A-cells of cat islets of Langerhans following sympathetic stimulation of glucagon secretion, *J. Cell Biol.* **46:**593–599.

92. Frohman, L. A., and Bernardis, L. L., 1971, Effect of hypothalamic stimulation on plasma glucose, insulin, and glucagon levels, *Am. J. Physiol.* **221:**1596–1603.

93. Frohman, L. A., Bernardis, L. L., and Stachura, M. E., 1974, Factors modifying plasma insulin and glucose responses to ventromedial hypothalamic stimulation, *Metabolism* **23:**1047–1056.

94. Porte, D., Jr., Graber, A. L., Kuzuya, T., and Williams, R. H., 1966, The effect of epinephrine on immunoreactive insulin levels in man, *J. Clin. Invest.* **45:**228–236.

95. Lerner, R. L., and Porte, D., Jr., 1971, Epinephrine: Selective inhibition of the actue insulin response to glucose, *J. Clin. Invest.* **50:**2453–2457.

96. Cerasi, E., Luft, R., and Efendić, S., 1971, Antagonism between glucose and epinephrine regarding insulin secretion; a dose–response study in man, *Acta Med. Scand.* **190:**411–417.

97. Gerich, J. E., Karam, J. H., and Forsham, P. H., 1973, Stimulation of glucagon secretion by epinephrine in man, *J. Clin, Endocrinol. Metab.* **37:**479–481.

98. Gerich, J. E., Langlois, M., Noacco, C., Schneider, V., and Forsham, P. H., 1974, Adrenergic modulation of pancreatic glucagon secretion in man, *J. Clin. Invest.* **53:**1441–1446.

99. Kaneto, A., Miki, E., and Kosaka, K., 1975, Effect of beta and beta₂ adrenoreceptor stimulants infused intrapancreatically on glucagon and insulin secretion, *Endocrinology* **97:**1166–1173.

100. Vance, J. E., Buchanan, K. D., O'Hara, D., Williams, R. H., and Porte, D., Jr., 1969, Insulin and glucagon responses in subjects with pheochromocytoma: Effect of alpha adrenergic blockade, *J. Clin. Endocrinol. Metab.* **29:**911–916.

101. Colwell, J. A., 1969, Inhibition of insulin secretion by catecholamines in pheochromocytoma, *Ann. Intern. Med.* **71:**251–256.

102. Coore, H. G., and Randle, P. J., 1964, Regulation of insulin secretion studied with pieces of rabbit pancreas incubated *in vitro, Biochem. J.* **93:**66–78.

103. Malaisse, W., Malaisse-Lagae, F., Wright, P. H., and Ashmore, J., 1967, Effects of adrenergic and cholinergic agents upon insulin secretion *in vitro, Endocrinology* **80:**975–978.

104. Leclercq-Meyer, V., Brisson, G. R., and Malaisse, W. J., 1971, Effect of adrenaline and glucose on release of glucagon and insulin *in vitro, Nature (London) New Biol.* **231:**248–249.

105. Iversen, J., 1971, Secretion of glucagon from the isolated, perfused canine pancreas, *J. Clin. Invest.* **50:**2123–2136.

106. Iversen, J., 1973, Adrenergic receptors and the secretion of glucagon and insulin from the isolated, perfused canine pancreas, *J. Clin. Invest.* **52:**2102–2116.

107. Weir, G. C., Knowlton, S. D., and Martin, D. B., 1974, Glucagon secretion from the perfused rat pancreas; studies with glucose and catecholamines, *J. Clin. Invest.* **54:**1403–1412.

108. Jarrousse, C. and Rosselin, G., 1975, Interaction of amino acids and cyclic AMP on the release of insulin and glucagon by newborn rat pancreas, *Endocrinology* **96:**168–177.

109. Young, J. B., and Landsberg, L., 1976, Pancreatic and hepatic norepinephrine (NE) turnover in the rat: A method for assessing sympathetic regulation of carbohydrate metabolism, *Clin. Res.* **24:**640A.

110. Walter, R. M., Dudl, R. J., Palmer, J. P., and Ensinck, J. W., 1974, The effect of adrenergic blockade on the glucagon responses to starvation and hypoglycemia in man, *J. Clin. Invest.* **54:**1214–1220.

111. Brodows, R. G., Campbell, R. G., Al-Aziz, A. J., and Pi-Sunyer, F. X., 1976, Lack of central autonomic regulation of substrate during early fasting in man, *Metabolism* **25:**803–807.

112. Bloom, S. R., Edwards, A. V., Hardy, R. N., Malinowska, K., and Silver, M., 1975, Cardiovascular and endocrine responses to feeding in the young calf, *J. Physiol. (London)* **253:**135–155.

113. Frohman, L. A., Muller, E. E., and Cocchi, D., 1973, Central nervous system mediated inhibition of insulin secretion due to 2-deoxyglucose, *Horm. Metab. Res.* **5:**21–26.

114. Miller, R. E., Waid, T. H., and Joyce, M. P., 1976, Direct neural inhibition of insulin secretion in response to systemic hypoglycemia, *Am. J. Physiol.* **230:**1090–1094.

115. Ensinck, J. W., Walter, R. M., Palmer, J. P., Brodows, R. G., and Campbell, R. G., 1976, Glucagon responses to hypoglycemia in adrenalectomized man, *Metabolism* **25:**227–232.

116. Palmer, J. P., Henry, D. P., Benson, J. W., Johnson, D. G., and Ensinck, J. W., 1976, Glucagon response to hypoglycemia in sympathectomized man, *J. Clin. Invest.* **57:**522–525.

117. Lindsey, A., Santeusanio, F., Braaten, J., Faloona, G. R., and Unger, R. H., 1974, Pancreatic alpha-cell function in trauma, *J. Am. Med. Assoc.* **227:**757.-761.

118. Baum, D., and Porte, D., Jr., 1969, Effect of acute hypoxia on circulating insulin levels, *J. Clin. Endocrinol. Metab.* **29:**991–994.

119. Blackard, W. G., Nelson, N. C., and Labat, J. A., 1967, Insulin secretion in hypothermic dogs, *Am. J. Physiol.* **212:**1185.-1187.

120. Baum, D., Dillard, D. H., and Porte, D., Jr., 1968, Inhibition of insulin release in infants undergoing deep hypothermic cardiovascular surgery, *N. Engl. J. Med.* **279:**1309–1314.

121. Baum, D., and Porte, D., Jr., 1971, Alpha-adrenergic inhibition of immunoreactive insulin release during deep hypothermia, *Am. J. Physiol.* **221:**303–311.

122. Kervran, A., Gilbert, M., Girard, J. R., Assan, R., and Jost, A., 1976, Effect of environmental temperature on glucose-induced insulin response in the newborn rat, *Diabetes* **25:**1026–1030.

123. Allison, S. P., Hinton, P., and Chamberlain, M. J., 1968, Intravenous glucose-tolerance, insulin, and free-fatty-acid levels in burned patients, *Lancet* **2:**1113–1116.

124. Wilmore, D. W., Lindsey, C. A., Moylan, J. A., Faloona, G. R., Pruitt, B. A., and Unger, R. H., 1974, Hyperglucagonaemia after burns, *Lancet* **1:**73–75.

125. Orton, C. I., Segal, A. W., Bloom, S. R., and Clarke, J., 1975, Hypersecretion of glucagon and gastrin in severely burnt patients, *Br. Med. Jr.* **2:**170–172.
126. Cerchio, G. M., Moss, G. S., Popovich, P. A., Butler, E., and Siegel, D. C., 1971, Serum insulin and growth hormone response to hemorrhagic shock, *Endocrinology* **88:**138–143.
127. Hiebert, J. M., Sixt, N., Soeldner, J. S., and Egdahl, R. H., 1973, Altered insulin and glucose metabolism produced by epinephrine during hemorrhagic shock in the adrenalectomized primate, *Surgery* **74:**223–234.
128. Hiebert, J. M., Celik. Z., Soeldner, J. S., and Egdahl, R. H., 1973, Insulin response to hemorrhagic shock in the intact and adrenalectomized primate, *Am. J. Surg.* **125:**501–507.
129. Lindsey, C. A., Faloona, G. R., and Unger, R. H., 1975, Plasma glucagon levels during rapid exsanguination with and without adrenergic blockade, *Diabetes* **24:**313–316.
130. Rocha, D. M., Santeusanio, F., Faloona, G. R., and Unger, R. H., 1973, Abnormal pancreatic alpha-cell function in bacterial infections, *N. Engl. J. Med.* **288:**700–703.
131. Dykes, J. R. W., Saxton, C., and Taylor, S. H., 1969, Insulin secretion in cardiogenic shock, *Br. Med. J.* **2:**490.
132. Taylor, S. H., Saxton, C., Majid, P. A., Dykes, J. R. W., Ghosh, P., and Stoker, J. B., 1969, Insulin secretion following myocardial infarction; with particular respect to the pathogenesis of cardiogenic shock, *Lancet* **2:**1373–1378.
133. Christensen, N. J., and Videbaek, J., 1974, Plasma catecholamines and carbohydrate metabolism in patients with acute myocardial infarction, *J. Clin. Invest.* **54:**278–286.
134. Willerson, J. T., Hutcheson, D. R., Leshin, S. J., Faloona, G. R., and Unger, R. H., 1974, Serum glucagon and insulin levels and their relationship to blood glucose values in patients with acute myocardial infarction and acute coronary insufficiency, *Am. J. Med.* **57:**747–753.
135. Bloom, S. R., Daniel, P. M., Johnston, D. I., Ogawa, O., and Pratt, O. E., 1973, Release of glucagon, induced by stress, *Q. J. Exp. Physiol.* **58:**99–108.
136. Shah, J. H., Wongsurawat, N., Aran, P. P., Motto, G. S., and Bowser, E. N., 1977, A method for studying acute insulin secretion and glucose tolerance in unanesthetized and unrestrained rats; the effect of mild stress on carbohydrate metabolism, *Diabetes* **26:**1–6.
137. Galbo, H., Holst, J. J., and Christensen, N. J., 1975, Glucagon and plasma catecholamine responses to graded and prolonged exercise in man, *J. Appl. Physiol.* **38:**70–76.
138. Luyckx, A. S., Dresse, A., Cession-Fossion, A., and Lefebvre, P. J., 1975, Catecholamines and exercise-induced glucagon and fatty acid mobilization in the rat, *Am. J. Physiol.* **229:**376–383.
139. Luyckx, A. S., and Lefebvre, P. J., 1974, Mechanisms involved in the exercise-induced increase in glucagon secretion in rats, *Diabetes* **23:**81–93.
140. Melander, A., Ericson, L. E., Ljunggren, J.-H., Norberg, K.-A., Persson, B., Sundler, F., Tibblin, S., and Westgren, U., 1974, Sympathetic innervation of the normal human thyroid, *J. Clin. Endocrinol. Metab.* **39:**713–718.
141. Melander, A., Ericson, L. E., Sundler, F., and Ingbar, S. H., 1974, Sympathetic innervation of the mouse thyroid and its significance in thyroid hormone secretion, *Endocrinology* **94:**959–966.
142. Tice, L. W., and Creveling, C. R., 1975, Electron microscopic identification

of adrenergic nerve endings on thyroid epithelial cells, *Endocrinology* **97**:1123–1129.

143. Maayan, M. L., and Ingbar, S. H., 1970, Effects of epinephrine on iodine and intermediary metabolism in isolated thyroid cells, *Endocrinology* **87**:588–595.

144. Maayan, M. L., Shapiro, R., and Ingbar, S. H., 1973, Epinephrine precursors: Effects on the iodine and intermediary metabolism of isolated calf thyroid cells, *Endocrinology* **92**:912–916.

145. Marshall, N. J., von Borcke, S., and Malan, P. G., 1975, Studies on isoproterenol stimulation of adenyl cyclase in membrane preparations from the bovine thyroid, *Endocrinology* **96**:1520–1524.

146. Melander, A., Nilsson, E., and Sundler, F., 1972, Sympathetic activation of thyroid hormone secretion in mice, *Endocrinology* **90**:194–199.

147. Ericson, L. E., Melander, A., Owman, C., and Sundler, F., 1970, Endocytosis of thyroglobulin and release of thyroid hormone in mice by catecholamines and 5-hydroxytryptamine, *Endocrinology* **87**:915–923.

148. Melander, A., and Sundler, F., 1972, Interactions between catecholamines, 5-hydroxytryptamine and TSH on the secretion of thyroid hormone, *Endocrinology* **90**:188–193.

149. Melander, A., Ranklev, E., Sundler, F., and Westgren, U., 1975, Beta$_2$-adrenergic stimulation of thyroid hormone secretion, *Endocrinology* **97**:332–336.

150. Coleoni, A. H., 1972, Effects of the administration of catecholamine-depleting drugs on the thyroid function of the rat, *Pharmacology* **8**:300–310.

151. Hollands, B. C. S., and Vanov, S., 1965, Localization of catechol amines in visceral organs and ganglia of the rat, guinea-pig and rabbit, *Br. J. Pharmacol.* **25**:307–316.

152. Jacobowitz, D., 1965, Histochemical studies of the autonomic innervation of the gut, *J. Pharmacol. Exp. Ther.* **149**:358–364.

153. Hayes, J. R., Ardill, J., Kennedy, T. L., Shanks, R. G., and Buchanan, K. D., 1972, Stimulation of gastrin release by catecholamines, *Lancet* **1**:819–821.

154. Stadil, F., and Rehfeld, J. F., 1973, Release of gastrin by epinephrine in man, *Gastroenterology* **65**:210–215.

155. Christensen, K. C., and Stadil, F., 1976, Effect of epinephrine and norepinephrine on gastrin release and gastric secretion of acid in man, *Scand. J. Gastroenterol. Suppl.* **37**:87–92.

156. Brandsborg, O., Brandsborg, M., and Christensen, N. J., 1976, The role of the beta-adrenergic receptor in the secretion of gastrin: Studies in normal subjects and in patients with duodenal ulcers, *Eur. J. Clin. Invest.* **6**:395–401.

157. Kronborg, O., 1975, The effect of beta-adrenergic blockade upon basal and pentagastrin-stimulated gastric acid secretion and upon gastrin response to food, *Scand. J. Gastroenterol.* **10**:757–762.

158. Brandsborg, O., Brandsborg, M., and Christensen, N. J., 1975, Plasma adrenaline and serum gastrin: Studies in insulin-induced hypoglycemia and after adrenaline infusions, *Gastroenterology* **68**:455–460.

159. Christensen, K. C., and Stadil, F., 1976, On the beta-adrenergic contribution to the gastric acid and gastrin responses to hypoglycaemia in man, *Scand. J. Gastroenterol. Suppl.* **37**:81–86.

160. Kronborg, O., Pedersen, T., Stadil, F., and Rehfeld, J. F., 1974, The effect of beta-adrenergic blockade upon gastric acid secretion and gastrin secretion

during hypoglycaemia before and after vagotomy, *Scand, J. Gastroenterol.* **9:**173–176.

161. Kaess, H., Utz, G., Techentrup, U., Hauck, A. M., and Dörner, M., 1975, The effect of propranolol and phentolamine on serum gastrin concentration in response to respiratory acidosis in normal man, *Eur. J. Clin. Invest.* **5:**401–408.

162. Stadil, F., and Rehfeld, J. F., 1974, Effect of insulin injection on serum gastrin concentrations in duodenal ulcer patients and normal subjects, *Scand. J. Gastroenterol.* **9:**143–147.

163. Foster, G. V., 1968, Calcitonin (thyrocalcitonin), *N. Engl. J. Med.* **279:**349–360.

164. Hirsch, P. F., and Munson, P. L., 1969, Thyrocalcitonin, *Physiol. Rev.* **49:**548–622.

165. Queener, S. F., and Bell, N. H., 1975, Calcitonin: A general survey, *Metabolism* **24:**555–567.

166. Avioli, L. V., Shieber, W., and Kipnis, D. M., 1971, Role of glucagon and adrenergic receptors in thyrocalcitonin release in the dog, *Endocrinology* **88:**1337–1340.

167. Bates, R. F. L., Phillippo, M., and Lawrence, C. B., 1970, The effect of propranolol on calcitonin secretion, *J. Endocrinol.* **48:**viii–ix.

168. Bates, R. F. L., Bruce, J. B., and Care, A. D., 1970, The effect of catecholamines on calcitonin secretion in the pig, *J. Endocrinol.* **46:**xi–xii.

169. Care, A. D., Bates, R. F. L., and Gitelman, H. J., 1970, A possible role for the adenyl cyclase system in calcitonin release, *J. Endocrinol.* **48:**1–15.

170. Bell, N. H., and Queener, S., 1974, Stimulation of calcitonin synthesis and release *in vitro* by calcium and dibutyryl cyclic AMP, *Nature (London)* **248:**343–344.

171. Bell, N. H., 1970, Effects of glucagon, dibutyryl cyclic 3',5'-adenosine monophosphate, and theophylline on calcitonin secretion in vitro, *J. Clin. Invest.* **49:**1368–1373.

172. Phillippo, M., Lawrence, C. B., Bruce, J. B., and Donaldson, D. R., 1972, Feeding and calcitonin secretion in sheep, *J. Endocrinol.* **53:**419–424.

173. Milhaud, G., Perault-Staub, A.-M., and Staub, J.-F., 1972, Diurnal variation of plasma calcium and calcitonin function in the rat, *J. Physiol. (London)* **222:**559–567.

174. Swaminathan, R., Bates, R. F. L., Bloom, S. R., Ganguli, P. C., and Care, A. D., 1973, The relationship between food, gastro-intestinal hormones and calcitonin secretion, *J. Endocrinol.* **59:**217–230.

175. Altenähr, E., 1971, Electron microscopical evidence for innervation of chief cells in human parathyroid gland, *Experientia* **27:**1077.

176. Norberg, K.-A., Persson, B., and Granberg, P.-O., 1975, Adrenergic innervation of the human parathyroid glands, *Acta Chir, Scand.* **141:**319–322.

177. Kukreja, S. C., Banerjee, P., Ayala, G., Bowser, E. N., Hargis, G. K., Henderson, W. J., and Williams, G. A., 1976, Selective β_1 receptor mediation of parathyroid hormone secretion, *Clin. Res.* **24:**363A.

178. Williams, G. A., Hargis, G. K., Bowser, E. N., Henderson, W. J., and Martinez, N. J., 1973, Evidence for a role of adenosine 3',5'-monophosphate in parathyroid hormone release, *Endocrinology* **92:**687–691.

179. Kukreja, S. C., Johnson, P. A., Ayala, G., Banerjee, P., Bowser, E. N., Hargis, G. K., and Williams, G. A., 1976, Role of calcium and beta-adrenergic system

in control of parathyroid hormone secretion, *Proc. Soc. Exp. Biol. Med.* **151:**326–328.

180. Kureja, S. C., Hargis, G. K., Bowser, E. N., Henderson, W. J., Fisherman, E. W., and Williams, G. A., 1975, Role of adrenergic stimuli in parathyroid hormone secretion in man, *J. Clin. Endocrinol. Metab.* **40:**478–481.

181. Fischer, J. A., Blum, J. W., and Binswanger, U., 1973, Acute parathyroid hormone response to epinephrine *in vivo, J. Clin. Invest.* **52:**2434–2440.

182. Shah, J. H., Motto, G. S., Kukreja, S. C., Hargis, G. K., and Williams, G. A., 1975, Stimulation of the secretion of parathyroid hormone during hypoglycemic stress, *J. Clin. Endocrinol. Metab.* **41:**692–696.

183. Morey, E. R., and Kenny, A. D., 1964, Effects of catecholamines on urinary calcium and phosphorus in intact and parathyroidectomized rats, *Endocrinology* **75:**78–85.

184. Swinton, N. W., Clerkin, E. P., and Flint, L. D., 1972, Hypercalcemia and familial pheochromocytoma; correction after adrenalectomy, *Ann. Intern. Med.* **76:**455–457.

185. Finlayson, J. F., and Casey, J. H., 1975, Hypercalcaemia and multiple pheochromocytomas, *Ann. Intern. Med.* **82:**810–811.

186. Miller, S. S., Sizemore, G. W., Sheps, S. G., and Tyce, G. M., 1975, Parathyroid function in patients with pheochromocytoma, *Ann. Intern. Med.* **82:**372–375.

187. Fisher, J. W., 1972, Erythropoietin: Pharmacology, biogenesis and control of production, *Pharmacol. Rev.* **24:**459–508.

188. Fisher, J. W., Samuels, A., and Langston, J., 1968, Effects of angiotensin, norepinephrine and renal artery constriction on erythropoietin production, *Ann. N. Y. Acad. Sci.* **149:**308–317.

189. Bradley, J. E., Young, J. D., Jr., and Lentz, G., 1961, Polycythemia secondary to pheochromocytoma, *J. Urol.* **86:**1–6.

190. Waldmann, T. A., and Bradley, J. E., 1961, Polycythemia secondary to a pheochromocytoma with production of an erythropoiesis stimulating factor by the tumor, *Proc. Soc. Exp. Biol. Med.* **108:**425–427.

191. Takaku, F., Hirashima, K., and Okinaka, S., 1962, Studies on the mechanism of erythropoietin production. II. Effect of bilateral section of the splanchnic nerves, *J. Lab. Clin. Med.* **59:**821–825.

192. Halvorsen, S., 1964, Effects of hypothalamic lesions on the erythropoietic response to hypoxia in rabbits, *Acta Physiol. Scand.* **61:**1–19.

193. Fink, G. D., Paulo, L. G., and Fisher, J. W., 1975, Effects of beta adrenergic blocking agents on erythropoietin production in rabbits exposed to hypoxia, *J. Pharmacol. Exp. Ther.* **193:**176–181.

194. DeQuattro, V., and Chan, S., 1972, Raised plasma-catecholamines in some patients with primary hypertension, *Lancet* **1:**806–809.

195. Louis, W. J., Doyle, A. E., and Anavekar, S., 1973, Plasma norepinephrine levels in essential hypertension, *N. Engl. J. Med.* **288:**599–601.

196. Louis, W. J., Doyle, A. E., Anavekar, S. N., Johnston, C. I., Geffen, L. B., and Rush, R., 1974, Plasma catecholamine, dopamine-beta-hydroxylase, and renin levels in essential hypertension, *Circ. Res. (Suppl. I)* **34-35:**I-57–I-63.

197. Doyle, A. E., 1975, Sympathetic nervous activity in hypertension, *Hosp. Pract.* **10**(11):87–95.

198. Peart, W. S., 1966, Catecholamines and hypertension, *Pharmacol. Rev.* **18:**667–672.

199. DeQuattro, V., and Sjoerdsma, A., 1968, Catecholamine turnover in normotensive and hypertensive man: Effects of antiadrenergic drugs, *J. Clin. Invest.* **47:**2359–2373.
200. Chalmers, J. P., 1975, Brain amines and models of experimental hypertension, *Circ. Res.* **36:**469–480.
201. Yamori, Y., 1976, Neurogenic mechanisms of spontaneous hypertension, in: *Regulation of Blood Pressure by the Central Nervous System* (G. Onesti, M. Fernandes, and K. E. Kim, eds.), pp. 65–76, Grune & Stratton, New York.
202. Judy, W. V., Watanabe, A. M., Henry, D. P., Besch, H. R., Murphy, W. R., and Hockel, G. M., 1976, Sympathetic nerve activity; role in regulation of blood pressure in the spontaneously hypertensive rat, *Circ. Res. (Suppl. II)* **38:**II-21–II-29.
203. Louis, W. J., Krauss, K. R., Kopin, I. J., and Sjoerdsma, A., 1970, Catecholamine metabolism in hypertensive rats, *Circ. Res.* **27:**589–594.
204. Nagatsu, T., Kato, T., Numata (Sudo), Y., Ikuta, K., Umezawa, H., Matsuzaki, M., and Takeuchi, T., 1974, Serum dopamine β-hydroxylase activity in developing hypertensive rats, *Nature (London)* **251:**630–631.
205. Saavedra, J. M., Grobecker, H., and Axelrod, J., 1976, Adrenaline-forming enzyme in brainstem: Elevation in genetic and experimental hypertension, *Science* **191:**483–484.
206. Ebihara, A., and Martz, B. L., 1970, Comparative effects of currently available antihypertensive agents on spontaneously and renal hypertensive rats, *Am. J. Med. Sci.* **259:**257–261.
207. Shiono, K., and Sokabe, H., 1976, Renin–angiotensin system in spontaneously hypertensive rats, *Am. J. Physiol.* **231:**1295–1299.
208. Buñag, R. D., Riley, E., and Montello, M., 1976, Sustained pressor responsiveness to prolonged hypothalamic stimulation in awake rats, *Am. J. Physiol.* **231:**1708–1715.
209. Brown, A. M., Saum, W. R., and Tuley, F. H., 1976, A comparison of aortic baroreceptor discharge in normotensive and spontaneously hypertensive rats, *Circ. Res.* **39:**488–496.
210. Spector, S., Fleisch, J. H., Maling, H. M., and Brodie, B. B., 1969, Vascular smooth muscle reactivity in normotensive and hypertensive rats, *Science* **166:**1300–1301.
211. Hermsmeyer, K., 1976, Electrogenesis of increased norepinephrine sensitivity of arterial vascular muscle in hypertension, *Circ. Res.* **38:**362–367.
212. Hermsmeyer, K., 1976, Cellular basis for increased sensitivity of vascular smooth muscle in spontaneously hypertensive rats, *Circ. Res. (Suppl. II)* **38:**II-53–II-57.
213. McRitchie, R. J., Vatner, S., F., Heyndrick. G. R., and Braunwald, E., 1976, The role of arterial baroreceptors in the regulation of arterial pressure in conscious dogs, *Circ. Res.* **39:**666–670.
214. DeQuattro, V., Nagatsu, T., Maronde, R., and Alexander, N., 1969, Catecholamine synthesis in rabbits with neurogenic hypertension, *Circ. Res.* **24:**545–555.
215. Ripley, R. C., Hollifield, J. W., and Nies, A. S., 1977, Sustained hypertension after section of the glossopharyngeal nerve, *Am. J. Med.* **62:**297–302.
216. Doba, N., and Reis, D. J., 1973, Acute fulminating neurogenic hypertension produced by brainstem lesions in the rat, *Circ. Res.* **32:**584–593.
217. Doba, N., and Reis, D. J., 1974, Role of central and peripheral adrenergic

mechanisms in neurogenic hypertension produced by brainstem lesions in rat, *Circ. Res.* **34**:293–301.

218. Nathan, M. A., and Reis, D. J., 1975, Fulminating arterial hypertension with pulmonary edema from release of adrenomedullary catecholamines after lesions of the anterior hypothalamus in the rat, *Circ. Res.* **37**:226–235.

219. de Champlain, J., Mueller, R. A., and Axelrod, J., 1969, Turnover and synthesis of norepinephrine in experimental hypertension in rats, *Circ. Res.* **25**:285–291.

220. de Champlain, J., Krakoff, L. R., and Axelrod, J., 1968, Relationship between sodium intake and norepinephrine storage during the development of experimental hypertension, *Circ. Res.* **23**:479–491.

221. Krakoff, L. R., de Champlain, J., and Axelrod, J., 1967, Abnormal storage of norepinephrine in experimental hypertension in the rat, *Circ. Res.* **21**:583–591.

222. de Champlain, J., Farley, L., Cousineau, D., and van Ameringen, M.-R., 1976, Circulating catecholamine levels in human and experimental hypertension, *Circ. Res.* **38**:109–114.

223. Reid, J. L., Zivin, J. A., and Kopin, I. J., 1975, Central and peripheral adrenergic mechanisms in the development of deoxycorticosterone–sali hypertension in rats, *Circ. Res.* **37**:569–579.

224. de Champlain, J., and van Ameringen, M. R., 1972, Regulation of blood pressure by sympathetic nerve fibers and adrenal medulla in normotensive and hypertensive rats, *Circ. Res.* **31**:617–628.

225. Lewis, P. J., Dargie, H. J., and Dollery, C. T., 1975, Role of saline consumption in the prevention of deoxycorticosterone hypertension in rats by central 6-hydroxydopamine, *Clin. Sci. Mol. Med.* **48**:327–330.

226. Grewal, R. S., and Kaul, C. L., 1971, Importance of the sympathetic nervous system in the development of renal hypertension in the rat, *Br. J. Pharmacol.* **42**:497–504.

227. Lewis, P. J., Reid, J. L., Chalmers, J. P., and Dollery, C. T., 1973, Importance of central catecholaminergic neurones in the development and maintenance of renal hypertension, *Clin. Sci. Mol. Med.* **45**(Suppl. 1):115s–118s.

228. Douglas, J. R., Jr., Johnson, E. M., Jr., Heist, J. F., Marshall, G. R., and Needleman, P., 1976, Is the peripheral sympatho-adrenal nervous system necessary for renal hypertension?, *J. Pharmacol. Exp. Ther.* **196**:35–43.

229. Goldstein, B. M., and Brody, M. J., 1976, Pressor response to intravertebral angiotensin II: Abolition by central catecholamine depletion, in: *Regulation of Blood Pressure by the Central Nervous System* (G. Onesti, M. Fernandes, and K. E. Kim. eds.), pp. 183–189, Grune & Stratton, New York.

230. Ferrario, C. M., Gildenberg, P. L., and McCubbin, J. W., 1972, Cardiovascular effects of angiotensin mediated by the central nervous system, *Circ. Res.* **30**:257–262.

231. Severs, W. B., and Daniels-Severs, A. E., 1973, Effects of angiotensin on the central nervous system, *Pharmacol. Rev.* **25**:415–449.

232. Brunjes, S., 1964, Catecholamine metabolism in essential hypertension, *N. Engl. J. Med.* **271**:120–124.

233. Berglund, G., Tibblin, G., and Aurell, M., 1975, Urinary noradrenaline excretion and renal function in normal and hypertensive 50-year-old men, *Clin. Sci. Mol. Med.* **49**:485–493.

234. Nestel, P. J., and Esler, M. D., 1970, Patterns of catecholamine excretion in urine in hypertension, *Circ. Res. (Suppl. II)* **26-27**:II-75–II-81.
235. Weidmann, P., Hirsch, D., Beretta-Piccoli, C., Reubi, F. C., and Ziegler, W. H., 1977, Interrelations among blood pressure, blood volume, plasma renin activity and urinary catecholamines in benign essential hypertension, *Am. J. Med.* **62**:209–218.
236. Cuche, J.-L., Kuchel, O., Barbeau, A., and Genest, J., 1975, Urinary homovanillic acid, dopamine and norepinephrine excretion in patients with essential hypertension, *Can. Med. Assoc. J.* **112**:443–446.
237. Landsberg, L., 1971, L-3,4-Dihydroxyphenylalanine-induced release of norepinephrine from the rat heart, *Biochem. Pharmacol.* **20**:3452–3457.
238. Landsberg, L., and Bruno, S. J., 1973, 3,4-Dihydroxyphenylalanine, dopamine and norepinephrine storage in the rat heart after L-dopa—further evidence for norepinephrine release, *Biochem. Pharmacol.* **22**:417–425.
239. Gitlow, S. E., Mendlowitz, M., Bertani, L. M., Wilk, E. K., and Glabman, S., 1969, Tritium excretion of normotensive and hypertensive subjects after administration of tritiated norepinephrine, *J. Lab. Clin. Med.* **73**:129–134.
240. Landsberg, L., de Champlain, J., and Axelrod, J., 1969, Increased biosynthesis of cardiac norepinephrine after hypophysectomy, *J. Pharmacol. Exp. Ther.* **165**:102–107.
241. Naftchi, N. E., Wooten, G. F., Lowman, E. W., and Axelrod, J., 1973, Increased serum dopamine-β-hydroxylase activity during neurogenic hypertension in quadriplegia, in: *Frontiers in Catecholamine Research* (E. Usdin and S. Snyder, eds.), pp. 1143–1147, Pergamon Press, New York.
242. Engelman, K., Portnoy, B., and Sjoerdsma, A., 1970, Plasma catecholamine concentrations in patients with hypertension, *Circ. Res. (Suppl. I)* **26-27**:I-141–I-145.
243. DeQuattro, V., Miura, Y., Lurvey, A., Cosgrove, M., and Mendez, R., 1975, Increased plasma catecholamine concentrations and vas deferens norepinephrine biosynthesis in men with elevated blood pressure, *Circ. Res.* **36**:118–126.
244. Lake, C. R., Ziegler, M. G., Coleman, M. D., and Kopin, I. J., 1977, Age-adjusted plasma norepinephrine levels are similar in normotensive and hypertensive subjects, *N. Engl. J. Med.* **296**:208–209.
245. Christensen, M. S., and Christensen, N. J., 1972, Plasma catecholamines in hypertension, *Scand. J. Clin. Lab. Invest.* **30**:169–173.
246. Chodakowska, J., Nazar, K., Wocial, B., Jarecki, M., and Skórka, B., 1975, Plasma catecholamines and renin activity in response to exercise in patients with essential hypertension, *Clin. Sci. Mol. Med.* **49**:511–514.
247. Mathias, C. J., Christensen, N. J., Corbett, J. L., Frankel, H. L., and Spalding, J. M. K., 1976, Plasma catecholamines during paroxysmal neurogenic hypertension in quadriplegic man, *Circ. Res.* **39**:204–208.
248. Schanberg, S. M., Stone, R. A., Kirshner, N., Gunnells, J. C., and Robinson, R. R., 1974, Plasma dopamine β-hydroxylase: A possible aid in the study and evaluation of hypertension, *Science* **183**:523–525.
249. Schanberg, S. M., and Kirshner, N., 1976, Serum dopamine-β-hydroxylase as an indicator of sympathetic activity and primary hypertension, *Biochem. Pharmacol.* **25**:617–621.
250. Stone, R. A., Gunnells, J. C., Robinson, R. R., Schanberg, S. M., and

Kirshner, N., 1974, Dopamine-beta-hydroxylase in primary and secondary hypertension, *Circ. Res. (Suppl. I)* **34-35:**I-47–I-56.

251. Rockson, S. G., Stone, R. A., Gunnells, J. C., Schanberg, S. M., Kirshner, N., and Robinson, R. R., 1975, Plasma dopamine-β-hydroxylase activity in oral contraceptive hypertension, *Circulation* **51:**916–923.
252. Horwitz, D., Alexander, R. W., Lovenberg, W., and Keiser, H. R., 1973, Human serum dopamine-β-hydroxylase; relationship to hypertension and sympathetic activity, *Circ. Res.* **32:**594–599.
253. Freedman, L. S., Roffman, M., and Goldstein, M., 1973, Changes in human dopamine-β-hydroxylase activity in various physiological and pathological states, in: *Frontiers in Catecholamine Research* (E. Usdin and S. Snyder, eds.), pp. 1109–1114, Pergamon Press, New York.
254. Alexandre, J. M., London, G. M., Chevillard, C., Lemaire, P., Safar, M. E., and Weiss, Y., 1975, The meaning of dopamine β-hydroxylase in essential hypertension, *Clin. Sci. Mol. Med.* **49:**573–579.
255. Geffen, L. B., Rush, R. A., Louis, W. J., and Doyle, A. E., 1973, Plasma dopamine β-hydroxylase and noradrenaline amounts in essential hypertension, *Clin. Sci.* **44:**617–620.
256. Laragh, J. H., 1973, Vasoconstriction–volume analysis for understanding and treating hypertension: The use of renin and aldosterone profiles, *Am. J. Med.* **55:**261–274.
257. Hollenberg, N. K., Epstein, M., Basch, R. I., Couch, N. P., Hickler, R. B., and Merrill, J. P., 1969, Renin secretion in essential and accelerated hypertension, *Am. J. Med.* **47:**855–859.
258. Esler, M. D., Julius, S., Randall, O. S., Ellis, C. N., and Kashima, T., 1975, Relation of renin status to neurogenic vascular resistance in borderline hypertension, *Am. J. Cardiol.* **36:**708–715.
259. Esler, M., Julius, S., Zweifler, A., Randall, O., Harburg, E., Gardiner, H., and DeQuattro, V., 1977, Mild high-renin essential hypertension: Neurogenic human hypertension?, *N. Engl. J. Med.* **296:**405–411.
260. Frohlich, E. D., 1971, Beta adrenergic blockade in the circulatory regulation of hyperkinetic states, *Am. J. Cardiol.* **27:**195–199.
261. Esler, M., Zweifler, A., Randall, O., Julius, S., Bennett, J., Rydelek, P., Cohen, E., and DeQuattro, V., 1976, Suppression of sympathetic nervous function in low-renin essential hypertension, *Lancet* **2:**115–118.
262. Julius, S., and Esler, M., 1975, Autonomic nervous cardiovascular regulation in borderline hypertension, *Am. J. Cardiol.* **36:**685–696.
263. Frohlich, E. D., 1977, Cardiac participation in hypertension, *Cardiovasc. Med.* **2:**109–111.
264. Korner, P. I., and Fletcher, P. J., 1977, Role of the heart in causing and maintaining hypertension, *Cardiovasc. Med.* **2:**139–155.
265. Pfeffer, M. A., Frohlich, E. D., Pfeffer, J. M., and Weiss ,A. K., 1974, Pathophysiological implications of the increased cardiac output of young spontaneously hypertensive rats, *Circ. Res. (Suppl. I)* **34-35:**I-235–I-244.
266. Safar, M. E., Weiss, Y. A., London, G. M., Frackowiak, R. F., and Milliez, P. L., 1974, Cardiopulmonary blood volume in borderline hypertension, *Clin. Sci. Mol. Med.* **47:**153–164.
267. Tarazi, R. C., Ibrahim, M. M., Dustan, H. P., and Ferrario, C. M., 1974, Cardiac factors in hypertension, *Circ. Res. (Suppl. 1)* **34-35:**I-213–I-221.

268. Simon, G., 1976, Altered venous function in hypertensive rats, *Circ. Res.* **38**:412–418.
269. Hollenberg, N. K., and Adams, D. F., 1976, The renal circulation in hypertensive disease, *Am. J. Med.* **60**:773–784.
270. Laverty, R., 1973, The mechanisms of action of some antihypertensive drugs, *Br. Med. Bull.* **29**:152–157.
271. Haeusler, G., 1973, Central adrenergic neurons and the control of blood pressure, in: *Frontiers in Catecholamine Research* (E. Usdin and S. Snyder, eds.), pp. 879–881, Pergamon Press, New York.
272. Kobinger, W., 1976, Central modulation of cardiovascular activity by clonidine and other adrenergic substances, in: *Regulation of Blood Pressure by the Central Nervous System* (G. Onesti, M. Fernandes, and K. E. Kim, eds.), pp. 283–292, Grune & Stratton, New York.
273. van Zwieten, P. A., 1976, The centrally mediated action of α-methyldopa, in: *Regulation of Blood Pressure by the Central Nervous System* (G. Onesti, M. Fernandes, and K. E. Kim, eds.), pp. 293–301, Grune & Stratton, New York.
274. Laubie, M., Delbarre, B., Bogaievsky, D., Bogaievsky, Y., Tsoucaris-Kupfer, D., Senon, D., Schmitt, H., and Schmitt, H., 1976, Pharmacological evidence for a central α-sympathomimetic mechanism controlling blood pressure and heart rate, *Circ. Res. (Suppl. II)* **38**:II-35–II-41.
275. Myers, M. G., Lewis, P. J., Reid, J. L., and Dollery, C. T., 1975, Brain concentration of propranolol in relation to hypotensive effect in the rabbit with observations on brain propranolol levels in man, *J. Pharmacol. Exp. Ther.* **192**:327–335.
276. Garvey, H. L., and Ram, N., 1975, Comparative antihypertensive effects and tissue distribution of beta adrenergic blocking drugs, *J. Pharmacol. Exp. Ther.* **194**:220–233.
277. Lewis, P. J., and Haeusler, G., 1975, Reduction in sympathetic nervous activity as a mechanism for hypotensive effect of propranolol, *Nature (London* **256**:440.
278. Lorimer, A. R., Dunn, F. G., Jones, J. V., and Lawrie, T. D. V., 1976, Beta-adrenoreceptor blockade in hypertension, *Am. J. Med.* **60**:877–885.
279. Bühler, F. R., Laragh, J. H., Baer, L., Vaughan, E. D., Jr., and Brunner, H. R., 1972, Propranolol inhibition of renin secretion; a specific approach to diagnosis and treatment of renin-dependent hypertensive diseases, *N. Engl. J. Med.* **287**:1209–1214.
280. Bühler, F. R., Laragh, J. H., Vaughan, E. D., Jr., Brunner, H. R. Gavras, H., and Baer, L., 1973, Antihypertensive action of propranolol; specific anti-renin responses in high and normal renin forms of essential, renal, renovascular and malignant hypertension, *Am. J. Cardiol.* **32**:511–522.
281. Laragh, J. H., 1976, Modern system for treating high blood pressure based on renin profiling and vasoconstriction–volume analysis; A primary role for beta blocking drugs such as propranolol, *Am. J. Med.* **61**:797–810.
282. Karlberg, B. E., and Tolagen, K., 1976, Different antihypertensive effect of beta-blocking drugs in low and normal–high renin hypertension, *Am. J. Med.* **60**:891–896.
283. Menard, J., Bertagna, X., N'Guyen, P. T., Degoulet, P., and Corvol, P., 1976, Rapid identification of patients with essential hypertension sensitive to acebutolol (a new cardioselective beta-blocker), *Am. J. Med.* **60**:886–890.
284. Stumpe, K. O., Kolloch, R., Vetter, H., Gramann, W., Krück, F., Ressel, C.,

and Higuchi, M., 1976, Acute and long-term studies of the mechanisms of action of beta-blocking drugs in lowering blood pressure, *Am. J. Med.* **60:**853–865.

285. Lewis, P., 1976, The essential action of propranolol in hypertension, *Am. J. Med.* **60:**837–852.

286. Holland, O. B., and Kaplan, N. M., 1976, Propranolol in the treatment of hypertension, *N. Engl. J. Med.* **294:**930–936.

287. Bravo, E. L., Tarazi, R. C., and Dustan, H. P., 1975, β-Adrenergic blockade in diuretic-treated patients with essential hypertension, *N. Engl. J. Med.* **292:**66–70.

288. Woods, J. W., Pittman, A. W., Pulliam, C. C., Werk, E. E., Jr., Waider, W., and Allen, C. A., 1976, Renin profiling in hypertension and its use in treatment with propranolol and chlorthalidone, *N. Engl. J. Med.* **294:**1137–1143.

289. Hollifield, J. W., Sherman, K., Zwagg, R., V., and Shand, D. G., 1976, Proposed mechanisms of propranolol's antihypertensive effect in essential hypertension, *N. Engl. J. Med.* **295:**68–73.

290. Mookherjee, S., Eich, R. H., Obeid, A. I., and Smulyan, H., 1977, Hemodynamic and plasma renin effects of propranolol in essential hypertension, *Arch. Intern. Med.* **137:**290–295.

291. Weber, M. A., Lopez-Ovejero, J. A., Drayer, J. I., Case, D. B., and Laragh, J. H., 1977, Renin reactivity as a determinant of responsiveness to antihypertensive treatment, *Arch. Intern. Med.* **137:**284–289.

292. Atterhög, J.-H., Dunér, H., and Pernow, B., 1976, Experience with pindolol, a betareceptor blocker, in the treatment of hypertension, *Am. J. Med.* **60:**872–876.

293. Gutmann, M. C., and Benson, H., 1971, Interaction of environmental factors and systemic arterial blood pressure: A reveiw, *Medicine* **50:**543–553.

294. Benson, H., Rosner, B. A., Marzetta, B. R., and Klemchuk, H. M., 1974, Decreased blood pressure in pharmacologically treated hypertensive patients who regularly elicited the relaxation response, *Lancet* **1:**289–291.

295. Benson, H., Rosner, B. A., Marzetta, B. R., and Klemchuk, H. P., 1974, Decreased blood pressure in borderline hypertensive subjects who practiced meditation, *J. Chronic Dis.* **27:**163–169.

296. Editorial, 1975, *Lancet* **1:**1230–1231.

297. Stone, R. A., and De Leo, J., 1976, Psychotherapeutic control of hypertension, *N. Engl. J. Med.* **294:**80–84.

298. Bevan, R. D., 1975, Effect of sympathetic denervation on smooth muscle cell proliferation in the growing rabbit ear artery, *Circ. Res.* **37:**14–19.

299. Bevan, J. A., Bevan, R. D., Chang, P. C., Pegram, B. L., Purdy, R. E., and Su, C., 1975, Analysis of changes in reactivity of rabbit arteries and veins two weeks after induction of hypertension by coarctation of the abdominal aorta, *Circ. Res.* **37:**183–190.

300. Lee, T. C., Coffey, R. J., Mackin, J., Cobb, M., Routon, J., and Canary, J. J., 1973, The use of propranolol in the surgical treatment of thyrotoxic patients, *Ann. Surg.* **177:**643–647.

301. Michie, W., Hamer-Hodges, D. W., Pegg, C. A. S., Orr, F. G. G., and Bewsher, P. D., 1974, Beta-blockade and partial thyroidectomy for thyrotoxicosis, *Lancet* **1:**1009–1011.

302. Toft, A. D., Irvine, W. J., McIntosh, D., MacLeod, D. A. D., Seth, J.,

Cameron, E. H. D., and Lidgard, G. P., 1976, Propranolol in the treatment of thyrotoxicosis by subtotal thyroidectomy, *J. Clin. Endocrinol. Metab.* **43:**1312–1316.

303. Marshall, N. J., von Borcke, S., and Malan, P. G., 1975, Studies on inhibition of TSH stimulation of adenyl cyclase activity in thyroid plasma membrane preparations by propranolol, *Endocrinology* **96:**1513–1519.

304. Eriksson, M., Rubenfeld, S., Garber, A. J., and Kohler, P. O., 1977, Propranolol does not prevent thyroid storm, *N. Engl. J. Med.* **296:**263–264.

305. Williams, L. T., Lefkowitz, R. J., Watanabe, A. M., Hathaway, D. R., and Besch, H. R., Jr., 1977, Thyroid hormone regulation of β-adrenergic receptor number, *J. Biol. Chem.* **252:**2787–2789.

306. Ciaraldi, T., and Marinetti, G. V., 1977, Thyroxine and propylthiouracil effects *in vivo* on alpha and beta adrenergic receptors in rat heart, *Biochem. Biophys. Res. Commun.* **74:**984–991.

307. Rastogi, R. B., and Singhal, R. L., 1976, Influence of neonatal and adult hyperthyroidism on behavior and biosynthetic capacity for norepinephrine, dopamine and 5-hydroxytryptamine in rat brain, *J. Pharmacol. Exp. Ther.* **198:**609–618.

308. DeLellis, R. A., Wolfe, H. J., Gagel, R. F., Feldman, Z. T., Miller, H. H., Gang, D. L., and Reichlin, S., 1976, Adrenal medullary hyperplasia; a morphometric analysis in patients with familial medullary thyroid carcinoma, *Am. J. Pathol.* **83:**177–196.

309. Carney, J. A., Sizemore, G. W., and Sheps, S. G., 1976, Adrenal medullary disease in multiple endocrine neoplasia, type 2; pheochromocytoma and its precursors, *Am. J. Clin. Pathol.* **66:**279–290.

310. Horton, W. A., Wong, V., and Eldridge, R., 1976, Von Hippel–Lindau disease; clinical and pathological manifestations in nine families with 50 affected members, *Arch. Intern. Med.* **136:**769–777.

311. Carney, J. A., Go, V. L. W., Sizemore, G. W., and Hayles, A. B., 1976, Alimentary-tract ganglioneuromatosis, a major component of the syndrome of multiple endocrine neoplasia, type 2b, *N. Engl. J. Med.* **295:**1287–1291.

312. Dunn, F. G., De Carvalho, J. G. R., Kem, D. C., Higgins, J. R., and Frohlich, E. D., 1976, Pheochromocytoma crisis induced by saralasin; relation of angiotensin analogue to catecholamine release, *N. Engl. J. Med.* **295:**605–607.

313. Vetter, H., Vetter, W., Warnholz, C., Bayer, J.-M., Käser, H., Vielhaber, K., and Krück, F., 1976, Renin and aldosterone secretion in pheochromocytoma; effect of chronic alpha-adrenergic receptor blockade, *Am. J. Med.* **60:**866–871.

314. Hansen, O. P., Hansen, M., Hansen, H. H., and Rose, B., 1976, Multiple endocrine adenomatosis of mixed type, *Acta Med. Scand.* **200:**327–331.

315. Lake, C. R., Ziegler, M. G., and Kopin, I. J., 1976, Use of plasma norepinephrine for evaluation of sympathetic neuronal function in man, *Life Sci.* **18:**1315–1326.

316. Cryer, P. E., 1976, Isotope-derivative measurements of plasma norepinephrine and epinephrine in man, *Diabetes* **25:**1071–1085.

317. Cryer, P. E., Haymond, M. W., Santiago, J. V., and Shah, S. D., 1976, Norepinephrine and epinephrine release and adrenergic mediation of smoking-associated hemodynamic and metabolic events, *N. Engl. J. Med.* **295:**573–577.

318. Ziegler, M. G., Lake, C. R., and Kopin, I. J., 1976, Deficient sympathetic nervous response in familial dysautonomia, *N. Engl. J. Med.* **294:**630–633.
319. Ziegler, M. G., Lake, C. R., and Kopin, I. J., 1977, The sympathetic-nervous-system defect in primary orthostatic hypotension, *N. Engl. J. Med.* **296:**293–297.

Autoimmunity in Endocrine Disease

Jay Silverberg and Robert Volpé

11.1. Introduction

It is a truism that developments in one discipline often unexpectedly illuminate a second area. Thus, recent illuminating advances in immunology have led to new understandings of the pathogenetic mechanisms of many hitherto obscure endocrine disorders. When an endocrine organ is the target of an immune assault, the dysfunction usually manifests itself as gland failure; however, in at least one disorder, Graves' disease, the aberration in immune function is expressed as hyperfunction of the target endocrine gland. In the following discussion, we will detail the evidence that favors an immune basis for certain disorders affecting the thyroid gland, the adrenal cortex, the endocrine pancreas, the gonads, the parathyroid glands, and even the pituitary gland.

JAY SILVERBERG and ROBERT VOLPÉ • Endocrinology Research Laboratory, The Wellesley Hospital; Department of Medicine, University of Toronto, Toronto, Ontario, Canada. Dr. Silverberg is a Fellow of the Medical Research Council of Canada.

11.2. Basic Considerations

The immune system probably evolved in vertebrates to protect the organism from invading foreign elements (primarily microbial) in the environment. To be effective, the basic immune response must first recognize the invader, and then process it and dispose of it in the most efficient manner. Substances recognized as foreign by the immune system are termed *antigens;* for the most part, these are peptides, but they may be other substances, such as polysaccharides. The inability to recognize an antigen as foreign is termed *tolerance,*[1] and no immune response results; on the other hand, should a natural component of an organism be mistaken as foreign and an immune response be mounted against this component, an *autoimmune disturbance* occurs.[2] In this discussion, we are concerned with alterations in the immune system that cause an immune response to be mounted against the endocrine glands.

The components of the immune system consist of both cellular and humoral elements.[3] The cellular elements can be thought of as specific and nonspecific. Specific cellular components such as lymphocytes have the ability to recognize a specific target and respond accordingly. Nonspecific cellular components such as macrophages are recruited into the immune response; they will be discussed further below. The humoral elements of the immune system can similarly be divided into specific (antibody) and nonspecific (complement) components. Most endocrine disorders with an immune basis involve both cellular and humoral, as well as specific and nonspecific, elements.

The lymphocyte is the cornerstone of the immune system in man. Currently, there appear to be at least two well-defined populations of lymphocytes: the thymus-dependent (T) lymphocyte and the bursa-equivalent (B) lymphocyte.[4] These two populations of cells are probably derived from a stem cell situated in the bone marrow. The precursors of the T lymphocytes undergo maturation in the thymus, whereas the precursors of the B lymphocytes undergo maturation in the bursa of Fabricius above the cloaca in birds; in mammals, the area for B-cell maturation is not well defined, but probably is in the bone marrow.

The maturation of T lymphocytes within the thymus probably takes place under the influence of a thymic hormone, thymopoietin,[5] secreted by the thymic epithelial cells. The emergent T lymphocytes can be identified by several means; the best-known method, however, relates to their ability to form rosettes with sheep red blood cells (E rosettes).[6] The T lymphocytes perform several important immune functions: (1) They may kill target cells directly.[7] (2) They may cooperate with B lymphocytes in antibody production ("helper" T lymphocytes).[8] (3) They may secrete low-molecular weight substances (lymphokines) that mediate certain immune phenomena; these substances include migration-inhibition factor (MIF), transfer factor, and interferon.[3] (4) Finally, T lymphocytes may function as suppressor cells alone,[9] or in conjunction with other types of cells: suppressor T lymphocytes block immune responses by other T and B lymphocytes. When a suppressor T lymphocyte blocks an immune response against a foreign antigen, immune tolerance to that antigen is produced. Suppressor T lymphocytes may also block a misdirected immune response against normal organs (immune surveillance), and hence may save the organism from an immune assault against its own tissues.

B lymphocytes are precursors of the cells that secrete antibody.[3] They can be identified by their ability to form rosettes with sheep red blood cells only in the presence of antibody and complement (EAC rosettes).[6] They may also be identified by their surface markers; B lymphocytes have immunoglobulin on their surface as well as receptors for the third component of the complement system and for the Fc portion of the immunoglobulin molecule.[10] For B lymphocytes to produce antibody in response to an antigen, it is usually necessary for them to interact with a specific helper T lymphocyte, which has become sensitized to the same antigen.

The macrophage has a rather nonspecific role in the immune system, in that macrophages by themselves cannot single out specific targets for immune attack. The macrophage appears to have a role in processing antigen into a form that allows lymphoid cells to mount an immune response.[11] In addition, by the process of phagocytosis, macrophages digest foreign protein and cells injured by the more specific lymphoid and humoral elements.[12] Furthermore, macrophages, like B lymphocytes, also possess receptors for the Fc component of immunoglobulin.[10] They can therefore be "armed" by antibody.[13] The role of these armed macrophages is not yet apparent.

Other cellular elements in the immune system have roles that are even less well defined. Killer (K) cells[14] attack and destroy certain cells that are coated with antibody; this cellular destruction is not mediated by phagocytosis. The origin of K cells may be either the macrophage or lymphocyte population, or perhaps both populations. Null cells[15] resemble lymphocytes morphologically, but lack the characteristics of either T or B lymphocytes; they may represent a more primitive precursor of T or B lymphocytes.

The role of granulocytes and nonspecific humoral elements such as the complement system will not be discussed further, although undoubtedly they play a role in the immune response.

How do these complex cellular and humoral elements of the immune system interact to produce autoimmune disease in the endocrine system? According to Burnet,[16] in the normal course of differentiation of the immune system, lymphocytes undergo spontaneous mutations to produce clones of cells capable of interacting with all the foreign antigens the organism is likely to encounter. Occasionally, a clone of lymphocytes will evolve that has the capability of directing an immune response against a normal tissue component. Under normal circumstances, this "forbidden clone"[2] would be held in check by surveillance mechanisms consisting of suppressor T lymphocytes and perhaps other cells; hence, no self-directed immune response would result. It is postulated that in autoimmune disease, there is a specific defect in the surveillance function of certain suppressor T lymphocytes; this allows a clone of self-directed T lymphocytes that has arisen by random mutation to survive and propagate. This surviving "forbidden clone" of T lymphocytes then interacts with its complementary antigen in or on the target organ, initiating a localized cellular immune response. There is no apparent need for any antigenic change in the target organ for this interaction to take place. The consequences of this cellular immune response may or may not result in organ destruction. The same organ-directed clone of T lymphocytes may then act as helper T lymphocytes directing appropriate already-present B lymphocytes to produce the organ-directed antibody. These organ-directed antibodies may result in organ dysfunction or organ stimulation, as in Graves' disease, or they may result in no apparent change in the physiology of the organ, serving only as a marker for the immune response. K cells may also be involved in this immune response by attacking antibody-coated target cells. This general schema for a localized autoimmune response against an endocrine organ is portrayed in Fig. 1.

Table I lists the endocrine as well as other frequently associated nonendocrine organ-specific disorders believed to have an autoimmune basis. It is well known that these disorders tend to occur together in certain patients and in their relatives.[17–19] It is also known that certain histocompatibility antigens are associated with more than random frequency with certain autoimmune endocrine disorders,[20] e.g., HLA-B8 with diabetes mellitus,[21] idiopathic Addison's disease,[22] and Graves' disease in Caucasians.[23] Since many patients with these conditions do *not* have the appropriate HLA antigen, it would seem that these histocompatibility antigens themselves may not have a role in the expression of autoimmune disease; they may serve, however, as markers of those genes that *do* control immune responses and are presumably nearby the aforementioned *HLA* genes; i.e., a defective gene governing immunosuppression over thyroid-directed immunocytes and the gene for histocompatibility antigen HLA-B8 may be close enough on the same chromosome to be inherited together in many cases of organ-specific autoimmune disease. At this time, however, this relationship is speculative.

Graves' disease, as well as the other autoimmune endocrine diseases,

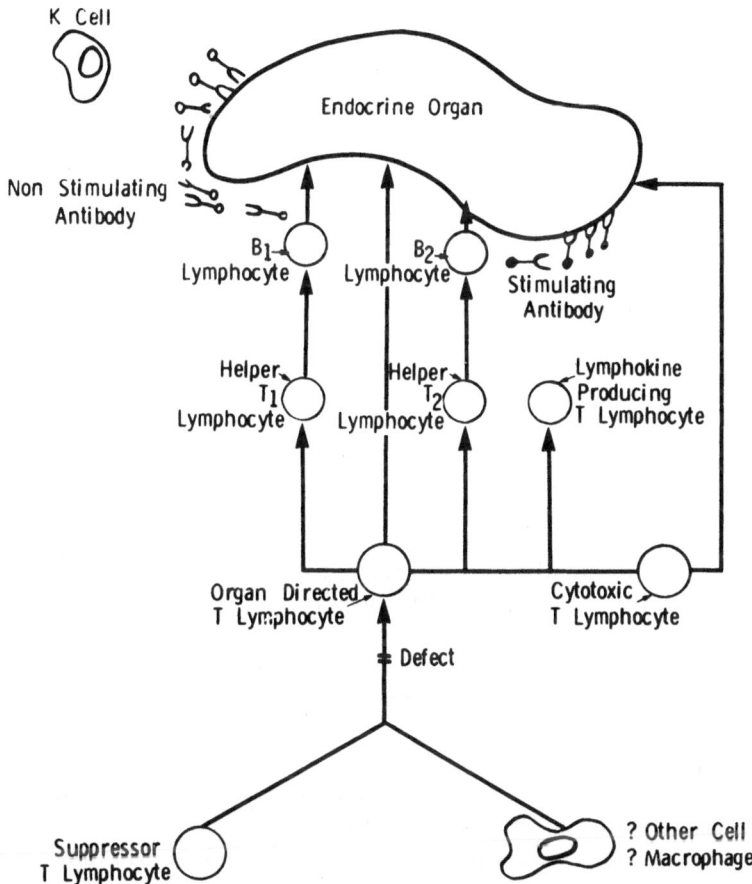

Fig. 1. General model for autoimmune endocrine disease. The model illustrates the various immune alterations that take place in autoimmune endocrine disease. The basic defect is a failure of immune surveillance mediated by suppressor T lymphocytes and perhaps other cells. This allows a clone of organ-directed T lymphocytes that has arisen by normal random mutation to survive and proliferate. Some of these T lymphocytes may act as helper T lymphocytes and interact with organ-directed B lymphocytes in antibody production; T_1 and B_1 are involved in nonstimulating immunoglobulin production, T_2 and B_2 are involved in organ-directed stimulating immunoglobulin production (as occurs in Graves' disease). The organ-directed T lymphocyte may also participate in a direct cytotoxic response (cytotoxic T) or produce low-molecular-weight substances, lymphokines, that aid in the mediation of the immune response. Killer cells (K cells) may interact with immunoglobulin-coated target cells to bring about target-cell destruction. The extent to which each of these events takes place in any given autoimmune endocrine disease is variable.

Table I. Organ-Specific Diseases of Humans Considered to Be of an
Autoimmune Nature

Endocrine	Non-endocrine-associated disorders
Thyroid	Pernicious anemia
Hashimoto's thyroiditis	Vitiligo
Graves' disease	Rheumatoid arthritis
Islet	Idiopathic thrombocytopenic purpura
Juvenile diabetes mellitus	Myasthenia gravis
Adrenal cortex	Sjögren's syndrone
Idiopathic Addison's disease	Chronic active hepatitis
Gonad	Alopecia areata
Autoimmune oophoritis	Predisposition to mucocutaneous
Autoimmune orchitis	candidiasis
Some cases of infertility	
Parathyroid	
Idiopathic hypoparathyroidism	
Pituitary	
Autoimmune hypophysitis	

do not appear to be inherited according to simple Mendelian laws;[18,24,25] either polygenic inheritance with variable expressivity occurs or the expression of the gene for the defect resulting in autoimmune disease is modified by some further factor. Viral infection is one environmental factor that has been suggested by some as a possible influence on the development of autoimmune disease in the endocrine system.[19,26,28] Another possible "environmental" factor is the random mutation of specific "forbidden" clones of lymphocytes in an organism lacking the inherited ability to suppress one or more of them.[19]

Three possible mechanisms have been suggested whereby viruses may interact with an organism to set up an autoimmune response: (1) Viral infection may modify the host tissue in such a manner that there is an antigenic change ("self" to nonself") sufficient to incite an immune response directed at that tissue. This seems unlikely in autoimmune endocrine conditions, since, as will be discussed further below, there is no evidence of any antigenic disturbance in these disorders. (2) Viruses may modify genes controlling immune responses such as surveillance. This could account for sporadic cases of autoimmune endocrine disease, but could not account for familial cases unless it could be shown that these families possess a hereditary predisposition to develop such a viral infection. (3) Viruses may modify lymphocytes in such a way as to affect the frequency of "forbidden clone" formation. Hence, such an organ-directed clone of T lymphocytes may not arise "spontaneously" by mutation, but as the result of an environmental influence such as a viral infection. Data adequate to establish these hypotheses or any hypothesis involving viruses in the mediation of autoimmune endocrine disease are lacking, and any role for viruses in these disorders must be considered speculative.[19]

11.3. Autoimmunity and the Thyroid

Graves' disease was described over 150 years ago and Hashimoto's disease over 60 years ago, but only recently has there been any understanding of their pathogenesis. On clinical inspection, patients with these conditions were found to have certain features suggestive of an immune process. Patients with Graves' disease occasionally have an enlarged spleen and lymphadenopathy. Patients with Hashimoto's disease commonly have hypergammaglobulinemia, while patients with Graves' disease often have lymphocytosis. Moreover, in both these conditions, there is thymic enlargement and a lymphocytic infiltrate in the thyroid stroma.[25] In addition, other autoimmune diseases (e.g., pernicious anemia, diabetes mellitus, myasthenia gravis, rheumatoid arthritis) frequently coexist, or occur in relatives of patients with either Graves' disease or Hashimoto's diseases.[19] However, the first important evidence that a disordered immune system may cause thyroid disease was reported in 1956 by Roitt et al.,[29] who discovered antibodies to thyroglobulin in the sera of patients with Hashimoto's disease. In the same year, Rose and Witebsky[30] produced lesions similar to those of Hashimoto's disease in the thyroid gland of rabbits by immunizing them with extracts of thyroid tissue. About 15 years later, Twarog and Rose[31] were able to induce autoimmune thyroiditis by transfer of lymphoid cells. The immune nature of Graves' disease became evident after 1956, when Adams and Purvis[32] detected the presence of in the sera of some patients with Graves' disease an abnormal thyroid stimulator that stimulated the thyroid for a much longer period than did TSH; this substance was termed *long-acting thyroid stimulator* (LATS). About a decade later, Kriss et al.[33] found that LATS was an immunoglobulin belonging to the IgG class.

Current views of the role of humoral and cell-mediated immunity in Hashimoto's and Graves' diseases will be explained more fully below.

11.3.1. Humoral Immunity in Thyroid Disease

Antibody may be produced to a number of antigens in thyroid tissue; these include thyroglobulin[29] microsomal antigen,[34] a second antigen in the colloid,[34] a nonreceptor cell-surface antigen,[35] the thyroid hormones, thyroxine (T_4) and triiodothyronine (T_3),[36] and the thyrotrophin (TSH) receptor on the cell surface.[37] Polyclonal antibodies to each of these antigens may be produced. The role of these antibodies in inducing thyroid disease is not yet completely understood. It would appear that some of these antibodies have no role in producing pathological lesions in the thyroid, but some do interfere with the function of the thyroid cell, and at least one type of antibody stimulates thyroid cells.

It was once believed that thyroglobulin is a "sequestered antigen" within the thyroid follicles that is not recognizable to the organism as "self," and that disruption of the follicles with escape of the thyroglobulin might lead to autoimmune thyroiditis.[38] It is now known, however, that thyroglobulin begins to leak into the circulation *in utero* in all persons, and in fact is a normal constituent of the blood. Thus, the "secluded antigen" theory can be dismissed.[25]

Plasma thyroglobulin is increased in patients with thyroid malignancy, colloid goiter, and subacute thyroiditis, as well as in the sera of patients with Graves' and Hashimoto's diseases.[39] Increased concentrations of plasma thyroglobulin are not necessarily associated, however, with the development of antibodies to thyroglobulin; they are, however, classically found in high titers in Hashimoto's and Graves' diseases and occasionally in lower titers in other diseases, some nonthyroidal autoimmune conditions, in asymptomatic relatives of patients with Graves' or Hashimoto's disease, and in some other apparently normal persons. These antibodies may be of any class, but precipitins belong mostly to class IgG.[34] Thyroglobulin antibodies are non-complement-fixing, and for the most part are species-specific, but do show some cross-reactivity with monkey thyroglobulin.[34] The tanned red cell agglutination test is the usual method for detecting these antibodies,[40] but the competitive binding radioimmunoassay of Mori and Kriss[41] is by far the most sensitive. The pathogenic significance of thyroglobulin antibodies in inducing thyroid lesions is probably minimal;[25] they may have a role, however, in "arming" macrophages or interacting with K cells. In this indirect manner, they may contribute to morphological damage of the thyroid.

Thyroid microsomal antigen is a lipoprotein found in the Golgi apparatus as well as in the smooth endoplasmic reticulum.[42] Antibodies to the microsomal antigen were shown to be complement-fixing[34] and have the ability to induce cytotoxic changes in monolayers of cultured thyroid cells.[43] Correlation exists between the titers of this antibody and the histological lesions in Hashimoto's disease. The titers of thyroglobulin antibodies do not correlate as well. Antimicrosomal antibodies can be detected by immunofluorescence, complement fixation, hemagglutination, or radioimmunoassay.[34] Hemagglutination is rapidly becoming the favored procedure.

Sera from some patients with Hashimoto's disease show a uniform immunofluorescence in the colloid of fixed sections of thyroid tissue even after absorption with thyroglobulin.[34] The antigen to which these antibodies are directed appears to be a protein that does not contain iodine. Antibodies to this nonthyroglobulin component of colloid may also be found in the serum of patients with Graves' disease, thyroid cancer, and subacute thyroiditis. The significance of this antibody is undertermined.

An antigen that is on the surface of the thyroid cell but distinct from the TSH receptor has been described. Fragraeus and Jonsson[35] showed that in some cases of Hashimoto's disease, antibodies to this antigen will produce a patchy immunofluorescent pattern on the thyroid cell surface. However, the role of this antibody–antigen system in thyroid disease is also unknown.

In Hashimoto's thyroiditis, antibodies are occasionally detected directed against the thyroid hormones, T_4 and T_3.[36] The titers of antibodies to T_4 and T_3 become important when measuring serum concentrations of these thyroid hormones. Depending on the extraction procedure, spuriously high or low T_4 or T_3 concentrations may result if these antibodies are present in sufficiently high titers. The presence of antibodies to T_4 and T_3 does not appear to affect the availability of thyroid hormones to tissues if thyroid reserve is adequate to respond to TSH.

Another, apparently unique, antibody is believed to be of pathogenic significance in the thyrotoxicosis of Graves' disease. This antibody (or rather a polyclonal family of antibodies that belong to the IgG class) is directed toward the TSH receptor on the human thyroid cell surface.[44] After binding to the TSH receptor, or closely contiguous sites, they stimulate thyroid hormone production through the adenylate cyclase–cyclic adenosine monophosphate (cAMP) system in a manner indistinguishable from the action of TSH (aside from a longer duration). The term *thyroid-stimulating immunoglobulin* (TSI) has been applied to these antibodies.[44] Actually, antibodies to receptors on cell surfaces have been described in other conditions, i.e., antibodies to the ACh receptor in sera of patients with myasthenia gravis[45] and to the insulin receptors in some rare forms of diabetes mellitus;[46] these latter antibodies are all of the blocking type and may impair cell function. In contrast, Graves' disease thus far appears to be unique, since TSI, after binding to the TSH receptor, is a stimulating antibody. Kahn,[47] however, recently reported evidence suggesting that an unusual type of hypoglycemia might be caused by a stimulating antibody directed toward the insulin receptor in peripheral tissues.

TSIs are known by several other terms, depending on their method of assay: long-acting thyroid stimulator (LATS),[32] LATS-protector (LATS-P),[48] human thyroid stimulator (HTS),[49] human thyroid adenylate cyclase stimulator (HTACS),[50] and thyrotropin displacement activity (TDA).[51] While TDA usually equates with TSI, it may also include nonsti-

mulating blocking or binding antibody to the thyrotropin receptor; this
will subsequently be discussed further.

The first assay system to measure thyroid-stimulating activity in
Graves' disease was a guinea pig system developed by Adams and Purvis;[32]
this method was later standardized by McKenzie,[52] using a mouse assay
system. In brief, mice are fed iodine-deficient diets and then given T_4 to
suppress endogenous TSH production; radioactive iodine is then
injected, which is rapidly taken up in the mouse thyroid glands. If serum
from a patient with Graves' disease is subsequently injected into these
mice, the amount of radioactive iodine released at 9 hr after injection is
greater than the amount of radioactive iodine released at 2 hr postinjection, indicating the presence of a LATS. TSH shows greater iodine release
2 hr postinjection than at later intervals. The active factor, LATS, is an
IgG.[33] LATS is detectable, however, in only about 50% of sera from
patients with Graves' disease,[53] and titers of LATS have no relationship to
the degree of thyrotoxicosis.[54] It was for this reason that the role of LATS
in the pathogenesis of Graves' disease was in doubt for some years.[24] With
the use of human thyroid cell or cell membrane preparations (to be
described below), however, it became possible to detect TSI in most, if not
all, cases of active, untreated Graves' disease.[37,51,55] It appears likely,
therefore, that all TSIs represent antibodies to the human TSH receptor
that stimulate the human thyroid cells; *some* of these *also* cross-react with
other mammalian thyroid glands, and are detectable by an animal assay
(such as the LATS assay). McKenzie and Zakarija[56] have now demonstrated this variable cross-reactivity.

It was in 1971 that Adams and Kennedy[48] were able to demonstrate
thyroid-stimulating potential in sera from patients with Graves' disease
who did not have detectable LATS using the "LATS-P" assay. In this
procedure, LATS-positive Graves' serum is incubated with human thyroid tissue prior to injection into mice. The LATS activity is absorbed by
the thyroid and thus seems to disappear. If one subsequently adds
another serum sample rich in LATS, it will not be absorbed by the human
thyroid tissue (presumably because all the binding sites have been occu-
pied by the first LATS sample). Thus, the LATS activity is "protected"
when finally assayed in the McKenzie mouse system. Similarly, if LATS-
negative serum from a patient with active untreated Graves' disease is first
incubated with human thyroid tissue and serum from a patient with a
high LATS titer is then incubated with the same thyroid tissue, the LATS
activity of the second serum is similarly "protected"; i.e., the LATS assay
remains positive. Normal serum will not "protect" LATS in this manner.
LATS-P is also an IgG. It is found in about 90% of sera from patients with
Graves' disease,[57] as well as in some cases of transient neonatal Graves'
disease.[58] While it is really a binding (not a stimulating) assay, in most
instances it equates with TSI.[57]

Other methods to detect TSI involve counting colloid droplet formation in thyroid cells[49] and measuring the generation of cAMP by thyroid slices or membranes after incubation with sera of patients with Graves' disease.[49,55]

A more recent method of detecting TSI is a radioreceptor assay. This method utilizes the ability of TSI to displace radioactively labeled TSH from the TSH receptor of human thyroid membranes.[44] When sera from patients with Graves' disease are examined by this method, the displacement of labeled TSH from thyroid membranes is usually, but not invariably, due to TSI; however, blocking (or merely binding) antibodies, capable of binding to the TSH receptor but not capable of inducing thyroid-cell stimulation, are also detected. Hence, a suitable term was suggested by O'Donnell *et al.*[51] for the active principle in this assay: *TSH-displacing activity* (TDA).

The detection of TSI in the sera of patients with Graves' disease has some practical applications to clinical medicine. First, it is a sensitive procedure for diffentiating Graves' disease from other forms of thyrotoxicosis. Since the treatment for hyperthyroidism in Graves' disease differs from that in other forms of hyperthyroidism, making an accurate diagnosis is of some importance. Second, TSI determinations can be used to detect true immunological remissions in patients with Graves' disease on antithyroid drug therapy;[51] if even a well-controlled patient on such medication still has evidence of TSI, the risk of a relapse after cessation of treatment appears to be considerable, whereas the probability is much less when TSI is not detected.[51] Finally, measurements of TSI have been of some interest in relation to the pathogenesis of endocrine exophthalmos.[51,59] About 50% of euthyroid patients with exophthalmos have no detectable TSI. This suggests that the ophthalmopathy of Graves' disease is a separate but overlapping condition, with no dependence on a thyroid abnormality for the development of the oculopathy.

Finally, it should be noted that some patients with Hashimoto's disease, or "euthyroid opthalmic Graves' disease," or Graves' disease in remission, are euthyroid, yet have detectable TSI.[51,54,59] This apparent paradox can be accounted for by the possibility that coincident thyroiditis is present in the thyroid glands of those patients, and the cell destruction induced by this lesion may limit the expression of thyrotoxicosis. Alternatively, this finding of TDA may be accounted for by blocking or binding (but not stimulating) antibodies, as previously mentioned. It is of interest that some patients with classic Graves' thyrotoxicosis have no detectable TDA,[51] probably due to limitations of the assay system (rather than TSI actually being absent), since in the TDA assay system, these "false-negative" patients have a statistically higher TDA than non-Graves' controls (although still within normal limits). Using the cAMP assay in human thyroid slices, McKenzie and Zakarija[55] detected TSI in virtually all sera from patients with active untreated Graves' disease examined. This may also suggest that there are some TSIs that do not bind any more effectively to the TSH receptor than nonspecific normal IgG, yet are still capable of specific stimulation. Thus, they may be negative in the TDA assay, but positive in a stimulatory assay.

11.3.2. Cell-Mediated Immunity in Thyroid Disease

Thus far, we have examined just one arm of the immune system in thyroid disease, humoral immunity; however, the other element of the immune system, cell-mediated immunity, is also important. Tests of cell-mediated immunity are primarily concerned with a T-lymphocyte function, but recently a role for killer or K cells in thyroid disease has also been explored.

Although lymphocytosis is common in Graves' disease and to a lesser extent in Hashimoto's thyroiditis,[25] proportions of T lymphocytes (as determined by E-rosette formation) and B lymphocytes (as determined by EAC-rosette formation) are normal.[60,61]

The procedure most commonly employed in measuring cell-mediated immune responses *in vitro* is the migration-inhibition factor (MIF) production test. MIF is a lymphokine secreted by T lymphocytes when exposed to an antigen to which they have previously been sensitized. This lymphokine inhibits the migration of white cells from the site of an immune response. The test is carried out *in vitro* by packing capillary tubes with peripheral blood leukocytes and setting them in a planchet containing medium. If a nonspecific antigen is added to the medium, the white cells will freely migrate out of the capillary tube; if, however, the medium contains an antigen to which the T lymphocytes in the capillary tube have previously been sensitized, cell migration from the tube is impeded. This reduction in cell migration is an index of MIF production.

MIF has been detected in most patients with Hashimoto's disease when crude thyroid extract,[62,63] thyroglobulin,[62,64] thyroid microsomes,[62,63,65] or thyroid mitochondria[62] were used as the antigen. Similarly, most patients with Graves' disease show MIF production when crude thyroid[63] or thyroid microsomes[63,65] are used as antigen. Healthy control patients, patients with nonimmune thyroid disease such as nontoxic colloid goiter or thyroid carcinoma, and patients with other autoimmune diseases such as systemic lupus erythematosis or rheumatoid arthritis do not show evidence of MIF production to various thyroid antigens.[63] Higher responses in the MIF test have been found in patients with Hashimoto's disease whose goiters would not regress with thyroid hormone, whereas in those patients whose goiters were easily suppressible on thyroid hormone, there were lower levels of MIF production.[65] In both Graves' disease and Hashimoto's disease, MIF production does not correlate with levels of various circulating thyroid antibodies.[65] It is of interest that mitochondrial antigen, whether from human thyroid, liver, or kidney, or even rat liver, will also elicit increased MIF production by leukocytes from Graves' and Hashimoto's diseases;[62,66,67] hence, mitochondrial antigen in this test is not completely organ- or species-specific. While the test does represent sensitization of T lymphocytes to thyroid and other antigens, under some circumstances immune complexes may also play some role in MIF production.[68,69]

T-lymphocyte function may also be tested by the lymphocytic response to certain plant lecithins, such as phytohemagglutinin (PHA). PHA stimulates T lymphocytes only, not B lymphocytes.[70] If lymphoctye preparations from patients with Graves' disease are cultured with PHA and the culture medium is removed after 6 days and then incubated with thyroid slices, these slices will show evidence of increased cAMP production.[71] This implies that PHA stimulated thyroid-directed "helper" T lymphocytes, which then interacted with thyroid-directed B lymphocytes; these B lymphocytes then responded by releasing TSI into the culture medium. Patients with nonimmune thyroid disease and healthy controls do not show increased cAMP production in this system.

When lymphocytes are cultured with an antigen to which they are sensitized, they undergo blast transformation; this can be detected morphologically or by uptake of tritiated thymidine ($[^3H]T$). Unfortunately, this has not proved to be a useful method of detecting cell-mediated immune responses in Graves' and Hashimoto's diseases. Conflicting evidence concerning blast transformation when lymphocytes from patients with Graves' disease or Hashimoto's disease are cultured with thyroglobulin or crude thyroid extract allow no firm conclusions to be drawn.[72]

Finally, T lymphocytes may be tested *in vitro* by direct cytotoxicity of target cells coated with appropriate antigen. Lymphocytes of patients with Hashimoto's disease have been shown to be cytotoxic for chicken red blood cells coated with thyroglobulin.[73] Also, lymphocytes from about 50% of patients with this disease will damage thyroid cell monolayers;[74] this effect can be abolished by antithymocyte globulin, suggesting that T lymphocytes mediate the phenomenon. Whether T-lymphocyte-mediated cytotoxicity is a function of direct cell-to-cell interaction or is the result of a soluble factor released from sensitized T lymphocytes is presently unknown.

K cells, as previously mentioned, are nonphagocytic cells of possible lymphoid or monocytic origin, but they do not appear to be T lymphocytes, B lymphocytes, or macrophages. K cells have the capacity to destroy target cells coated with antigen–antibody complexes.[72] Peripheral blood lymphocyte suspensions contain 5–15% of K cells.[14,72] If a suspension of normal human lymphocytes is incubated with isotope-labeled, thyroglobulin-coated chicken red blood cells, significant cytotoxicity, measured by release of the isotope, results if serum from patients with Hashimoto's disease, primary hypothyroid, or Graves' disease is added to the medium.[75] When control serum is added, isotope is not released. It is thought that normal human peripheral blood lymphocytes contain K cells capable of destroying target cells coated with thyroglobulin–antithyroglobulin immune complexes. These complexes form on the target-cell surface because the abnormal sera contain thyroglobulin antibody that binds to the thyroglobulin on the target-cell surface. Cytotoxicity is thought to be mediated by attachment of the K cell to the Fc portion of the immunoglobulin in the immune complex. The role of this *in vitro* phenomenon in the development of Hashimoto's disease is as yet unresolved.

It is of interest to consider how these altered immune responses might be initiated. The two obvious possibilities are that the immune phenomena are either primary or secondary to an antigenic stimulus. Previously, it was considered that a specific antigen, previously unknown to the lymphocytes, made its appearance and consequently sensitized the lymphocytes. Such a mechanism might explain the appearance of the sensitized lymphocytes and the various immunoglobulins if there were (1) a change in the antigenicity of the thyroid constituents or (2) injury to the thyroid that could expose antigenic determinants to which there was no immune tolerance—the latter mechanism being described as the "secluded antigen" etiology (see above), and previously favored as a probable explanation of Hashimoto's thyroiditis.[38] As pointed out earlier in this discussion, however, the most suspect antigen, thyroglobulin, normally begins to leak out from its "secluded" follicles into the circulation, commencing before birth in most (if not all) persons. Thyroglobulin-binding B lymphocytes are present in all persons from before birth.[76]

There is very little evidence that thyroid injury with consequent thyroid antigenic change is a prerequisite for Graves' disease, or indeed for Hashimoto's thyroiditis.[19, 77,78] When thyroid injury is produced under various circumstances, e.g., the thyroid injury of subacute thyroiditis, only rarely does either Graves' disease or Hashimoto's thyroiditis occur.[78,79] Actually, in subacute thyroiditis, there is an appropriate humoral and cell-mediated immune response to the extravasation of thyroid antigens during the period of inflammation, but as the outpouring of antigens gradually declines (as the inflammation subsides), the immune response declines as a consequence.[79,80] The immune response under these circumstances is appropriate and evanescent, almost invariably disappearing after some months. If such severe viral disease, as expressed in subacute thyroiditis, does not lead to Graves' disease or Hashimoto's thyroiditis, it is even more difficult to take seriously the suggestion that occult thyroid antigenic change (also possibly induced by viral infection) might result in the observed phenomena.[81] The latter suggestion presupposes a genetically based excessive immune response, not only to the thyroid antigen, but also to a few other specific organ antigens—to explain the overlap with other autoimmune diseases. Thus, there would have to be a genetically based hyperimmune response to a few organ antigens, but not to the vast majority of organ antigens, since generalized excessive immunological responsiveness is not a feature of patients with Graves' or Hashimoto's disease. Attempts to demonstrate actual antigenic alterations within the thyroid glands of Graves' and Hashimoto's diseases (as compared with normal glands) have not been successful.[82] Furthermore, an excessive immune responsiveness to minimal antigenic change would require some defect in the control of the lymphocytic response, since normal persons without such a defect would obviously respond only minimally, if at all, to such occult change.

Furthermore, Knox *et al.*[83] demonstrated that *normal* thyroid antigen is able to stimulate lymphocytes from patients with Graves' disease to produce TSI. It thus appears that thyroid antigenic change is not required for such a stimulus to take place. Moreover, the TSI produced under these circumstances or *in vivo* displaces TSH from *normal* thyroid cell membranes, and stimulates *normal* thyroid cells.[83] These observations are in accord with the view that no antigenic change is necessary to induce the disorder; they do not completely rule out this possibility, however, since cross-reactivity with normal antigens could be an alternative explanation.

Solomon and Chopra[84] suggested the possibility of a metabolic disturbance within the thyroid cells of patients with Graves' disease, to which the observed immunological changes might be secondary. There is now good evidence, however, that there is no such metabolic disturbance within the thyroid cells;[25] furthermore, such a concept would face the same philosophical objections as those cited above.

11.3.3. Genetics of Graves' Disease and Hashimoto's Disease

There is very considerable evidence that both Graves' disease and Hashimoto's disease occur with increased frequency in specific families, and thus appear to be genetically induced; indeed, these two disorders tend to occur in the *same* families. In fact, as has been noted above, Hashimoto's and Graves' diseases can coexist with the same thyroid gland. Moreover, there are several reports of homozygous twins of whom one has classic Hashimoto's thyroiditis, while the other has Graves' disease.

In addition, and as mentioned earlier, there is also an increased incidence of other autoimmune diseases in patients with Graves' disease and Hashimoto's thyroiditis, as well as in their families; these include diabetes mellitus, pernicious anemia, myasthenia gravis, rheumatoid arthritis, and others. Moreover, functional thyroid disturbances and thyroid antibodies occur in about half the first-order relatives of patients with autoimmune thyroid disease.[85]

Studies of the concordance rates of Graves' disease in twins have indicated a concordance of about 30–70% in homozygous twins, and 3–9% in heterozygous twins.[24] This strong concordance in the homozygous group is compelling evidence of a genetic basis for this disorder. It is of interest, however, that there is *no* concordance in 40–70% (at least during the time of study), and that the time the disease occurs in one twin may vary widely from the time of onset in the second twin. Thus, it would appear that other than purely genetic influences are necessary before the disease is expressed.

Studies of the age-specific incidence rates in both Graves' and Hashimoto's diseases have shown clearly that the diseases do occur at random in the genetically predisposed populations.[18,24] This, together with the observations about concordance rates in twins, is in accord with the possibility that the genetic defect is one of a defect in immune surveillance, whereas the secondary influence could be the random appearance (by normal mutation) of the appropriate thyroid-directed "forbidden clone" of T lymphocytes. Such a clone of lymphocytes, having escaped normal suppression, would then proceed to initiate the immune disorder.

It was shown recently that there is a relationship of the histocompatibility genes to Graves' disease, although this relationship has not been so clear for Hashimoto's thyroiditis. Thus, among patients with Graves' disease, there is an increased incidence of HLA-B8 in Caucasians[23] and of HLA-BW35 in Japanese.[86] The majority of patients with Graves' disease, however, do not bear this HLA antigen. Furthermore, their first-order relatives, despite having functional disturbances of the thyroid gland, have no increased incidence of HLA-B8 (in Caucasians).[85] In Hashimoto's thyroiditis, only one study has suggested a relationship of HLA-B8 to the disorder, whereas three other studies have not shown such a relationship.[19]

It would thus appear likely that the histocompatibility genes are not the precise genes responsible for the disorders. They apparently act as markers, however, suggesting a nearby locus for the truly appropriate immune reactive gene that may be responsible. Studies of mixed lymphocyte reaction genes may soon illuminate this area.[85]

11.3.4. Possible Role of Stress in the Induction of Hyperthyroidism

For generations, many authors have pointed out that emotional stress may induce Graves' disease. Indeed, in the patient seen by Parry in 1786 (but published in 1825),[87] hyperthyroidism was precipitated by an emotional trauma. It has not yet been possible, however, to prove a cause-and-effect relationship between such stresses and the onset of the hyperthyroidism.[88] The problem in such studies may have to do with the selection of improper control populations. Recently, for example, a study of Graves' disease in Northern Ireland compared per capita rates of antithyroid drugs utilized before and after the civil disorders that developed in 1968;[89] this study failed to show any increase in the use of antithyroid medications following the development of the conflict. Moreover, persons studied under stressful situations have generally failed to show any change in thyroid status.[88] On the other hand, an apparent epidemic of Graves' disease occurred in Denmark during the German occupation.[90] The problem with all these observations probably relates to the resistance (in terms of thyroid status) of normal persons to the influence of such stresses. The appropriate study would be in the population that is genetically predisposed, namely, in the families of patients with Graves' disease; such a population should then be compared to an unselected population in response to equivalent stresses.

The authors are nevertheless prejudiced to the view that stress can and does percipitate hyperthyroidism, presumably in predisposed persons. The mechansim by which this could occur is unknown. However, lines of speculation have suggested possible alternative pathways. First, suggestions that this effect might be mediated through the hypothalamic–pituitary–thyroid axis (i.e., TRH–TSH) have not been verified. Indeed, TSH in untreated Graves' disease is almost invariably low, with flat responses to TRH,[91] and florid Graves' disease has occurred in patients following apparently complete hypophysectomy.[92] Thus, in the hyperthyroidism of Graves' disease, pituitary secretion of TSH is inhibited. When patients become hypothyroid following treatment of hyperthyroidism, TSH increases; i.e., pituitary function seems normal in Graves' disease.

Another alternative and more attractive possibility is that stress may mediate its effects through the CRH–ACTH–cortisol axis, with its ultimate effects on suppressor T lymphocytes and immune surveillance. The well-known effect of corticosteroids in reducing T-lymphocyte function is in accord with this possibility.[93] It might be suggested, therefore, that if a person had a genetic partial isolated defect in suppressor T lymphocytes, stress might further reduce his surveillance capacity; thus, the defect that had been only minimal or partial would be temporarily converted into a complete (but still isolated) defect, rendering it impossible for the particular clone of thyroid-directed T lymphocytes to be suppressed. The latter, "forbidden clone" of T lymphocytes would then initiate the disease in the manner already suggested.

It is of interest that Graves' disease has appeared in patients taking immunosuppressive or corticosteroid therapy.[94,95] Since such medication in high dosage may suppress the manifestations of Graves' disease, it may be difficult to concede that it may also precipitate the condition.[96] It may be that levels of cortisol or immunosuppressive drugs that are required to inhibit the thyroid-directed "helper" T lymphocytes inducing the cell-mediated immunity within the thyroid gland, i.e., dosages that would suppress the disease itself, may prove to be much larger than those necessary to suppress those suppressor T lymphocytes with a partial defect in their functional capacity.

Once the hyperthyroidism commences, it seems to be a self-perpetu-ating disorder, remitting only when interrupted by nonspecific or specific therapy. This self-perpetuation is not understood. It is possible, however, that hyperthyroidism itself may be seen by the organism as a "stress"; in hyperthyroidism, there are increased cortisol secretion rates and increased adrenocortical size.[97] In addition, there is some evidence that thyroxine itself may affect T-lymphocyte function.[98]

11.3.5. Remissions in Graves' Disease

While even long-term remissions have been recognized for many years as occurring in Graves' disease (and occasionally in Hashimoto's thyroiditis), there has been little understanding of the nature of these remissions. In some cases, increasing thyroid destruction (possibly of autoimmune nature) may bring about such remissions. In many patients in remission, however, all evidence of the disease disappears, including the immunological stigmata. Thus, at least one form of remission in Graves' disease could be considered an "immunological remission." It is possible that this form of remission may occur only in those whose Graves' disease was initiated by "stress," i.e., only in persons with a *partial* defect in immune surveillance. The restoration of a euthyroid status by antithyroid drugs or other means, or the reduction of stress, may allow the immune mechanism to be restored to its former capacity, suppressing the "forbid-den clone" of lymphocytes once again. This is consistent with the disap-pearance of TSI in patients in long-term remissions.[51] MIF responses to thyroid antigen also become negative. Those patients with a presumed complete isolated defect in immune surveillance would not be expected to go into remission, no matter how long antithyroid drug therapy may be continued. It may be noted, however, that there is at least a suggestion that antithyroid drug therapy itself can be immunosuppressive,[99] although this could not explain long-term remissions. In any event, prolonged remissions in the group with continuing immunological activity could be brought about only as a result of continued thyroid destruction.

11.3.6. Nature of the Ophthalmopathy

Infiltrative ophthalmopathy associated with Graves' disease is charac-terized by two pathological processes: (1) myositis of the extraocular muscles with edema, lymphocytic infiltration, muscle necrosis, and fibrosis in the late stages; and (2) proliferation of retroorbital fat and connective tissue.[100] This form of ophthalmopathy is responsible for the clinical manifestations of proptosis, periorbital edema, and diplopia. It is common knowledge that ophthalmopathy may not relate temporally to the onset of hyperthyroidism; it may precede, coincide with, or follow the hyperthyroid phase. In almost half the patients with Graves' disease and hyperthyroidism, no ophthalmopathy will occur during their course. Occasionally, patients with Hashimoto's disease and primary idiopathic myxedema will have typical "endocrine ophthalmophathy," and this condition may also occur in persons with no clinical evidence of thyroid disease; some of the latter may have laboratory evidence of thyroid involvement, but in some there is no evidence whatsoever of thyroid disease, even by quite sophisticated testing.[101]

It seems clear that the ocular lesions are immune in nature. Patients with ophthalmopathy associated with hyperthyroidism can be shown to have cellular immunity in response to both retroorbital muscle antigens and thyroid antigens by means of the MIF test.[101] If thyrotoxicosis in Graves' disease occurs without ophthalmopathy, MIF is usually demonstrable only against thyroid antigen. Conversely, in patients with euthyroid exophthalmos manifesting no evidence of thyroid disease whatever, MIF is produced only against retroorbital muscle antigen, not against thyroid antigen.

Estimations of TSI in patients with euthyroid ophthalmic Graves' disease, by either the LATS-P assay or the TSH displacement assay, have shown variable results. In some of these patients, TSI is present; in these, there is invariably evidence of thyroid disease. In others, however, who may have either no demonstrable thyroid disease or clinical Hashimoto's thyroiditis, TSI is absent.[51,59]

From the studies of cell-mediated immunity and TSI cited above, it would appear that exophthalmos may not always relate to the presence of thyroid disease, and thus perhaps should be considered a separate, albeit closely related, overlapping autoimmune disorder.[25]

Humoral immunoglobulins probably play a cooperative role in the development of exophthalmos, as it has been observed that an IgG from the serum of patients with exophthalmos is exophthalmogenic experimentally, and Fakhri and Hobbs[102] showed cooperation between antibody and lymphocytes in the production of exophthalmos.

Other theories for the production of exophthalmos must be mentioned. Konishi et al.[103] demonstrated that retroorbital muscle has affinity for both thyroglobulin and thyroglobulin–antibody immune complexes, and Kriss[104] demonstrated lymphatic connections between the thyroid region and the retroorbital area. These investigators postulated that there must be a transport of thyroid antigens, antibodies, antigen–antibody complexes, and/or immunologically competent cells from the thyroid region to the retroorbital space through the lymphatics, where affinity to retroorbital muscle then initiates an immune reaction.[103] Mullin *et al.*[105] confirmed the affinity of retroorbital muscle for these complexes and found thyroglobulin within even normal retroorbital muscle. Konishi *et al.*[103] therefore postulated a direct relationship of the exophthalmos to the thyroid by means of the transport by lymphatics of the aforenamed factors. This hypothesis fails, however, to explain the lack of temporal relationship of ophthalmopathy to hyperthyroidism, and does not account for the fact that ophthalmopathy may occur with no evidence of hyperthyroidism, or indeed of any thyroid disease, in some patients. Thus, this hypothesis cannot explain all cases of ophthalmic Graves' disease, although it cannot be excluded as a cause of some cases of the disorder.

Another theory was advanced by Kohn and Winand,[106] who showed that TSH and fragments of TSH (the latter devoid of thyroid-stimulating ability) can produce experimental exophthalmos, and they extrapolated from the data to suggest that these are factors in the genesis of human exophthalmos. However, both TSH and TSH subunits are suppressed in Graves' disease when hyperthyroidism coexists with ophthalmopathy.[91,107] Furthermore, the disorder was reported to occur after apparent total hypophysectomy.[92] Finally, TSH did not seem to act as either an antigen or an antigenic enhancer in the MIF studies of Munro *et al.*[101] From these observations, it does not seem necessary to invoke TSH as a factor in the human disease.

It is the view of the authors that the ophthalmopathy and the thyroid disorder of Graves' disease, are two closely related organ-specific autoimmune diseases; they frequently coexist, but either may occur alone.

11.4. Autoimmunity and the Pancreas

There is increasing evidence suggesting that certain types of diabetes mellitus may result from an autoimmune assault on pancreatic islet-cell tissue. Features that suggest this possibility include the association of insulinopenic diabetes with other autoimmune conditions, the presence in such diabetics of humoral and cell-mediated immunity to islet-cell antigens, and the pathology of the endocrine pancreas in this disorder. The role of viruses in the development of diabetes has been much discussed and will be given special attention below.

Diabetes associated with failure of other endocrine glands has long been recognized. Diabetes has now been shown to occur in about 14% of patients with Addison's disease; the association is primarily between insulinopenic diabetics and autoimmune adrenal failure.[108] Conversely, the prevalence of Addison's disease in a diabetic population is 5-fold that in the general population.[109] Associations between pernicious anemia, Graves' disease, Hashimoto's disease, primary hypothyroidism, and myasthenia gravis have also been established.[109] Moreover, many diabetics have antibodies to various endocrine tissues in the absence of overt gland failure. Thyroid and gastric parietal cell microsomal antibodies have been found most commonly in young, female, insulinopenic diabetics.[109,110] There is a suggestion that the presence of such antibodies may be a risk factor for significantly shortened longevity in such a population.[111] Curiously, there is only a poor association between diabetes and the presence of thyroglobulin antibodies.[112] Intrinsic factor antibodies are found in a small percentage of middle-aged female insulinopenic diabetics, half of whom have latent pernicious anemia.[113] An association also exists between diabetes and the presence of adrenocortical antibodies, but this association is weak, despite the stronger association of diabetes with idiopathic Addison's disease.[114]

The search for islet-cell antibody in diabetics was somewhat elusive until recently, when a complement-fixing IgG, probably directed to lipoprotein antigens in the microsomal fraction of islet tissue, was found in the sera of insulinopenic diabetics.[115,116] This islet-cell antibody will produce immunofluorescence with alpha, beta, and delta islet-cell subtypes. It is independent of insulin administration, and is present only if the diabetes coexists with one or more autoimmune diseases. In the latter population, islet-directed antibody is found in 30% of sera tested. It is uncertain whether this immunoglobulin is a mediator of islet dysfunction or merely a marker for a subset of diabetes, probably caused by disordered immunity.

Insulin antibodies have been found in virtually all diabetics taking insulin,[117] but they are almost never found in sera of diabetics prior to insulin administration. A rare syndrome, termed the *insulin autoimmune syndrome* was recently reported, in which such insulin antibodies were found independent of prior insulin administration.[118,119,120] These patients have glucose intolerance, reactive hypoglycemia, circulating hyperinsulinemia, and islet-cell hyperplasia. Their serum contains an insulin-binding immunoglobulin, of class IgG, with only κ light chains (diabetics receiving exogenous insulin have IgG, IgM, and IgA insulin antibodies with both κ and λ light chains).[109] This suggests that the glucose intolerance in this unusual type of diabetes is due to a single type of insulin-directed antibody produced by a single clone of lymphocytes and plasma cells. The reactive hypoglycemia may result from the inappropriate release of insulin bound by the immunoglobulin.

Another rare antibody-mediated form of diabetes was documented by Flier *et al.*[46] Their patients, all nonobese females, have acanthosis nigricans and extreme insulin resistance, requiring up to 1000 times the usual daily dosage of insulin to control blood glucose. These patients have decreased binding of insulin to insulin receptors in peripheral tissue such as monocytes. The immunoglobulin fraction from these patients produces an identical insulin-binding defect on insulin receptors of normal tissue. This suggests that such patients have glucose intolerance because blocking antibodies compete with receptors in peripheral tissue.

Cell-mediated immune responses have also been studied extensively in diabetes mellitus. The proportions of circulating T and B lymphocytes are normal.[121] Altered lymphocyte responses to mitogens such as PHA have been documented in some diabetics;[122] this appears to be the result of poor diabetic control, however, rather than a primary immune defect, since the depression of lymphocyte transformation to PHA disappears once metabolic control is achieved.[121] The MIF test, however, has proved most useful in detecting altered cell-mediated immune responses in diabetes. Leukocytes from about 30% of all diabetics have significant MIF production when exposed to pancreatic islet-cell antigens,[109] whereas increased MIF production is found in 65% of insulin-dependent patients tested; this phenomenon occurs independently of prior insulin administration.[123] The antigen required to elicit MIF production is contained in a particulate fraction of islet tissue, but is apparently not species-specific. As with Hashimoto's thyroiditis, MIF production by diabetic leukocytes is also observed using liver mitochondrial antigen;[124] this antigen may be a nonspecific marker of some localized autoimmune diseases, since it also elicits MIF production from leukocytes from patients with Hashimoto's disease,[62] pernicious anemia,[125] and primary biliary cirrhosis.[66] In addition, lymphocytes of insulinopenic diabetic patients (some of whom have not yet received insulin) show increased uptake of [³H]T when cultured with porcine or bovine insulin, another evidence of cell-mediated immunity. The B chain of the insulin molecule seems to be the antigen necessary for this response.[109] In contrast, the A chain of insulin appears to be the major antigenic component for antibody production in diabetics taking exogenous insulin.[126] It is thus possible that cellular and humoral immune responses may recognize different sites of some molecules as antigenic.

Histological examination of the pancreases of juvenile insulin-requiring diabetics, if made within 1 year of diagnosis, will often show lymphocytic infiltration in the islets, termed *insulitis* by Von Meyenburg;[127] this lesion is almost never seen in maturity-onset diabetics. A probable explanation for this pathological lesion is that it represents evidence of an immune lesion in the islets, although some workers have suggested that it may result from a viral infection of islet tissue.

Viruses have been suspected as potential etiological agents in diabetes for over 50 years.[128] Experimentally, M-variant of encephalomyocarditis virus and Coxsackie B virus have been shown to induce diabetes in laboratory animals.[129,130] In man, mumps, rubella, infectious mononucleosis, and group B Coxsackie viruses can all invade the pancreas.[131] Gamble et al.[132] showed that insulinopenic diabetics have higher titers of antibodies to Coxsackie B4 virus than controls do, if tested within 3 months of diagnosis. Despite this, a virus has never been cultured from the pancreas, blood, or excreta of newly diagnosed diabetic patients. Furthermore, more recent studies regarding the relationship of viral antibodies to the onset of insulinopenic diabetes have been conflicting, and there is no convincing evidence linking viruses to islet-cell destruction in man.[19] It is also possible that viruses may produce diabetes by altering immune responses. This could occur by either interfering with immune surveillance or inducing an islet-cell-directed clone of T and B lymphocytes; these possibilities are likewise speculative.

The HLA system of tissue antigens has been studied extensively in diabetes. Nerup et al.[21] found that two-thirds of diabetics have either HLA-B8 or HLA-BW15 antigen. HLA-BW15 is found in juvenile and some maturity-onset diabetics; antigen B8 is found primarily in nonobese insulinopenic diabetics.

It may be added parenthetically that there is currently no evidence of an immunological basis for the development of the angiopathy or any of the other complications of diabetes.

It thus appears that a proportion of young insulin-dependent diabetics probably have beta-cell destruction on an autoimmune basis. However, this may not represent the etiological basis of many of the cases of maturity-onset diabetes mellitus. It may be concluded that diabetes mellitus may be due to several causes, but that autoimmune isletitis leads to a severe insulinopenic form of the disease.

11.5. Autoimmunity and the Adrenal

Between 1904 and 1923, at Guy's Hospital, London, 76% of all cases of Addison's disease were caused by tuberculosis;[133] the remainder were considered idiopathic in etiology. At the same institution between 1948 and 1957, 60% of the cases of primary adrenal failure were "idiopathic,"[134] and today the proportion is even higher. It now appears evident that idiopathic Addison's disease represents an autoimmune disorder resulting in adrenal cortical failure. Evidence favoring this view is summarized below.

Animals immunized with homologous or heterologous adrenal tissue mixed with Freund's adjuvant develop adrenal antibodies, as well as adrenal lesions similar to those of idiopathic Addison's disease in humans, namely, lymphocytic infiltration in the adrenal parenchyma.[135] Furthermore, this adrenal lesion can be induced in a normal recipient animal by transfer of lymphocytes.[136] These observations suggest that destruction of the adrenal cortex can be achieved by immune manipulations in animals.

Idiopathic adrenal failure in humans has many epidemiological characteristics of an autoimmune disease. First, there is a female preponderance.[108] When idiopathic Addison's disease occurs with other autoimmune diseases, the sex distribution is predominantly female for all decades of life; when this condition occurs alone, the female predominance is evident only after the first three decades.[135] Moreover, in common with other autoimmune conditions, Addison's disease occurs more frequently in certain families.[137] Occasionally it is seen in identical twins,[135] and in some families it has the characteristics of an autosomal recessive trait.[138, 139] Finally, idiopathic Addison's disease often coexists with other autoimmune conditions; about 40% of cases occur together with one or more other autoimmune disorders. For example, Nerup reported that in idiopathic Addison's disease, the prevalence rate of diabetes mellitus was 14%; for gonadal insufficiency, 13%; for myxedema and Hashimoto's disease (the concurrence of Addison's disease with hypothyroidism is known as Schmidt's syndrome), 9% for Graves' disease, 9% for pernicious anemia, 3%; and for hypoparathyroidism, 2%.[108] The prevalence rates for any of these conditions in the control population are much lower. Additionally, antibodies to parathyroid, ovary, gastric mucosa, intrinsic factor, and thyroid antigens may be found in patients with idiopathic Addison's disease, without clinically overt abnormalities in these organs.[108] These epidemiological associations are true only for idiopathic adrenal failure, and not for tuberculous or other types of adrenal insufficiency.

There is abundant evidence of humoral immune phenomena in idiopathic Addison's disease. In 1957, one year after the discovery of antibodies to thyroglobulin in Hashimoto's disease, Anderson et al.[140] demonstrated adrenal antibodies in two patients with idiopathic Addison's disease. Since that time, adrenal antibodies have been found in this condition by immunofluorescence, complement fixation, tanned red cell agglutination, and gel diffusion.[108] They belong to the IgG class of immunoglobulins, and titers are generally low, seldom greater than 1:64.[108] Of patients with idiopathic Addison's disease, 65% have detectable adrenal antibody, while patients with unequivocal tuberculous adrenal failure for the most part do not have adrenal antibodies.[135] Antibody is found more frequently in female patients, early in the course of their disease; antibody titers are generally lower in elderly patients.[135] Idiopathic hypoparathyroidism is the only other autoimmune condition in which a high prevalence of adrenal cortical antibody is found (25–30% of cases).[108] The antigens against which the adrenal antibody is directed are found not only in human adrenal tissue, both fetal and adult, but also in the adrenals of many animals.[135] The antigens are found in all layers of the adrenal cortex, but are particularly abundant in the zona fasciculata.[108] They are deficient in the adrenals of patients who have undergone steroid therapy. The antigens are localized in the microsomal fraction. Biochemically, they are probably a carbohydrate-containing lipoprotein.[108]

The role of adrenal antibodies in mediating the destruction of adrenal cortical tissue is unclear. Patients with other autoimmune diseases (e.g., idiopathic hypoparathyroidism) may have adrenal antibody and yet manifest no defect in adrenal cortical function as assessed by corticotropin stimulation tests.[108] Women with idiopathic Addison's disease and detectable titers of adrenal antibody have given birth to infants with adrenal antibody in their cord blood, yet these infants showed no impairment in adrenal function.[108] It appears that adrenal antibody is not destructive to adrenal cortical tissue *per se,* although it may have a role in K-cell-mediated cytotoxicity.

Evidence for cellular immune responses is also found in idiopathic Addison's disease. In 1969, Nerup *et al.*[141] demonstrated that leukocytes from patients with this condition produced MIF when exposed to adrenal antigens. Although a small number of patients with tuberculous Addison's disease show a response in this assay, up to 80% of patients with idiopathic Addison's disease show evidence of cellular immunity directed toward adrenal tissue by the MIF test.[142] Although idiopathic Addison's disease, as previously mentioned, occurs more commonly in females, cellular immune responses to adrenal antigens are more frequent in males with this condition.[141] MIF production shows no correlation with the age of onset of the adrenal failure, the duration of the disease, or the presence of antibodies. Of patients with idiopathic Addison's disease, however, 90% have adrenal antibodies in their sera or cell-mediated immune responses to adrenal tissue.[108].The antigen responsible for MIF production is species-nonspecific and is found in the mitochondrial fraction of adrenal cell homogenates.[143] The response in the MIF test in idiopathic Addison's disease correlates well with intradermal skin testing with adrenal antigen, another test of cell-mediated immunity.[144] It would appear that cell-mediated immunity plays an important part in producing adrenocortical destruction in idiopathic Addison's disease; however, the precise manner in which adrenocortical-directed T lymphocytes mediate the lesion is unresolved.

11.6. Autoimmunity and the Gonad

The human gonad consists of two functional units, one concerned with the production of steroid sex hormones, the other with germ cell production. Both these units can be the target of immune destruction. In women, autoimmune oophoritis results in the destruction of the steroid-producing cells as well as the germ cells, with subsequent hypogonadism and infertility. Similarly, in men, autoimmune orchitis may result in the destruction of both Leydig and germ cell elements. However, a selective immune attack may be mounted against spermatozoa. A man may make antibody against his own spermatozoa, or a woman may produce antibody directed against the spermatozoa of her sexual partner; infertility without hypogonadism may result in both these situations. Pure infertility due to immune mechanisms probably has a different pathogenesis than the general model for autoimmune disease in endocrine organs outlined earlier in this review. On the other hand, autoimmune oophoritis and orchitis probably do follow this model, and the gonadal lesions result from damage induced by gonad-directed T and B lymphocytes, once again secondary to a defect in immune surveillance.

11.6.1. Autoimmune Oophoritis

In 1933, Duff and Bernstein[145] described two Addisonian women with atrophic ovaries. Since that time, numerous women have been described with primary amenorrhea or premature menopause, high serum levels of gonadotropins, and one or more coexistent autoimmune diseases. The vast majority of these patients also have idiopathic Addison's disease; occasionally, such patients do not have adrenocortical dysfunction, but have another autoimmune condition such as idiopathic hypoparathyroidism.[146] Conversely, menstrual abnormalities were found in 25% of patients with idiopathic Addison's disease by Irvine and Barnes.[135]

With the development of immunofluorescent techniques, many women with idiopathic Addison's disease and menstrual abnormalities were found to have ovarian antibodies; patients with other autoimmune diseases and menstrual abnormalities occasionally had ovarian antibodies, while on the other hand, such antibodies were only rarely detectable in patients with pure premature menopause (or idiopathic primary amenorrhea).[146] When ovarian failure occurs in the absence of a second autoimmune disorder, an immune basis is difficult to document.

In patients with autoimmune oophoritis, ovarian antibodies may show binding to antigens on granulosa cells of human Graafian follicles as well as to antigens in the corpus luteum, the interstitial cells of human testis, or the trophoblastic tissue of the placenta.[147] Such patients may have antibodies to a variety of antigens or to different steroid-hormone-producing organs (presumably containing common antigens). Since the majority of patients with autoimmune oophoritis have coexistent idiopathic Addison's disease, such patients have antibody to adrenocortical antigens as well.[146] It is of interest that adrenocortical tissue can usually absorb antibodies to extra adrenal steroid-producing tissue, but extracts of ovary, testis, and placenta may not absorb antibody reactive to antigens in the adrenal cortex.[135] This implies that most but not all antigens found in extragonadal steroid-producing tissue are also found in the adrenal cortex.

The role of ovarian antibody in producing the pathological lesions in autoimmune oophoritis is uncertain. Some patients with idiopathic Addison's disease and ovarian antibodies have no evidence of menstrual dysfunction.[148] McNatty and Short[149] found, however, that sera from some patients with idiopathic Addison's disease and ovarian failure that contained antibody against corpus luteum and adrenocortical antigens produced cytotoxic changes in granulosa cells in culture, paralleled by a fall in their progesterone production. The cytotoxicity of the sera was complement-dependent and correlated with the immunofluorescent staining pattern: a clumping staining pattern with sections of corpus luteum invariably produced cytotoxicity, and sera giving a confluent staining pattern failed to produce cytotoxic changes. In contrast, Edmonds et al.[150] described a patient with autoimmune thyroiditis, adrenalitis, and premature ovarian failure who had no detectable ovarian antibodies. The patient's leukocytes produced MIF, however, when exposed to ovarian antigen (as well as thyroid, adrenal, and testicular antigen.) From these observations, it may be that some types of ovarian antibody help bring about the pathological lesion in autoimmune oophoritis, whereas others may merely serve as markers for this condition. Cell-mediated immunity probably has an important role in premature ovarian failure, and it is not clear whether or not this is independent of humoral influences.

In autoimmune oophoritis, the ovaries are small and shrunken. Histologically, lymphocytic infiltration is seen,[151] but occasionally the ovaries appear as fibrous streaks,[152] almost identical to the streak ovaries in Turner's syndrome. (This may be analogous to the atrophied thyroid seen in "idiopathic myxedema," which is now believed to be a variant of autoimmune thyroiditis.) If a woman is seen who has primary ovarian failure, with "streak" ovaries and a normal female karyotype, investigation for a coexistent autoimmune disease is warranted.

11.6.2. Autoimmune Orchitis

Autoimmune disease in general is less common in males. Occasionally, men are encountered with primary hypogonadism and antibodies to testicular antigens. Many of these patients have idiopathic Addison's disease as well. Irvine and Barnes[135] described a 15-year-old Addisonian male with testicular atrophy, bilateral gynecomastia, and antibodies in his serum reactive against Leydig cell antigens; however, they described two additional Addisonian men with such antibodies but no gonadal deficit. Murthy *et al.*[153] reported a male patient with autoimmune destruction of both thyroid and adrenal cortex, pernicious anemia, vitiligo, and primary testicular failure. Histologically, the testis showed areas of fibrosis but no lymphocytic infiltrate. The patient's serum was shown by immunofluorescence to contain an antibody toward the basement membrane around the seminiferous tubules. Some immunofluorescence was also seen in the nuclei of cells in the germinal epithelium.

Clearly, more studies must be undertaken before the relationship between cell-mediated and humoral immunity in autoimmune orchitis and in oophoritis is fully understood.

11.6.3. Infertility

The mechanism whereby the immune system produces infertility without hypogonadism appears to be different from the general model for autoimmune endocrine disease previously outlined. The pathogenesis of autoimmune disease in the thyroid, adrenal, islets of the pancreas, gonads, parathyroids, and perhaps the pituitary, does not seem to relate to any change or peculiarity of the antigenicity of some component of these tissues, but rather to a defect in immune surveillance that allows organ-directed clones of lymphoid cells (arising normally by random mutation) to survive, and then function without being normally suppressed. Unlike the organs referred to above, spermatozoa acquire new antigens during spermatogenesis, which begins after puberty.[154] Since these sperm antigens were not present in the neonatal period, no tolerance exists toward them; they are regarded as "nonself." Normal males do not produce immune responses to their own spermatozoa only because spermatozoa are segregated from antibody-forming tissue by a "blood–testis barrier" at the basement membrane of the seminiferous tubules and conducting system (the epididymis, the vas deferens, and the urethra). This barrier is disrupted in patients who have undergone vasectomy, and half of such patients have in their blood antibody to sperm.[155]

The pioneer observations were made in 1922 by Meaker,[156] who showed that sera from two sterile women could agglutinate and immobilize the spermatozoa of their husbands. However, sperm agglutinins were not defined as having a possible role in infertility until the independent observations of Wilson[157] and Rünke.[158] The ability to agglutinate sperm has been found in the serum of many men and women with idiopathic infertility. Sperm agglutinins have also been found, however, in unmarried women and even in pregnant women.[159] High titers of sperm agglutinins measured by various methods seem to correlate well with infertility;[160] low titers are nonspecific and may be due to nonimmunoglobulin factors in serum, such as steroids bound to β-lipoproteins.[161] Infertile men may have detectable agglutinins in their semen, which may result in clumps of spermatozoa bound together on examination of an ejaculate.[162] A second sperm-directed antibody is the complement-fixing sperm-immobilizing antibody.[163] This antibody may be found in both infertile men and women.[159,163] It is not found quite as frequently in infertile patients as sperm-agglutinating antibody, but it appears to be more specific, not being found in patients with documented fertility.[159]

The mechanism whereby sperm antibodies produce infertility is not entirely understood. The most likely possibility is that sperm agglutinins and sperm-immobilizing antibodies decrease the ability of spermatozoa to penetrate cervical mucus.[160] Sperm antibodies generally do not cause azoospermia or alter testicular histology, but spermatotoxic complement-dependent antibodies have been found in the sera of some infertile men;[164] their importance remains to be precisely determined.

The role of cell-mediated immunity in infertility is poorly understood. Lymphocyte stimulation in response to sperm antigen has been observed in some infertile men, primarily those with azoospermia and a history of testicular injury.[165] MIF production by leukocytes in response to spermatozoal antigen has been explored in infertile women. Unfortunately, this test has proved to be very insensitive in this situation; many positive responses have also occurred in fertile women.[166]

Why sperm antibody forms in some males is not known. It is likely that most men will form antibody to their sperm if their immune system is exposed to sperm antigens. Titers of such antibody have been found in patients with lesions that result in the breakdown of the "blood–testis barrier": obstructive azoospermia, prostatovesiculitis, gonorrheal or tuberculous epididymytis, vasectomy, and trauma to the testis.[162, 167,168] However, about half of all males with antibodies to sperm will not have any history suggestive of these initiating factors. Perhaps some of these patients have a genetic predisposition toward sperm antibody formation, possibly related to a defect in surveillance, analogous to mechanisms in other autoimmune endocrine disease; at present, however, there is no evidence to support this suggestion.

Why some women develop antibody to sperm in also poorly understood. It is felt that various enzyme systems in the female genital tract degrade sperm antigens before they can come into contact with the immune system. A defective enzyme system may be present in women with sperm antibodies and may lead to female immunological infertility.[159]

Immune mechanisms thus appear to have some role in infertility. As much as 30% of unexplained infertility may have an immune basis.[169]

Consequently, manipulation of the immune system may provide an effective means of fertility control in the near future.

11.7. Autoimmunity and the Parathyroids

It has been proposed that many cases of idiopathic hypoparathyroidism may be caused by an immune disturbance. Frequently, this condition is preceded by mucocutaneous and ungual candidiasis;[170] idiopathic Addison's disease and pernicious anemia are common accompanying disorders.[171] Pathologically, the parathyroid glands are infiltrated with lymphocytes.[172]

These observations prompted investigators to search for evidence of humoral and cell-mediated immunity in idiopathic hypoparathyroidism. Blizzard et al.[173] detected antibodies to parathyroid tissue by immunofluorescence in 33% of patients with idiopathic hypoparathyroidism alone; when idiopathic hypoparathyroidism was associated with another autoimmune condition, parathyroid antibodies were found in 41% of cases. These antibodies may also be detected in sera of patients without hypoparathyroidism: they have been found in 26% of patients with idiopathic Addison's disease, in 12% of patients with Hashimoto's thyroiditis, and, surprisingly, in 6% of the general population. The antigen to which these antibodies are directed is more abundant in normal parathyroid tissue than in adenomatous parathyroids; it is also found in both oxyphil and chief cells.[174] Patients with idiopathic hypoparathyroidism are also likely to have antibodies to adrenal, gastric, and thyroid tissue, even in the absence of overt disease in these organs.[173]

Studies concerned with cell-mediated immunity in idiopathic hypoparathyroidism are sparse. Moulias et al.,[175] however, found MIF production by leukocytes from 5 of 8 patients with idiopathic hypoparathyroidism, using a human parathyroid antigen; 10 control patients were negative in this test. MIF production to adrenal and thyroid antigens is occasionally found in patients with idiopathic hypoparathyroidism without clinical disease in those organs.

Some cases of parathyroid failure therefore appear to belong to the family of organ-specific autoimmune diseases. Interestingly, the age of onset is earlier than in most of the other autoimmune diseases, cases often appearing in childhood and adolescence.[135] Also, for unclear reasons, mucocutaneous and ungual candidiasis and perhaps vitiligo may be more common in this condition than in other autoimmune endocrine disorders.[170] The parathyroid antibodies that are seen in about a third of these cases probably have little if any role in causing the destructive lesions in these glands, since these antibodies may be found in "euparathyroid" patients with other autoimmune disease, as well as in the normal population.[173] Cell-mediated immune mechanisms may assume more importance.

11.8. Autoimmunity and the Pituitary

The evidence that disordered immunity produces some forms of pituitary disease is sparse. Part of the reason is the relative inaccessibility of the gland to biopsy and, until recently, the difficulty in distinguishing primary from secondary failure of the endocrine glands served by the trophic hormones of the pituitary. Nevertheless, certain cases of hypopituitarism possibly have an immune basis.

In 1967, Goudie and Pinkerton[176] described a young woman with Hashimoto's disease who died in adrenal crisis. Necropsy findings disclosed a small pituitary gland with a lymphocytic infiltrate in the pars anterior. Lymphocytes may be observed in the pituitaries of normal accident or suicide victims, but they are found near the pars intermedia, never in the pars anterior.[177] Lack[179] reported a patient with a lymphocytic infiltrate with germinal follicle formation in the pars anterior of the pituitary; secondary hypothyroidism and adrenal cortical atrophy were found as well. Arvanitakis and Knouss[179] described a patient with candidiasis, hypoparathyroidism, and loss of several pituitary trophic hormones; a second patient was described with candidiasis and corticotropin deficiency. Pituitary antibodies sought by indirect immunofluorescence were undetectable in these two cases. It seems possible that these cases may have been examples of autoimmune hypophysitis. In the future, as more sensitive means of testing immune function become available, more definite evidence for autoimmune hypophysitis will probably accumulate.

11.9. Conclusions

Through epidemiological and pathological evidence, as well as by specific tests for humoral and cell-mediated immunity, it seems clear that disorders of immunity can produce endocrine disease. For the most part, this is manifested as gland failure, but in at least one example, Graves' disease, the immune disorder is expressed as overstimulation of the endocrine gland. The pathogenesis of such autoimmune endocrine disorders does not seem to be related to any antigenic change in the glandular tissue, but is probably the result of specific defects in immune surveillance, which is a function of suppressor T lymphocytes and perhaps other cells in the immune system. This allows organ-specific clones of T lymphocytes (arising normally by random mutation) to survive, interact with their appropriate B-lymphocyte counterparts, and subsequently attack the target gland, unsuppressed by the usual regulatory control mechanisms. Macrophages and K cells may assist in the mediation of the immune response as well. The autoimmune endocrine diseases seem to cluster in some families, indicating that the immune defects responsible for these conditions are inherited. Certain HLA tissue antigens, especially HLA-B8, may serve as a marker for the immune defect responsible for some autoimmune endocrine diseases, but probably do not represent the precise gene responsible for these disorders. The coexistence of two or more autoimmune diseases would presumably depend on two variables: first, the magnitude of the surveillance defect (to two or more "forbidden clones" of lymphocytes), and second, the randomized rate of appearance of the appropriate clone.

ACKNOWLEDGMENT

Work cited from this laboratory was supported by a grant from the Medical Research Council of Canada (MT859).

References

1. Burnet, F. M. (ed.), 1972, Tolerance and paralysis, in: *Autoimmunity and Autoimmune Disease*, pp. 59–71, Medical and Technical Publishing Co., Lancaster, Great Britain.
2. Burnet, F. M. (ed.), 1972, Introduction, in: *Autoimmunity and Autoimmune Disease*, pp. 1–8, Medical and Technical Publishing Co., Lancaster, Great Britain.
3. Playfair, J. H. L., 1975, Introduction, in: *Autoimmunity in Endocrine Disease, Clinics in Endocrinology and Metabolism*, Vol. 4 (W. J. Irvine, ed.), pp. 229–239, W. B. Saunders Co, London.
4. Roitt, I. M., Greaves, M. F., Torrigiani, G., Brostoff, J., and Playfair, J. H. L., 1969, The cellular basis of immunological response, *Lancet* **2:**367–371.
5. Goldstein, G., 1976, The thymus as an endocrine organ, *Proceedings of the 5th International Congress of Endocrinology*, July 18–24, 1976, Hamburg, Excerpta Medica, Amsterdam, International Congress Series, No. 402, 1977.
6. Mendes, N. F., Tolnai, M. E. A., Silveira, N. P. A., Gilbertsen, R. B., and Metzgar, R. S., 1973, Technical aspects of the rosette tests used to detect human complement receptor (B) and sheep erythrocyte-binding (T) lymphocytes, *J. Immunol.* **111:**860–867.
7. Burnet, F. M. (ed.), 1972, Modern immunological theory, in: *Autoimmunity and Autoimmune Disease*, pp. 33–57, Medical and Technical Publishing Co., Lancaster, Great Britain.
8. Allison, A. C., 1974, Interactions of T and B lymphocytes in self-tolerance and autoimmunity, in: *Immunological Tolerance—Mechanisms of Potential Ther-*

apeutic Applications (D. H. Katz and B. Benacerraf, eds), pp. 25–29, Academic Press, New York and London.

9. Asherson, G. L., and Zembala, M., 1976, Suppressor "T" cells in cell-mediated immunity, *Br. Med. Bull.* **32:**158–164.

10. Rowlands, D. T., and Daniele, R. P., 1975, Surface receptors in the immune response, *N. Engl. J. Med.* **293:**26–32.

11. Holan, V., Hasek, M., Bubenik, J., and Chutna, J., 1974, Antigen-mediated macrophage adherence inhibition, *Cell. Immunol.* **13:**107–116.

12. Lessin, L. S., and Besses, M., 1972, Morphology of monocytes and macrophages, in: *Hematology* (W. J. Williams, E. Beutler, A. J. Erslev, and R. W. Rundy, eds.), pp. 731–740, McGraw-Hill Book Co., Toronto.

13. Marti, J. H., Grosser, N., and Thomson, D. M. P., 1976, Leucocyte adherence inhibition assay for the detection of anti-tumor immunity. II. Monocyte reacts with tumour antigen via cytophilic anti-tumour antibody, *Int. J. Cancer* **18:**48–57.

14. Calder, E. A., Urbaniak, S. J., Penhale, W. J., and Irvine, W, J, 1974, Characterization of human lymphoid cell-mediated antibody-dependent cytotoxicity (LDAC), *Clin. Exp. Immunol.* **18:**579–593.

15. Gelfand, M. C., Elfenbein, G. J., Frank, M. M., and Paul, W. E., 1974, Ontogeny of B lymphocytes. II. Relative rates of appearance of lymphocytes bearing surface immunoglobulin and complement receptors, *J. Exp. Med.* **139:**1125–1141.

16. Burnet, F. M. (ed.), 1959, The clonal selection theory of antibody production, in: *The Clonal Selection Theory of Acquired Immunity*, pp. 49–68, Cambridge University Press, Cambridge.

17. Block, M. B., Pachman, L. M., Windhorst, D., and Goldfine, I. D., 1971, Immunological findings in familial juvenile endocrine deficiency syndrome associated with mucocutaneous candidiasis, *Am. J. Med. Sci.* **261:**213–218.

18. Volpé, R., Clarke, P. V., and Row, V. V., 1973, Relationship of age-specific incidence rates to immunological aspects of Hashimoto's thyroiditis, *Can. Med. Assoc. J.* **109:**898–901.

19. Volpé, R., 1977, The role of autoimmunity in hypoendocrine and hyperendocrine function, *Ann. Intern. Med.* **87:**86–99.

20. McDevitt, H. O., and Bodmer, W. F,, 1972, Histocompatibility antigens, immune responsiveness and susceptibility to disease, *Am. J. Med.* **52:**1–8.

21. Nerup, J. Platz, P., Andersen, O. O., Christy, M., Lynsgøe, J., Poulsen, J. E., Ryder, L. P., Thomsen, M., Nielsen, L. S., and Svejgaard, A., 1974, *HL-A* antigens and diabetes mellitus, *Lancet* **2:**864–866.

22. Platz, P., Ryder, L., Nielsen, L. S., Svejgaard, A., Thomsen, M., Christy, M., and Nerup, J., 1974, *HL-A* and idiopathic Addison's disease, *Lancet* **2:**289.

23. Grumet, C., Konishi, J., Payne, R. O., and Kriss, J. P., 1973, Association of Graves' disease with *HL-A8*, *Clin. Res.* **21:**493 (abstract).

24. Volpé, R., Edmonds, M., Lamki, L., Clarke, P. V., and Row, V. V., 1972, The pathogenesis of Graves' disease: A disorder of delayed hypersensitivity?, *Mayo Clin. Proc.* **47:**824–834.

25. Volpé, R., Farid, N. R., von Westarp, C., and Row, V. V., 1974, The pathogenesis of Graves' disease and Hashimoto's thyroiditis, *Clin. Endocrinol.* **3:**239–261.

26. Gamble, D. R., and Taylor, K. W., 1969, Seasonal incidence of diabetes mellitus, *Brit. Med. J.* **3:**631–633.

27. Freytag, G., 1974, Do viruses serve as mediators of immunological reac-

tions?, in: *Immunity and Autoimmunity in Diabetes Mellitus* (P. A. Bastenie and W. Gepts, eds.), pp. 241–251, Excerpta Medica, Amsterdam.

28. Joasoo, A., Robertson, P., and Murray, I. P. C., 1975, Viral antibodies in thyrotoxicosis, *Lancet* **2:**125.

29. Roitt, I. M., Doniach, D., Campbell, P. N., and Hudson, R. V., 1956, Auto-antibodies in Hashimoto's disease (lymphadenoid goitre), *Lancet* **2:**820–821.

30. Rose, N. R., and Witebsky, E., 1956, Studies on organ specificity. V. Changes in the thyroid gland of rabbits following active immunization with rabbit thyroid extracts, *J. Immuol.* **76:**417–427.

31. Twarog, F. J., and Rose, N. R., 1970, Transfer of autoimmune thyroiditis of the rat with lymph node cells, *J. Immunol.* **104:**1467–1475.

32. Adams, D. D., and Purvis, H. D., 1956, Abnormal response in the assay of thyrotrophin, *Proc. Univ. Otago Med. Sch.* **34:**11–12.

33. Kriss, J. P., Pleshakov, V., and Chien, J. R., 1964, Isolation and identification of the long-acting thyroid stimulator and its relation to hyperthyroidism and circumscribed pretibial myxedema, *J. Clin. Endocrinol. Metab.* **24:**1005–1028.

34. Doniach, D., 1975, Humoral and genetic aspects of thyroid autoimmunity in: *Autoimmunity in Endocrine Disease, Clinics in Endocrinology and Metabolism,* Vol. 4 (W. J. Irvine, ed.), pp. 267–285, W. B. Saunders Co., London.

35. Fagraeus, A., and Jonsson, J., 1970, Distribution of organ antibodies over the surface of thyroid cells as examined by the immunofluorescence test, *Immunology* **18:**413–416.

36. Ochi, Y., Shiomi, K., Hachiya, T., Yoshimura, M., and Miyazaki, T., 1972, Immunological analysis of abnormal binding of thyroid hormone in the gamma globulin, *J. Clin. Endocrinol. Metab.* **35:**743–752.

37. Mukhtar, E. D., Smith, B. R., Pyle, G. A., Hall, R., and Vice, R., 1975, Relation of thyroid stimulating immunoglobulins to thyroid function and effects of surgery, radioiodine, and antithyroid drugs, *Lancet* **1:**713–715.

38. Owen, C. A., Jr., 1958, A review of autoimmunization in Hashimoto's disease, *J. Clin. Endocrinol. Metab.* **18:**1015–1023.

39. Torrigiani, G., Doniach, D., and Roitt, I. M., 1969, Serum thyroglobulin levels in healthy subjects and in patients with thyroid disease, *J. Clin. Endocrinol. Metab.* **29:**305–314.

40. Anderson, J. R., Goudie, R. B., Gray, K. G., and Buchanan, W. W., 1961, Antibody to thyroglobulin in patients with collagen diseases, *Scott. Med. J.* **6:**449–456.

41. Mori, T., and Kriss, J. P., 1971, Measurement by competitive binding radioimmunoassay of serum anti-microsomal and anti-thyroglobulin antibodies in Graves' disease and other thyroid disorders, *J. Clin. Endocrinol. Metab.* **33:**688–698.

42. Roitt, I. M., Ling, N. R., Doniach, D., and Couchman, K. G., 1964, The cytoplasmic auto-antigen of the human thyroid. I. Immunological and biochemical characteristics, *Immunology* **7:**375–393.

43. Pulvertaft, R. J. V., Doniach, D., Roitt, I. M., and Hudson, R. V., 1959, Cytotoxic effects of Hashimoto's serum on human thyroid cells in tissue culture, *Lancet* **2:**214–216.

44. Smith, B. R., and Hall, R., 1974, Thyroid-stimulating immunoglobulins in Graves' disease, *Lancet* **2:**427–431.

45. Aharonov, A., Abramsky, O., Tarrab-Hazdai, R., and Fuchs, S., 1975, Humoral antibodies to acetylcholine receptors in patients with myasthenia gravis, *Lancet* **2:**340–342.

46. Flier, J. S., Kahn, C. R., Roth, J., and Bar, R. S., 1975, Antibodies that impair insulin receptor binding in an unusual diabetic syndrome with severe insulin resistance, *Science* **190**:63–65.
47. Kahn, C. R., 1976, Hypoglycemia associated with non-endocrine tumours, *Proceedings of the 58th Meeting of The Endocrine Society*, San Francisco, June 23–25.
48. Adams, D. D., and Kennedy, T. H., 1971, Evidence to suggest that LATS protector stimulates the human thyroid gland, *J. Clin. Endocrinol. Metab.* **33**:47–51.
49. Onaya, T., Kotani, M., Yamada, T., and Ochi, Y., 1973, New *in vitro* tests to detect the thyroid stimulator in sera from hyperthyroid patients by measuring colloid droplet formation and cyclic AMP in human thyroid slices, *J. Clin. Endocrinol. Metab.* **36**:859–866.
50. Orgiazzi, J., Williams, D. E., Chopra, I. J., and Solomon, D. H., 1976, Human thyroid adenyl cyclase stimulator in immunoglobulin G (IgG) of patients with Graves' disease, in: *Thyroid Research* (J. Robbins and L. E. Braverman, eds.), *Excerpta Med. Int. Congr. Ser.* **378**:407–410, Excerpta Medica, Amsterdam.
51. O'Donnell, J., Silverberg, J., Row, V. V., and Volpé, R., 1976, Thyrotrophin-displacement activity (TDA) of serum immunoglobulins in Graves' disease, Fifty-second Meeting of the American Thyroid Association, Toronto, September 15–18.
52. McKenzie, J. M., 1958, The bioassay of thyrotropin in serum, *Endocrinology* **63**:372–382.
53. Major, P. W., and Munro, D. S., 1962, Observations on the stimulation of thyroid function in mice by the injection of serum from normal subjects and from patients with thyroid disorders, *Clin. Sci.* **23**:463–475.
54. Kendall-Taylor, P., 1975, LATS and human-specific thyroid stimulator; their relation to Graves' disease, in: *Autoimmunity in Endocrine Disease, Clinics in Endocrinology and Metabolism*, Vol. 4 (W. J. Irvine, ed.), pp. 319–339, W. B. Saunders Co., London.
55. McKenzie, J. M., and Zakarija, M., 1976, A reconsideration of a thyroid-stimulating immunoglobulin as the cause of hyperthyroidism in Graves' disease, *J. Clin. Endocrinol. Metab.* **42**:778–781.
56. McKenzie, J. M., and Zakarija, M., 1976, Heterologous effects of human thyroid stimulating IgG, presented at the Vth International Congress of Endocrinology, Hamburg, July 18–24, Abstract No. 68.
57. Adams, D. D., Kennedy, T. H., and Stewart, R. D. H., 1974, Correlation between long-acting thyroid stimulator protector level and thyroid ^{131}I uptake in thyrotoxicosis, *Br. Med. J.* **2**:199–201.
58. Dirmikis, S. M., Munro, D. S., Hiller, E. J., Crawford, M. J., Wynne, J., and Purcell, M., 1974, Placental transmission of LATS-protector, *Lancet* **2**:1579–1580.
59. Solomon, D. H., Chopra, I. J., Chopra, U., and Smith, F. J., 1977, Identification of subgroups of euthyroid Graves's ophthalmopathy, *N. Engl. J. Med.* **296**:181–186.
60. Mulaisho, C., Abdon, N. I., and Utiger, R. D., 1975, Lack of T-cell immune abnormalities in peripheral blood lymphocytes in patients with Graves' disease or hypothyroidism, *J. Clin. Endocrinol. Metab.* **41**:266–270.
61. Volpé, R., and Row, V. V., 1975, Proportion of E rosettes normal in Graves's and Hashimoto's diseases: A retraction, *N. Engl. J. Med.* **293**:44.
62. Calder, E. A., McLeman, D., Barnes, E. W., and Irvine, W. J., 1972, The

effect of thyroid antigens on the *in vitro* migration of leucocytes from patients with Hashimoto thyroiditis, *Clin. Exp. Immunol.* **12**:428–438.
63. Lamki, L., Row, V. V., and Volpé, R., 1973, Cell-mediated immunity in Graves' disease and in Hashimoto's thyroiditis as shown by demonstration of migration inhibition factor (M.I.F.), *J. Clin. Endocrinol. Metab.* **36**:358–364.
64. Delespesse, G., Duchcateau, J., Collet, H., Govaerts, A., and Bastenie, P. A., 1972, Lymphocyte transformation with thyroglobulin in thyroid diseases, *Clin. Exp. Immunol.* **12**:439–445.
65. Wartenberg, J., Doniach, D., Brostoff, J., and Roitt, I. M., 1973, Leucocyte migration inhibition in thyroid disease, *Int. Arch. Allergy Appl. Immunol.* **44**:396–408.
66. Brostoff, J., 1970, Migration inhibition studies in human disease, *Proc. R. Soc. Med.* **63**:905–906.
67. Wartenberg, J., Doniach, D., Brostoff, J., and Roitt, I. M., 1973, Leucocyte migration inhibition with mitochondria in human autoimmune thyroid disorders, *Clin. Exp. Immunol.* **14**:203–212.
68. Packalen, T., and Wasserman, J., 1971, Inhibition of migration of normal guinea pig blood leukocytes by homologous immune gamma-2-globulin in the presence of specific antigen, *Int. Arch. Allergy Appl. Immunol.* **41**:790–796.
69. Kotkes, P., and Pick, E., 1975, Studies on the inhibition of macrophage migration induced by soluble antigen–antibody complexes, *Clin. Exp. Immunol.* **19**:105–120.
70. Greaves, M., Janossy, G., and Doenhoff, M., 1974, Selective triggering of T and B lymphocytes *in vitro* by polyclonal mitogens, *J. Exp. Med.* **140**:1–18.
71. Knox, A. J. S., von Westarp, C., Row, V. V., and Volpé, R., 1976, Demonstration of the production of human thyroid-stimulating immunoglobulins (HTSI) by Graves' lymphocytes cultured *in vitro* with phytohaemagglutinin (PHA), *Metabolism* **25**:1217–1223.
72. Calder, E. A., and Irvine, W. J., 1975, Cell-mediated immunity and immune complexes in thyroid disease, in: *Autoimmunity in Endocrine Disease, Clinics in Endocrinology and Metabolism*, Vol. 4 (W. J. Irvine, ed.), pp. 287–318, W. B. Saunders Co. London.
73. Calder, E. A., Penhale, W. J., Barnes, E. W., and Irvine, W. J., 1973, Cytotoxic lymphocytes in Hashimoto thyroiditis, *Clin. Exp. Immunol.* **14**:19–23.
74. Laryea, E., Row, V. V., and Volpé, R., 1973, The effect of blood leucocytes from patients with Hashimoto's disease on human thyroid cells in monolayer cultures, *Clin. Endocrinol.* **2**:23–25.
75. Calder, E. A., Penhale, W. J., McLeman, D., Barnes, E. W., and Irvine, W. J., 1973, Lymphocyte-dependent antibody-mediated cytotoxicity in Hashimoto thyroiditis, *Clin. Exp. Immunol.* **14**:153–158.
76. Roberts, I. M., Whittingham, S., and MacKay, I. R., 1973, Tolerance to an autoantigen-thyroglobulin. Antigen-binding lymphocytes in thymus and blood in health and autoimmune disease, *Lancet* **2**:936–940.
77. Volpé, R., 1975, Thyroiditis: Current views of the pathogenesis, in: *Current Concepts of Thyroid Disease* (G. N. Burrow, ed.), *Med. Clin. North Am.* **59**:1163–1175, W. B. Saunders Co., Philadelphia.
78. Volpé, R., 1976, The pathogenesis of Graves' disease, *Compr. Ther.* **2**:43–52.
79. Volpé, R., 1976, Acute and subacute thyroiditis, *Pharmacol. Ther. C* **1**:171–181.
80. Wall, J. R., Fang, S. L., Ingbar, S. H., and Braverman, L. E., 1976, Lympho-

cyte transformation in response to human thyroid extract in patients with subacute thyroiditis, *J. Clin. Endocrinol. Metab.* **43:**587–590.

81. Werner, S. C., and Fierer, J. A., 1972, Cell-mediated immunity in Graves' disease?, *N. Engl. J. Med.* **287:**1251.
82. von Westarp, C., Knox, A. J., Row, V. V., and Volpé, R., 1977, Comparison of thyroid antigens by the experimental production of precipitating antibodies to human thyroid fractions and the identification of an antibody which competes with long-acting thyroid stimulator (LATS) for thyroid binding, *Acta Endocrinol. (Copenhagen):* **84:**759–767.
83. Knox, A. J. S., von Westarp, C., Row, V. V., and Volpé, R., 1976, Thyroid antigen stimulates lymphocytes from patients with Graves' disease to produce thyroid-stimulating immunoglobulin (TSI), *J. Clin. Endocrinol. Metab.* **43:**330–337.
84. Solomon, D. H., and Chopra, I. J., 1972, Graves' disease—1972, *Mayo Clin. Proc.* **47:**803–813.
85. Chopra, I. J., Solomon, D. H., Chopra, U., Yoshihara, E., Terasaki, P. I., and Smith, F., 1977, Abnormalities in thyroid function in relatives of patients with Graves' disease and Hashimoto's thyroiditis: Lack of correlation with inheritance of *HLA-B8. J. Clin. Endocrinol. Metab.* **45:**45–54.
86. Grumet, F. C., Konishi, J., Payne, R. O., and Kriss, J. P., 1976, Association in Japanese of Graves' disease with the *HLA* specificity W5, in: *Thyroid Research* (J. Robbins and L. E. Braverman, eds.), *Excerpta Med. Int. Congr. Ser.* **378:**376–379, Excerpta Medica, Amsterdam.
87. Parry, C. H., 1825, *Collections from the Unpublished Medical Writings*, Vol. II, p. 11, Underwoods, London.
88. Volpé, R., Vale, J., and Johnston, M. W., 1960, The effects of certain physical and emotional tensions and strains on fluctuations in the level of serum protein-bound iodine, *J. Clin. Endocrinol. Metab.* **20:**415–428.
89. Hadden, D. R., and McDevitt, D. G., 1974, Environmental stress and thyrotoxicosis. Absence of association, *Lancet* **2:**577–578.
90. Iversen, K., 1949, An epidemic wave of thyrotoxicosis in Denmark during World War II, *Am. J. Med. Sci.* **217:**121–129.
91. Hershman, J. M., and Pittman, J. A., 1971, Utility of the radioimmunoassay of serum thyrotrophin in man, *Ann. Intern. Med.* **74:**481–490.
92. Furth, E. D., Becker, D. V., Ray, B. S., and Kane, J. W., 1962, Appearance of unilateral infiltrative exophthalmos of Graves' disease after the successful treatment of the same process in the contralateral eye by apparently total surgical hypophysectomy, *J. Clin. Endocrinol. Metab.* **22:**518–524.
93. Claman, H. N., 1972, Corticosteroids and lymphoid cells, *N. Engl. J. Med.* **287:**388–396.
94. Brown, D. M., and Lowman, J. T., 1964, Thyrotoxicosis occurring in two patients on prolonged high doses of steroids, *N. Engl. J. Med.* **270:**278–281.
95. McDougall, I. R., Greig, W. R., Gray, H. W., and Smith, J. F. B., 1971, Thyrotoxicosis developing during cyclophosphamide therapy, *Br. Med. J.* **4:**275–276.
96. Werner, S. C., and Platman, S. R., 1965, Remission of hyperthyroidism (Graves' disease) and altered pattern of serum-thyroxine binding induced by prednisone, *Lancet* **2:**751–755.
97. Kenny, F. M., Iturzaeta, N., Preeyasombat, C., Taylor, F. H., and Migeon, C., 1967, Cortisol production rate. VII. Hypothyroidism and hyperthyroidism in infants and children, *J. Clin. Endocrinol. Metab.* **27:**1616–1622.

98. Sorkin, E., and Desedovsky, H., 1976, Hormonal control of immune pro-
    cesses, *Proceedings of the 5th International Congress of Endocrinology*, Hamburg,
    July 18–24, Excerpta Medica, Amsterdam, International Congress Series,
    No. 402, 1977.
99. Wall, J. R., Manwar, G. L. Greenwood, D. M., and Walters, B. A., 1976, The
    in vitro suppression of lectin induced ^{3}H-thymidine incorporation into DNA
    of peripheral blood lymphocytes after the addition of propylthiouracil, *J.
    Clin. Endocrinol. Metab.* **43:**1406–1409.
100. Doniach, D., and Florin-Christensen, A., 1975, Autoimmunity in the patho-
    genesis of endocrine exophthalmos, in: *Autoimmunity in Endocrine Disease,
    Clinics in Endocrinology and Metabolism*, Vol. 4 (W. J. Irvine, ed.), pp. 341–350,
    W. B. Saunders Co., London.
101. Munro, R. E., Lamki, L., Row, V. V., and Volpé, R., 1973, Cell-mediated
    immunity in the exophthalmos of Graves' disease as demonstrated by the
    migration inhibition factor (MIF) test, *J. Clin. Endocrinol. Metab.* **37:**286–292.
102. Fakhri, O., and Hobbs, J. R., 1972, Detection of antibodies which can
    cooperate with lymphocytes, *Lancet* **2:**403–406.
103. Konishi, J., Herman, M. M., and Kriss, J. P., 1974, Binding of thyroglobulin
    and thyroglobulin–antithyroglobulin immune complex to extraocular mus-
    cle membrane, *Endocrinology* **95:**434–446.
104. Kriss, J. P., 1970, Radioisotopic thyroidolymphography in patients with
    Graves' disease, *J. Clin. Endocrinol. Metab.* **31:**315–324.
105. Mullin, B. R., Levinson, R. E., Friedman, A., Henson, D. E., Winand, R. J.,
    and Kohn, L. D., 1977, Delayed hypersensitivity in Graves' disease and
    exophthalmos: Identification of thyroglobulin in human orbital muscle,
    Endocrinology **100:**351–360.
106. Kohn, L. D., and Winand, R. J., 1971, Relationship of thyrotrophin to
    exophthalmos-producing substance, *J. Biol. Chem.* **246:**6570–6575.
107. Kourides, I. A., Weintraub, B. D., Ridgway, E. C., and Maloof, F., 1975,
    Pituitary secretion of free alpha and beta subunits of human thyrotropin in
    patients with thyroid disorders, *J. Clin. Endocrinol. Metab.* **40:**872–885.
108. Nerup, J., 1974, Addison's disease. A review of some clinical, pathological
    and immunological features, *Dan. Med. Bull.* **21:**201–217.
109. MacCuish, A. C., and Irvine, W. J., 1975, Autoimmunological aspects of
    diabetes mellitus, in: *Autoimmunity in Endocrine Disease, Clinics in Endocrinology
    and Metabolism*, Vol. 4 (W. J. Irvine, ed.), pp. 435–471, W. B. Saunders Co.,
    London.
110. Pettit, M. D., Landing, B. H., and Guest, G. M., 1961, Antithyroid antibody
    in juvenile diabetics, *J. Clin. Endocrinol. Metab.* **21:**209–210.
111. Whittingham, S., Mathews, J. D., Mackay, I. R., Stocks, A. E., Ungar, B., and
    Martin, F. I. R., 1971, Diabetes mellitus, autoimmunity and ageing, *Lancet*
    1:763–767.
112. Moore, J. M., and Neilson, J. McE., 1973, Antibodies to gastric mucosa and
    thyroid in diabetes mellitus, *Lancet* **2:**645–647.
113. Irvine, W. J., Clarke, B. F., Scarth, L., Cullen, D. R., and Duncan, L. J. P.,
    1970, Thyroid and gastric autoimmunity in patients with diabetes mellitus,
    Lancet **2:**163–168.
114. Nerup, J., and Binder, C., 1973, Thyroid, gastric and adrenal auto-immunity
    in diabetes mellitus, *Acta Endocrinol. (Copenhagen)* **72:**279–286.
115. Bottazzo, G. F., Florin-Christensen, A., and Doniach, D., 1974, Islet-cell
    antibodies in diabetes mellitus with autoimmune polyendocrine deficiency,
    Lancet **2:**1279–1283.

116. MacCuish, A. C., Barnes, E. W., Irvine, W. J., and Duncan, L. J. P., 1974, Antibodies to pancreatic islet cells in insulin-dependent diabetics with coexistent autoimmune disease, *Lancet* **2**:1529–1531.
117. Berson, S. A., and Yalow, R. S., 1965, Some current controversies in diabetes research, *Diabetes* **14**:549–572.
118. Ohneda, A., Matsuda, K., Sato, M., Yamagata, S., and Sato, T., 1974, Hypoglycemia due to apparent autoantibodies to insulin. Characterization of insulin-binding proteins, *Diabetes* **23**:41–50.
119. Følling, I., and Norman, N., 1972, Hyperglycemia, hypoglycemic attacks, and production of anti-insulin antibodies without previous known immunization. Immunological and functional studies in a patient, *Diabetes* **21**:814–826.
120. Hirata, Y., and Ishizu, H., 1972, Elevated insulin-binding capacity of serum proteins in a case with spontaneous hypoglycemia and mild diabetes not treated with insulin, *Tohoku J. Exp. Med.* **107**:277–286.
121. MacCuish, A. C., Urbaniak, S. J., Campbell, C. J., Duncan, L. J. P., and Irvine, W. J., 1974, Phytohemagglutinin transformation and circulating lymphocyte subpopulations in insulin-dependent diabetics, *Diabetes* **23**:708–712.
122. Brody, J. I., and Merlie, K., 1970, Metabolic and biosynthetic features of lymphocytes from patients with diabetes mellitus; similarities to lymphocytes in chronic lymphocytic leukaemia, *Br. J. Haematol.* **19**:193–201.
123. Nerup, J., Andersen, O. O., Bendixen, G., Egeberg, J., and Poulsen, J. E., 1971, Antipancreatic cellular hypersensitivity in diabetes mellitus, *Diabetes* **20**:424–427.
124. Richens, E. R., Ancill, R. J., Gough, K. R., and Hartog, M., 1973, Cellular hypersensitivity to mitochondrial antigens in diabetes mellitus, *Clin. Exp. Immunol.* **13**:1–7.
125. Goldstone, A. H., Calder, E. A., Barnes, E. W., and Irvine, W. J., 1973, The effect of gastric antigens on the *in vitro* migration of leucocytes from patients with atrophic gastritis and pernicious anaemia, *Clin. Exp. Immunol.* **14**:501–508.
126. Berson, S. A., and Yalow, R. S., 1959, Species-specificity of human anti-beef, pork insulin serum, *J. Clin. Invest.* **38**:2017–2025.
127. Von Meyenburg, H., 1940, Über "Insulitis" bei Diabetes, *Schweiz. Med. Wochenschr.* **21**:554–557.
128. Gundersen, E., 1927, Is diabetes of infectious origin?, *J. Infect. Dis.* **41**:197–202.
129. Craighead, J. E., and Steinke, J., 1971, Diabetes mellitus-like syndrome in mice infected with encephalomyocarditis virus, *Am. J. Pathol.* **63**:119–134.
130. Coleman, T. J., Gamble, D. R., and Taylor, K. W., 1973, Diabetes in mice after Coxsackie B4 virus infection, *Br. Med. J.* **3**:25–27.
131. Steinke, J., and Taylor, K. W., 1974, Viruses and the etiology of diabetes, *Diabetes* **23**:631–633.
132. Gamble, D. R., Kinsley, M. L., Fitzgerald, M. G., Bolton, R., and Taylor, K. W., 1969, Viral antibodies in diabetes mellitus, *Br. Med. J.* **3**:627–630.
133. Conybeare, J. J., and Millis, G. C., 1924, Observations on twenty-nine cases of Addison's disease treated at Guy's Hospital between 1904 and 1923, *Guy's Hosp. Rep.* **4**:369–375.
134. Maisey, I., and Stevens, A., 1969, Addison's disease at Guy's Hospital: A pathological study, *Guy's Hosp. Rep.* **118**:373–385.
135. Irvine, W. J., and Barnes, E. W., 1975, Addison's disease, ovarian failure,

and hypoparathyroidism, in: *Autoimmunity in Endocrine Disease, Clinics in Endocrinology and Metabolism,* Vol. 4 (W. J. Irvine, ed.), pp. 379–434, W. B. Saunders Co., London.

136. Levine, S., and Wenk, E. J., 1968, The production and passive transfer of allergic adrenalitis, *Am. J. Pathol.* **52:**41–53.

137. Frey, H. M. M., Vogt, J. H., and Nerup, J., 1973, Familial poly-endocrinopathy, *Acta Endocrinol. (Copenhagen)* **72:**401–416.

138. Spinner, M. W., Blizzard, R. M., and Childs, B., 1968, Clinical and genetic heterogeneity in idiopathic Addison's disease and hypoparathyroidism, *J. Clin. Endocrinol. Metab.* **28:**795–804.

139. Spinner, M. W., Blizzard, R. M., Gibbs, J., Abbey, H., and Childs, B., 1969, Familial distribution of organ-specific antibodies in the blood of patients with Addison's disease and hypoparathyroidism and their relatives, *Clin. Exp. Immunol.* **5:**461–468.

140. Anderson, J. R., Goudie, R. B, Gray, K. G., and Timbury, G. G., 1957, Autoantibodies in Addison's disease, *Lancet* **1:**1123–1124.

141. Nerup, J., Andersen, V., and Bendixen, G., 1969, Anti-adrenal cellular hypersensitivity in Addison's disease, *Clin. Exp. Immunol.* **4:**355–363.

142. Moulias, R., Goust, J. M., Deville, G., Chabrolle, A. D., Buffet, C., and Muller-Berat, C. N., 1970, Le test de migration des leucocytes du sang périphérique (TML). Un nouveau test d'hypersensibilite retardée *in vitro* chez l 'homme. II. Utisation dans les affections auto-immunes humaines. Résultats préliminaire et interprétation, *Presse Med.* **73:**2315–2318.

143. Nerup, J., and Bendixen, G., 1969, Antiadrenal cellular hypersensitivity in Addison's disease. III. Species-specificity and subcellular localization of the antigen, *Clin. Exp. Immunol.* **5:**355.-364.

144. Nerup, J., Andersen, V., and Bendixen, G., 1970, Anti-adrenal cellular hypersensitivity in Addison's disease. IV. *In vivo* and *in vitro* investigations on the mitochondrial fraction, *Clin. Exp. Immunol.* **6:**733–739.

145. Duff, G. L., and Bernstein, C., 1933, Five cases of Addison's disease with so-called atrophy of adrenal cortex, *Bull. Johns Hopkins Hosp.* **52:**67–83.

146. Ruehsen, M. de M., Blizzard, R. M., Garcia-Bunuel, R., and Jones, G. S., 1972, Autoimmunity and ovarian failure, *Am. J. Obstet. Gynecol.* **112:**693–703.

147. Irvine, W. J., Chan, M. M. W., and Scarth, L., 1969, The further characterization of autoantibodies reactive with extra-adrenal steroid-producing cells in patients with adrenal disorders, *Clin. Exp. Immunol.* **4:**489–503.

148. Kamp. P., Platz, P., and Nerup, J., 1974, "Steroid-cell" antibody in endocrine diseases, *Acta Endocrinol. (Copenhagen)* **76:**729–740.

149. McNatty, K. P., Short, R. V., Barnes, E. W., and Irvine, W. J., 1975, The cytotoxic effect of serum from patients with Addison's disease and autoimmune ovarian failure on human granulosa cells in culture, *Clin. Exp. Immunol.* **22:**378–384.

150. Edmonds, M., Lamki, L., Killinger, D. W., and Volpé, R., 1973, Autoimmune thyroiditis, adrenalitis, and oophoritis, *Am. J. Med.* **54:**782–787

151. Irvine, W. J., Chan, M. M. W., Scarth, L., Kolb, F. O., Hartog, M., Bayliss, R. I. S., and Drury, M. I., 1968, Immunological aspects of premature ovarian failure associated with idiopathic Addison's disease, *Lancet* **2:**883–887.

152. Drury, M. I., Keelan, D. M., Timoney, F. J., and Irvine, W. J., 1972, Juvenile familial endocrinopathy, *Clin. Exp. Immunol.* **7:**125–132.

153. Murthy, G. G., Peress, N. S., and Khan, S. A., 1976, Demonstration of

antibodies to testicular basement membrane by immunofluorescence in a patient with multiple primary endocrine deficiencies, *J. Clin. Endocrinol. Metab.* **42:**637–641.

154. Isojima, S., and Li, T. S., 1968, Stepwise appearance of sperm specific antigens in rats and their disappearance after fertilization, *Fertil. Steril.* **19:**999–1008.

155. Samuel, T., Kolk, A. H. J., Rümke, P., and Van Lis, J. M. J., 1975, Autoimmunity to sperm antigens in vasectomized men, *Clin. Exp. Immunol.* **21:**65–74.

156. Meaker, S. R., 1922, Some aspects of the problem of sterility, *Boston Med. Surg. J.* **187:**535–539.

157. Wilson, L., 1954, Sperm agglutinins in human semen and blood, *Proc. Soc. Exp. Biol. Med.* **85:**652–655.

158. Rümke, P., 1954, The presence of sperm antibodies in the serum of two patients with oligozoospermia, *Vox Sang.* **4:**135–140.

159. Li, T. S., 1974, Sperm immunology, infertility, and fertility control, *Obstet, Gynecol.* **44:**607–623.

160. Fjallbrant, B., 1968, Interrelation between high levels of sperm antibodies, reduced sperm penetration of cervical mucus by spermatozoa and sterility in men, *Acta Obstet. Gynecol. Scand.* **47:**102–118.

161. Boettcher, B., Hay, J., Kay, D. J., Baldo, B. A., and Roberts, T. K., 1970, Sperm agglutinating activity in some human sera, *Int. J. Fertil.* **15:**143–158.

162. Rümke, P., and Hellinger, G., 1959, Autoantibodies against spermatozoa in sterile men, *Am. J. Clin. Pathol.* **32:**357–363.

163. Rümke, P. H., and Hekman, A., 1975, Auto- and isoimmunity to sperm in infertility, in: *Autoimmunity and Endocrine Disease, Clinics in Endocrinology and Metabolism,* Vol. 4 (W. J., Irvine, ed.), pp. 473–496, W. B. Saunders Co., London.

164. Hamerlynck, J. V., and Rümke, P., 1968, Spermatoxic antibodies in man, in: *Proceedings of the Sixth World Congress of Fertility and Sterility,* pp. 287–294, The Israel Academy of Sciences and Humanities, Tel Aviv.

165. El-Alfi, O. S., and Bassili, F., 1970, Immunological aspermatogenesis in man. I. Blastoid transformation of lymphocytes in response to seminal antigen in cases of non-obstructive azoospermia, *J. Reprod. Fertil.* **21:**23–28.

166. Mettler, L., and Scheidel, P., 1973, Sensibilisierung gegen Sperma-antigene im zellgebundenen Immunsystem der Frau durch Nachweis des Migrations—Inhibitions Faktors, *Fortschr. Med.* **91:**1059–1061.

167. Haensch, R., 1969, Fluorescenzimmunologische Spermienautoantikörperbefunde bei männlichen Fertilitätsstörungen, *Arch. Gynaekol.* **208:**91–102.

168. Fjallbrant, B., 1968, Sperm antibodies and sterility in men, *Acta Obstet. Gynecol. Scand.* **47:** (Suppl.):5–38.

169. Shulman, S., 1972, Immunological barriers to fertility, *Obstet. Gynecol. Surv.* **27:**553–606.

170. Fields, J. P., Fragola, L., and Hadley, T. P., 1971, Hypoparathyroidism, candidiasis, alopecia and vitiligo, *Arch. Dermatol.* **103:**687–689.

171. Nusynowitz, M. L., Frame, B., and Kolb, F. O., 1976, The spectrum of the hypoparathyroidism states: A classification based on physiological principles, *Medicine (Baltimore)* **55:**105–119.

172. Irvine, W. J., 1971, Adrenalitis, hypoparathyroidism, and associated diseases, in: *Immunological Diseases,* Vol. 2, 2nd Ed. (M. Samter, ed.), pp. 1214–1227, Little, Brown, and Co., Boston.

173. Blizzard, R. M., Chee, D., and Davis, W., 1966, The incidence of parathyroid and other antibodies in the sera of patients with idiopathic hypoparathyroidism, *Clin. Exp. Immunol.* **1:**119–128.
174. Irvine, W. J., and Scarth, L., 1969, Antibody to the oxyphil cells of the human parathyroid in idiopathic hypoparathyroidism, *Clin. Exp. Immunol.* **4:**505–510.
175. Moulias, R., Goust, J. M., and Muller-Berat, C. N., 1971, Hypoparathyroidism and cell-mediated immunity, *Lancet* **1:**1239.
176. Goudie, R. B., and Pinkerton, P. H., 1962, Anterior hypophysitis and Hashimoto's disease in a young woman, *J. Pathol. Bacteriol.* **83:**584–585.
177. Shanklin, W. M., 1951, Lymphocytes and lymphoid tissue in the human pituitary, *Anat. Rec.* **111:**177–191.
178. Lack, E. E., 1975, Lymphoid "hypophysitis" with end organ insufficiency, *Arch. Pathol.* **99:**215–219.
179. Arvanitakis, C., and Knouss, R. F., 1973, Selective hypopituitarism. Impaired cell-mediated immunity and chronic mucocutaneous candidiasis, *J. Am. Med. Assoc.* **225:**1492–1495.

Index